ANEMIAS AND OTHER RED CELL DISORDERS

NOTICE

Medicine is an ever-changing science. As new research and clinical experience broaden our knowledge, changes in treatment and drug therapy are required. The authors and the publisher of this work have checked with sources believed to be reliable in their efforts to provide information that is complete and generally in accord with the standards accepted at the time of publication. However, in view of the possibility of human error or changes in medical sciences, neither the authors nor the publisher nor any other party who has been involved in the preparation or publication of this work warrants that the information contained herein is in every respect accurate or complete, and they disclaim all responsibility for any errors or omissions or for the results obtained from use of the information contained in this work. Readers are encouraged to confirm the information contained herein with other sources. For example and in particular, readers are advised to check the product information sheet included in the package of each drug they plan to administer to be certain that the information contained in this work is accurate and that changes have not been made in the recommended dose or in the contraindications for administration. This recommendation is of particular importance in connection with new or infrequently used drugs.

ANEMIAS AND OTHER RED CELL DISORDERS

Edited By:

Kenneth R. Bridges, MD

Medical Director, Supportive Care Oncology
Amgen, Inc.
Thousand Oaks, California

Former Position:
Associate Professor of Medicine
Hematology Division
Brigham and Women's Hospital
Boston, Massachusetts

Howard A. Pearson, MD

Professor Emeritus of Pediatrics
Yale University School of Medicine
Department of Pediatrics
Section of Pediatric Hematology/Oncology
Yale New Haven Hospital
New Haven, Connecticut

 Medical

MEDICAL PUBLISHING DIVISION

New York   Chicago   San Francisco   Lisbon   London   Madrid   Mexico City
New Delhi   San Juan   Seoul   Singapore   Sydney   Toronto

ANEMIAS AND OTHER RED CELL DISORDERS

1234567890   CTP/CTP   0987

ISBN 978-0-07-141940-6
MHID 0-07-141940-3

This book was set in Times Roman by Aptara Inc.
The editors were Joe Rusko and Christie Naglieri
The production supervisor was Sherri Souffrance
Project management was provided by Aptara Inc.
The designer was Marsha Cohen/Parallelogram Graphics
The cover designer was Perhsson Design
Cover Photo: Sickle cell anemia. Credit: Dr. Gopal Murti/Photo Researchers, Inc.
CTPS China was printer and binder.

This book is printed on acid-free paper.

Library of Congress Cataloging-in-Publication Data

Anemias and other red cell disorders/edited by Kenneth R. Bridges,
    Howard A. Pearson. – 1st ed.
p. ; cm.
Includes index.
ISBN 978-0-07-141940-6
1. Anemia. 2. Erythrocyte disorders. I. Bridges, Kenneth R. II. Pearson, Howard A.
[DNLM: 1. Anemia. 2. Bone Marrow Diseases. 3. Erythrocytes–pathology.
    WH 155 A5788 2007]
RC641.A499 2007
616.1′52–dc22
                    2007015659

DEDICATION

To Maria and Camille; sources of constant inspiration and support.

CONTENTS

PREFACE

Anemia is one of the conditions encompassed by "disorders of hematology" and consequently is reviewed in all medical textbooks devoted to this discipline. In recent years, the explosion of information relevant to the genetic, biochemical, and environmental factors that produce anemia has produced a parallel explosion in the breadth and complexity of overviews on the subject. The fact that knowledge of the processes involved in anemia often extends from molecules to man is a triumph of modern medical science. Expansive treatises exist that explore the complexities of anemia pathophysiology and the intricacies of its manifestations. However, the subtle nuances and unfortunately even the key messages of these works are sometimes apparent only to aficionados. More practically, many busy clinicians have neither the time nor the need to explore the fine points of esoteric anemias that may have little relevance to their medical practice.

Anemia is the most prevalent problem in hematology and is commonly encountered in routine medical care. This textbook aims to provide information on anemia for physicians who are neither hematologists nor anemia specialists. The goal is to create a working framework by which a practicing physician can reasonably evaluate a patient whose presenting complaint stems from an underlying anemia. The aim is to provide information that is practical but not simplistic. Common causes account for most anemias, and as such are the primary focus of this book.

Chapters are organized around the clinical features that most often prompt the initial encounter between doctor and patient. A table in each chapter lists the *Key Diagnostic Features* of particular types of anemia along with common identifying signs and possible approaches to distinguish and solidify the findings further. Characterization of this initial information allows the physician to collate the data and either begin treatment or consider referral to a specialist, as befits the clinical situation. A table of *Key Management Issues* provides a quick reference to important considerations in patient care. These tables are not meant to be all-inclusive guides. Rather, the object of these exercises is to provide a reasonable outline of the practical concerns involved in the care of the anemic patient.

In addition, the text discusses categories of anemia that are common in practice but are often absent from traditional textbooks of hematology. The anemia of pregnancy is an example of a common physiological condition that sometimes flies below the radar screen of hematology textbooks. The topic is prominent in textbooks of obstetrics and gynecology, but often is not well-appreciated outside that medical specialty. The same is true of anemia due to endocrine and metabolic conditions, such as anorexia nervosa. The goal is to provide a quick reference to support decisions about further work-up, evaluation, and treatment.

The book also addresses issues in anemia that commonly impact clinical practice but have no clear home in many textbooks on hematology. One such topic is age and anemia. The profound changes in the blood profile that occur between infancy and adolescence underlie the careful detail accorded to the issue in textbooks of pediatric hematology. By contrast, issues of age and anemia are not regularly discussed in texts on adult hematology. However, anemia in older people is a common and important clinical matter. Problems sometimes are attributed to "the anemia of old age." The clinician's perspective regarding the existence of such a phenomenon can profoundly affect the care of older people, and is addressed in the chapter on age and anemia. Additional sections of the book explore other common concerns in anemia that sometimes fall into a nosologic no man's land.

Ease and utility are the underlying tenets of the text. The background and overview discussions set the context for the problems that are examined. The information is not encyclopedic. Rather, the aim is to open the first door to the exploration of the medical edifice that is anemia. Sometimes examination of the atrium and a few adjacent rooms is sufficient to answer the questions at hand. At other times, more thorough mapping of nooks and crannies is needed. By opening the first door, this text sets the stage for that exploration.

Overview of Anemia

PRINCIPLES OF ANEMIA EVALUATION

Anemia, which is a red cell mass that is below the limit of normal, is probably the most common human pathological state worldwide. The condition is not a disease, but is instead the manifestation of an underlying pathological process. Anemia is a sign and not a diagnosis. Once recognized, however, the sign can serve as a road marker in the quest of cause. Although not a primary disease process, anemia can produce severe morbidity and occasionally even death. Chronic severe anemia strains the heart, for instance, and can produce high-output cardiac failure. Consequently, steps to correct the anemia should accompany the diagnostic evaluation.

■ DEFINING ANEMIA

Although red cell mass is the gold standard in the assessment of anemia, its measurement is cumbersome and rarely performed outside of research efforts. The procedure involves labeling a known quantity of red cells and returning them to the circulation.[1] The labeled cells equilibrate with the total population of erythrocytes. Plasma proteins tagged with a second label allow determination of the total plasma volume. The red cell mass calculation derives from the erythrocyte-specific activity of a subsequent blood sample. The process usually involves patient exposure to radiation, such as ^{51}Cr radiation. These hurtles make indirect assays preferable in the assessment of anemia. The two most common approaches are the determination of hemoglobin content per unit of blood and the hematocrit, which is the fraction of a quantity of blood composed of packed red cells.

Hemoglobin and hematocrit each is linked to the volume of a blood sample, which is the shortcoming of these approaches to anemia assessment. A change in the plasma portion of the blood volume changes both measures in the absence of a change in red cell mass. Dehydration, for instance, increases the values of the hematocrit and hemoglobin, meaning that it can mask anemia as defined by these variables. The clinician must factor conditions such as dehydration or pregnancy (which raises both the plasma volume and red cell mass) into considerations of anemia.

Errors in sample processing commonly produce spurious hemoglobin or hematocrit values. Automated blood analyzers greatly reduce mechanical counting errors. Problems in specimen handling are currently the primary culprits behind erroneous estimates of hemoglobin and hematocrit. Squeezing capillary blood during finger-stick collections, inaccurate filling of pipettes, failure to blot excess blood, and obtaining an even cell distribution in diluting fluid prior to sampling are common technique failures. These issues make repetition the correct first step when approaching a case of anemia based on a single laboratory determination.

The working definition of anemia is a blood hemoglobin value below the lower limit of a reference range. Reference ranges are generated by measuring hemoglobin values in hundreds or thousands of healthy subjects.[2] The plotted values approximate a Poisson distribution with the limits of normal defined as two standard deviations to either side of the mean. These 95% confidence limits assign "abnormal values" to 5% of healthy people, which must be considered in the anemia work-up. Marked anemia is always pathologic, but mild anemia can reflect individual variation. The

TABLE 1-1 | **RED CELL MEAN VALUES AT VARIOUS AGES**

Age	Erythrocyte Count ($\times\ 10^{-6}/\mu L$)	Hemoglobin (g/dL)	Mean Corpuscular Volume (fl)	Hematocrit (%)
1 day	5.6	21.2	106	56.1
1 month	4.7	15.6	91	44.6
1 year	4.6	11.6	77	35.2
4 years	4.7	12.6	80	37.1
8 years	4.7	12.9	80	38.9
14 years and older (female)	4.8 (4.2–5.4)	13.9 (11.9–16.0)	87	42 (37–47)
14 years and older (male)	5.4 (4.6–6.2)	15.8 (14.0–18.0)	87	47 (40–54)

The values shown exemplify the changes in erythrocyte count, hemoglobin, mean corpuscular volume, and hematocrit from birth to adolescence. Data sufficient to determine 95% confidence ranges exists only for females and males 14 years of age and older (95% range in parentheses).

hemoglobin value is quite constant for a single person, however. Someone with a hemoglobin value routinely at the high end of normal will not have values drop to the lower limit of normal without a perturbation in his or her physiology. The disturbance might be natural, such as the onset of pregnancy, or it might be pathologic, as with a bleeding peptic ulcer. Review of a patient's record to assess the hemoglobin profile should occur early in the work-up of anemia.

The reference range for hemoglobin is not fixed and must be adjusted for confounding variables, the most prominent of which are age and sex.[3] Table 1-1 highlights some of the age- and sex-specific differences in mean hemoglobin, red cell, and hematocrit values.[4] Much more detailed data exist in specialized discussions of these subjects. In the United States, the lower limits of normal hemoglobin values are 12.5 g/dL for adult females and 13.5 g/dL for adult males.

Knowing the definition of anemia leaves the issue of detecting the condition. Outward manifestations of anemia include findings such as pallor or glossitis. Symptoms include fatigue and dyspnea on exertion. None of these manifestations is specific to anemia, however, and often appear only in advanced cases. Evaluation of the blood itself is the sole unequivocal means of establishing the presence of an anemia.

■ **DETECTING ANEMIA**

Early in the history of medicine, people were designated as having anemia or "thin blood" because samples removed by bloodletting were pale and watery. This

TABLE 1-2 | **METHODS OF ASSESSING ANEMIA**

Method	Readout	Frequency of Use	Comment
^{51}Cr RBC labeling	Dilution of ^{51}Cr label in patient blood	Very low	• Most accurate approach to anemia determination • Cumbersome • Expensive • Involves patient exposure to radiation
Blood centrifugation	Volume of packed RBCs per volume of blood	High	• Fast • Accurate • Relatively labor intensive
Electrical current impedance assay	Impedance of electrical current by single cells	High	• Fast • Accurate • Low labor input • High throughput
Flow cytometry	Cell scattering of focused laser beam	Low	• Fast • Very accurate • Low labor input • High throughput
Finger-stick hemoglobin absorption	Hemoglobin light absorption by absorbimeter	Moderate	• Fast • Moderate accuracy • Moderate labor input

qualitative and unreliable approach was superseded over time by more quantitative methods. Currently several means exist to assess anemia as listed in Table 1-2. As noted, the gold standard is ^{51}Cr labeling of red cells to determine red cell mass. A second and more commonly used technique is centrifugation of a blood sample, which packs the red cells by centripetal force and leaves the plasma and white cells in an upper layer as shown schematically in Figure 1-1.[5]

Erythrocytes far outnumber other blood cells and account for the vast majority of the packed cell volume. White blood cells and platelets form a thin cream-colored layer at the interface between the packed red cells and the plasma called the "buffy

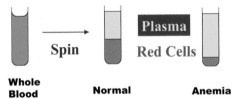

Spin

Whole Blood Normal Anemia

FIGURE 1–1 *The schematic shows the assessment of hematocrit by centrifugation. The tube containing the blood sample is centrifuged to pack the red cells at the bottom of the vessel. The plasma portion of the blood forms a clear supernatant while the packed red cells collect below. A thin milky line between the two is the buffy coat consisting of platelets and white cells. The hematocrit is the fraction of the entire sample comprised by packed red cells. Anemia reduces the volume of packed red cells to below normal.*

coat." The plasma supernatant portion of the centrifuged blood is pale yellow and easily distinguished from the packed red cells and the buffy coat. The percentage of the total blood volume occupied by the packed blood cells is called the hematocrit. The corrected hematocrit is the value of the apparent hematocrit obtained by centrifugation factored by 0.96, which compensates for the approximate 4% of the plasma that remains trapped between the packed red cells. The method is fast and accurate, but relatively labor intensive. The attractiveness of the spun hematocrit depends on both the number of samples processed and the cost of the labor input.

High-throughput information on anemia now commonly comes from an automated blood analyzer, several models of which are currently in widespread use. These devices provide CBC or "complete blood count," which contains a wealth of information pertinent to the nature of the anemia (Table 1-3). Proper interpretation of these data is paramount in the search for the cause of the anemia.

The most commonly used automated blood analyzer is the "impedance counter" shown schematically in Figure 1-2. An anticoagulant prevents the formation of fibrin clots in the blood sample that would interfere with the operation of the instrument as it draws cells through an aperture. The cell membrane is a high-resistance barrier to the electrical current flowing through the aperture. Each cell impedes the electric current as it passes through the aperture, producing a pulse that the instrument detects and amplifies. Adjustments in the sensitivity of the detector allow the relatively tiny platelets to pass without producing a signal. The instrument counts both white and red cells. The number of white cells (thousands/microliters) is too small to cause significant error in the red cell count (millions/microliters). Analyzers also determine the mean cell volume (MCV) of erythrocytes since the pulse amplitude is proportional to cell size.

The heme prosthetic group of hemoglobin conveys visible light absorption properties to the molecules that lend blood its red color. Hemoglobin concentration can be assessed in a hemolyzed blood sample by measuring the absorption at a specific wavelength. The shortcoming of this simple approach is that red cells contain various forms of hemoglobin that absorb light differently across the spectrum. Oxygenated hemoglobin (oxyhemoglobin) in which oxygen is linked noncovalently to

TABLE 1-3	AUTOMATED BLOOD ANALYZER READOUT (CBC)	
Variable	**Readout**	**Interpretation**
Red cell number	Millions/μL	The number of red cells per volume of blood.
MCV	Femtoliters	The mean volume of a single red cell.
Hb	g/dL	Quantity of hemoglobin in a volume of blood.
MCH	Picograms	The mean hemoglobin content of a single red cell.
MCHC	Percentage	Hemoglobin concentration within individual red cells. Calculated as (Hb/HCT)$\times$ 100
RDW	Percentage	Coefficient of size variation of red cells in a sample = (Standard deviation of red cell volume mean cell volume) $\times$ 100. A larger value indicates greater size variation.
HCT	Percentage	Mathematical derivation of the red cell fraction of the total blood volume.
WBC	Thousands/μL	Number of white cells per unit of blood.[a]
Plts	Hundreds of thousands per μL	Number of platelets per unit of blood.

Some analyzers give a simple WBC differential based on characteristics such as the size of the nucleus, granularity of the cell, and cell size.
MCV, mean red cell volume; Hb, hemoglobin; MCH, mean corpuscular hemoglobin; MCHC, mean corpuscular hemoglobin concentration; RDW, red cell distribution width; HCT, hematocrit; WBC, white cell count; Plts, platelet count.
[a] Peripheral blood nucleated red cells register as white cells and must be subtracted from the WBC total.

heme absorbs light differently than does hemoglobin in the absence of liganded oxygen (deoxyhemoglobin).[6] Carboxyhemoglobin, which often is a significant fraction of hemoglobin in smokers, has liganded carbon monoxide that produces a unique absorption spectrum. Hemoglobin can also exist in an oxidized form (methemoglobin), in which the valence state of iron in the heme group is Fe(III) rather than the usual

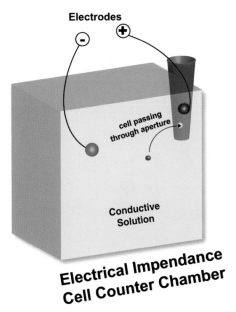

Electrodes

cell passing
through aperture →

**Conductive
Solution**

**Electrical Impendance
Cell Counter Chamber**

FIGURE 1-2 *Layout of an impedance blood cell analyzer. The two chambers are charged by electrodes, thereby establishing an electrical current in the conductive fluid that flows through the small aperture. A blood cell passing through the aperture interrupts the current flow for a duration that varies with cell size. The frequency of the interruptions provides the cell count while the magnitude of the disturbances gives the cell size. The red cell number and the mean cell volume are the primary readouts. The degree of variation in cell size gives the red cell distribution width.*

Fe(II). Methemoglobin's absorption profile differs dramatically from those of oxy- and deoxyhemoglobin.

Conversion of the various hemoglobin forms to cyanmethemoglobin circumvents possible errors due to these complex mixtures.[7] Hemoglobin and its derivatives (with the exception of the minute and unimportant amount of sulfhemoglobin) are oxidized to methemoglobin by adding blood to an alkaline potassium ferricyanide solution (Drabkin's solution). The methemoglobin then reacts with the potassium cyanide to form cyanmethemoglobin, a stable derivative with a maximum absorption at wavelength 540 nm. Interpolation from a standard curve provides the hemoglobin concentration in the sample unknown. Conditions that cause turbidity in the lysate, such as lipemia or Heinz bodies, can produce falsely high absorption readings and thereby an overestimation of the hemoglobin concentration.

With an automated counter, one aliquot of a blood sample passes through the counting apparatus of the analyzer, providing the red cell number and MCV. A separate lysed aliquot provides the hemoglobin determination. In theory, the use of two different samples to make primary measurements can introduce small errors into the calculations. This is particularly germane since many of the values commonly used by physicians are mathematical derivatives of these primary data (Table 1-3).

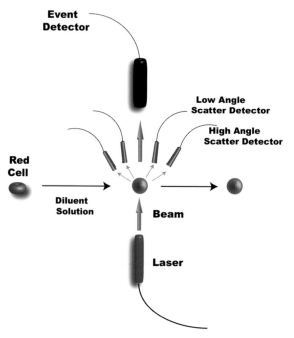

FIGURE 1-3 *A blood cell analyzer based on flow cytometry uses a laser beam focused on the cell aperture. The diluent solution converts the red cells to spheres from their typical toroid geometry. Cells flowing past the aperture interrupt the beam thereby providing a cell count. One group of photodetectors measures the low angle light scatter that correlates with cell size. Other detectors measure high-angle light scatter, which is a function of cellular protein content. This value is effectively the hemoglobin content since this molecule comprises the vast bulk of red cell protein.*

Newer methodology allows counting of erythrocytes by flow cytometry.[8] A diluent converts the red cells from their normal toroid shape into spheres that pass through a detection chamber containing a focused laser beam. The cells scatter the incident light at varying angles recorded by the instrument's detector (Figure 1-3). Interruption of the laser beam enumerates the cells in the sample. The instrument determines cell volume using low-angle light scatter while high-angle light scatter reflects internal protein content, which effectively is the hemoglobin concentration. Determination of red cell number, MCV, and hemoglobin content all on the same sample greatly reduces the risk of error.

Hematocrits reported by blood analyzers are derived numbers. The instrument uses the values for red cell number and MCV to calculate the hematocrit. Healthcare providers often discuss anemia using hematocrit values from blood analyzers because they harken back to the earlier centrifugation method. Although this approach is generally safe, conditions do arise that skew the hematocrit calculation. Either the hemoglobin value or the red cell number is a more reliable anemia indicator since the instrument directly measures both.

The red cell number quantifies erythrocytes per microliter of blood. As indicated in Table 1-1, normal values for an adult female range between 4.2×10^6 and 5.4×10^6 while those for a male are slightly higher. Anemia lowers the red cell number, making this value a key readout by the automated blood analyzer. Red cell number also varies markedly with the stage of life. The most dramatic differences occur during the neonatal period and infancy. A normal hemoglobin value for an adult female would represent significant anemia in a newborn.[9] Hemoglobin values decline modestly with advancing age.[10] Comorbid conditions in the elderly magnify this decline creating a perception of an "anemia of old age."[11] Anemia *should not* be written off to age without appropriately ruling out or at least considering serious and potentially deadly etiologies such as gastrointestinal malignancy.

The mean cell volume (MCV)—the average volume of the red cell in femtoliters—is a valuable information provided by every automated blood analyzer. Red cell sizes above or below the normal range (macrocytosis or microcytosis, respectively) help guide subsequent evaluation of anemia. Although microscopic observation gives a sense of red cell size, the blood analyzer provides a far superior determination. Anemias in which red cells are normal in both size and hemoglobin content are called "normochromic, normocytic." As with the red cell number, the MCV varies substantially with the stage of life. Newborns, for instance, have much larger red cells than do adults.

The red cell distribution width (RDW) is less familiar to most clinicians than are the variables discussed to this point. The RDW value reflects variation in red cell size. High RDW values mirror a large range in red cell size. Anemia due to combined iron and cobalamin deficiency, for instance, produces populations of large and small cells that are readily distinguished on microscopic examination of the blood smear. Anemia of this type also markedly elevates the RDW. The RDW can provide insight into the basis of an anemia because some processes increase its value while others do not. Microcytosis, for instance, exists with either iron deficiency or thalassemia. The former condition increases the RDW while the latter does not. Therefore, marked microcytosis with a normal RDW suggests thalassemia early in the work-up.

The automated blood analyzer also provides information on white cells and platelets in the blood sample. Consideration of these cells is central to the evaluation of anemia. Anemia in association with a low white cell count and low platelet count is usually more ominous than the one in which the values for these two constituents are normal. The morphology of the white cells and platelets is also important. Advanced blood analyzers provide information on the identities of the cells that comprise the population of white cells. These automated determinations of the components of the white cell population (also called the differential) are no substitute for manual blood examination. They can nonetheless guide the clinician who looks through the microscope. A single myeloblast in the white cell differential analysis, for example, makes leukemia a possible cause of the anemia in question.

Circulating red cells lack nuclei except under pathological conditions. Some disorders disturb bone marrow erythropoietic activity to such a degree that developing red cell precursors containing nuclei (normoblasts) escape into the blood stream. These "nucleated red cells" register as white cells with the blood analyzer. The total number of red cells in the circulation (millions/microliters) dwarfs the white cell population (thousands/microliters). Therefore, a small percentage of nucleated red cells in the peripheral blood can skew the white cell count tremendously. A manual count of nucleated red cells allows subtraction of these cells from the WBC total, giving the "corrected" white cell value.

The last method listed in Table 1-2 is the finger-stick hemoglobin absorption approach. Blood from the finger stick flows directly into a disposable cuvette allowing measurement of hemoglobin absorption. Internal adjustments include an allowance for the plasma in the sample. The accuracy of the approach is only moderate and subject to operator error. The approach is particularly suitable for screening blood donors who might be anemic since each donor receives substantial individual attention from a technician. Potential donors who fail the screening at this early point spare themselves and the institution subsequent expensive and time-consuming procedures.

■ RETICULOCYTE COUNT

The reticulocyte count is second only to the CBC in importance to the evaluation of anemia. The pathophysiology of anemia involves either the production of too few erythrocytes or the production of large numbers of red cells in concert with their rapid destruction or loss. The reticulocyte count is the arbiter of the type of anemia, being low in the former instance and high in the latter. This basic distinction allows the clinician to hone dramatically the search for the cause of the anemia.

Reticulocytes are newly formed red cells with residual strands of nuclear material called "reticulin" that remain following extrusion of the nucleus from bone marrow normoblasts. These new erythrocytes are 10–20% larger than red cells on average and have a faint bluish tint with Wright-Giemsa stain. Staining with a supravital dye such as brilliant cresol blue highlights the residual nuclear material and definitively identifies reticulocytes. These staining characteristics persist for only 1 or 2 days following release from the bone marrow. Thereafter, the erstwhile reticulocytes are identical to other red cells already in the circulation.

Reticulocytes provide unique insight into the operation of the bone marrow erythropoietic machinery. As a peripheral blood assay that reflects the activity of the bone marrow erythrocyte production system, the reticulocyte count is a powerful tool both for determining the cause of anemia and for the response to treatment. For example, a macrocytic anemia with a low reticulocyte count includes cobalamin deficiency in the differential diagnosis. The reticulocyte count achieves stratospheric levels with parenteral replacement of cobalamin in vitamin-deficient patients. The rise of the reticulocyte count substantially precedes an increase in the hemoglobin level, providing an early gauge of therapeutic response.

The lack of a reticulocyte response can indicate that the working diagnosis is incorrect. Moderate microcytosis and mild anemia are consistent with iron deficiency. For a person with a family history of thalassemia, however, the laboratory picture might represent thalassemia minor. A trial of iron replacement would correct the anemia only in the former case. The reticulocyte response to iron supplementation would give insight into the correct diagnosis even before more sophisticated test data are available.

No other component of the erythron has a similar window into the rate of cell production. A low platelet count, for instance, could reflect diminished production or a high rate of destruction of the cells. Only bone marrow examination can answer the question definitively. The peripheral blood platelet count provides the sole assessment of therapeutic response to an intervention for thrombocytopenia since no "reticulocyte equivalent" exists for platelets. Although theoretically possible to perform, serial bone marrow examinations to monitor the thrombopoietic system in this setting would be cruel and unusual punishment.

A terminological peculiarity sometimes confuses discussions of reticulocytes. The "reticulocyte count" reported by most clinical laboratories is given as a percentage of reticulocytes with respect to red cells in the sample. The normal value is about 1%. This reflects the practice of enumerating reticulocytes relative to erythrocytes in the early days of hematology when this work entailed manual counting of many microscopic fields. Expression of "reticulocyte count" as a percentage of red cells is a reasonable practice as long as the number of red cells is in the normal range. Anemias by definition have fewer red cells than normal. Consequently, the use of a percentage of red cells to determine reticulocyte production is invalid in the very circumstance where it is most needed. A normal "reticulocyte count" of 1% in the face of a hemoglobin value of 5 g/dL and 2.0×10^6 red cells/μL is patently abnormal. A number of formulae have been promulgated that purport to correct for the anemia and allow a clinician to assess whether the reticulocyte percentage value is elevated or depressed.

This semantic and conceptual trap is best avoided by using the true reticulocyte count, which is the number of reticulocytes per microliter of blood. This value is also termed the "reticulocyte number" to distinguish it from the percentage reticulocyte count. When the hemoglobin level is normal, blood contains between 40,000 and 50,000 reticulocytes/μL. An anemia with a reticulocyte number below this level is prima facie evidence of a hypoproliferative anemia.

Reticulocyte production should rise in the face of anemia as the low hemoglobin value triggers mechanisms that compensate for the deficit. With intact bone marrow hematopoietic machinery the reticulocyte number can easily supersede baseline values by 10-fold in response to a severe anemia. An anemia with a hemoglobin value of 5 g/dL and a reticulocyte number of 100,000/μL is a hypoproliferative anemia despite the "above normal" reticulocyte value since the increase in reticulocyte production is not commensurate with the degree of the anemia.

The automated blood analyzer red cell readout and the reticulocyte percentage value convert quickly into the reticulocyte number. The CBC provides the total number of red cells per microliter of blood, as previously noted. The reticulocyte percentage multiplied by the red cell number gives the reticulocyte number. For instance, an anemia with a red cell number of 3.1×10^6/μL and a reticulocyte count of 2% gives a reticulocyte number of 6.2×10^4 or 62,000/μL. The reticulocyte number is inordinately low for the degree of anemia. The anemia is hypoproliferative despite the normal reticulocyte percentage value.

■ PERIPHERAL BLOOD SMEAR

The peripheral blood smear gives valuable insight into the nature and possible causes of an anemia. The standard Wright-Giemsa stain highlights many characteristics of circulating erythrocytes, some of which are obvious while others are diaphanous. A careful review of the peripheral blood smear can pay large dividends to the clinician.

Red cells are roughly the size of lymphocyte nuclei, while their shape resembles a toroid. Thus there is a region of central pallor encompassing approximately one-third the diameter of the cell. Archetypal small red cells (microcytosis) occur with iron deficiency anemia. Iron-deficient erythrocytes also have exaggerated regions of central pallor. Some cells have only a thin rim of cytoplasm along their outer edge creating an appearance similar to hoop earrings. With extreme iron deficiency, many of the small red cells appear almost as cell fragments. Large erythrocytes in contrast are classically seen with deficiencies of cobalamin or folic acid. These macrocytic cells often assume an oval shape as well, producing quintessential macroovalocytes.

In some anemias the red cells have abnormal shapes or internal consistency rather than the normally bland interior with a smooth surface contour (Table 1-4). These changes can provide clues to the etiology of the condition. Erythrocytes with sharp, pointed projections of the plasma membrane are called "spur" cells and most commonly occur with severe liver failure. Sometimes the red cell membranes have a smooth, scalloped appearance. These "burr" cells are characteristic of anemia due to renal insufficiency. Red cell crescents that resemble sickles are eponymous for sickle cell disease. Schistocytes are misshapen cells that appear to have had their edges ripped from them. This sometimes is literally the case, as with the anemia due to disseminated intravascular coagulation. The red cells in this disorder tear apart as they whisk through microvasculature clogged with adhesive fibrin deposits.

Erythrocytes with regular contours can nonetheless have abnormalities that suggest an etiology for the anemia. Cells without central pallor are called "spherocytes" because they have a spheroidal rather than a toroidal shape. Hereditary spherocytosis is the archetype of an anemia with this red cell morphology. On average erythrocyte size is normal to slightly large in cases of hereditary spherocytosis.

Small spherocytes (microspherocytes) are characteristic of immune hemolytic anemia. In contrast to the cells in hereditary spherocytosis, microspherocytes reflect external assault on the red cells. Antibodies to erythrocyte membrane antigens accumulate and mark the cells for destruction by the reticuloendothelial system. Some of these targeted erythrocytes gain a second lease on life by literally tearing away from the grip of activated macrophages. The lost membrane reduces the surface area of the cells, creating microspherocytes that coexist with morphologically normal cells.

Hemoglobin is the predominant protein within erythrocytes. Red cells lack nuclei, mitochondria, and other subcellular structures seen in most mammalian cells. The uniform interior of these cells is altered with some anemias, producing visible inclusions. Howell-Jolly bodies are residual nuclear fragments seen in the erythrocytes of patients with dysfunctional spleens since the spleen normally removes these structures. Lead intoxication frequently produces basophilic particles composed of small

TABLE 1-4 | CELL MORPHOLOGY IN ANEMIA

Morphologic Characteristic	Basis of Finding	Special Stain	Comment
Howell-Jolly bodies	RBC nuclear remnants	N	• Increased with brisk hemolysis • Increased following splenectomy
Basophilic stippling	RNA remnants	N	• Impaired globin chain production (thalassemia; lead intoxication)
Pappenheimer bodies	Iron ferritin granules in cytoplasm	N	• Increased following splenectomy • Increased with transfusional iron overload
Heinz bodies	Hemoglobin aggregates	Y	• Unstable Hb • Enzymopathies • Hemoglobin H
Burr cells	Membrane perturbance	N	• Chronic renal failure • Common smear prep artifact
Acanthocytes (spur cells)	Membrane perturbance	N	• Severe hepatic insufficiency
Nucleated RBCs	Normoblast nuclei	N	• High with brisk hemolysis • Present with myelopthesis
Sickle cells	RBC distortion by hemoglobin polymers	N	• Sickle cell disease
Target cells	Low ratio of hemoglobin to red cell membrane; RBC dehydration	N	• Prominent in thalassemia • Present with iron deficiency
Spherocytes	Defective membrane protein	N	• Hereditary disorder • Immune hemolysis
Pseudo-Pelger-Huet cells	Neutrophils with bilobed nuclei	N	• Myelodysplasia

aggregates of residual RNA that lend a "stippled" appearance to the erythrocytes. Heinz bodies are hemoglobin aggregates common to enzymopathies such as G6PD deficiency. In contrast to the aforementioned structures, Heinz bodies are poorly visible by Wright-Giemsa stain and are best detected by a specific cell staining technique.

Occasionally, review of the peripheral smear reveals the definitive diagnosis in a case of anemia. Malaria is one of the most common causes of anemia worldwide afflicting nearly 400 million people each year. The malaria parasite is confined to the erythrocyte during one stage of its development. These malarial trophozoites are distinct entities that are readily visible with Wright-Giemsa staining of a peripheral smear. Searches for malarial parasites often require "thick" blood smears in which groups of red cells overlap. This smear technique increases the chance of detecting parasites over that employed with standard smears that spread red cells thinly to optimize their morphology.

White cell and platelet morphology can also provide clues to the etiology of an anemia. For instance, neutrophils that display the pseudo-Pelger-Huet anomaly point to myelodysplasia as a likely cause of anemia. Neutrophils on the smear containing few or no granules strengthen the case for this diagnosis. Large numbers of eosinophils on the peripheral smear suggest a parasitic infection. A far less common cause of anemia and eosinophilia is the hypereosinophilic syndrome.

White cells that normally are confined to the bone marrow appear in the peripheral blood with some forms of anemia. The misplaced white cells include myelocytes and metamyelocytes. When normoblasts (nucleated red blood cells) accompany the immature white cells in the peripheral blood, the picture is termed "leukoerythroblastic." Invasion of the bone marrow by foreign cells in a process called "myelophthesis" is commonly the basis of the problem. Bone marrow invasion is usually ominous with the intruders including entities such as metastatic breast cancer cells, abnormally proliferating fibroblasts, or bizarre macrophages such as those associated with sarcoidosis. A leukoerythroblastic peripheral blood picture places an anemia at a substantially greater level of seriousness.

Hematologists commonly lament the decline in review of peripheral smears by today's physicians. Automated blood analyzers provide a wealth of valuable data but elide much of the information available by a blood smear. Laboratory technicians who perform manual differential counts of white cells often are the sole source of comment on the nature of the blood smear. Jeremiads by hematologists are not simply the ranting of people obsessed with days of yore. No substitute exists for a careful review of the peripheral blood smear by the clinician. No technician should shoulder the burden of making critical diagnostic interpretations. In the review of the peripheral blood smear, the buck has a single stop.

■ BONE MARROW

Bone marrow examination has a special place in the anemia work-up since it is the organ of blood production. A key issue to be addressed by the physician is whether a bone marrow examination is needed to assess a particular case of anemia. The procedure changes the nature of the anemia evaluation because it requires the technical expertise of a hematologist or pathologist. The reticulocyte count often provides the basis for estimating the possible utility of a bone marrow examination. As a rule of thumb, bone marrow examination adds little useful data to the studies of anemias with high reticulocyte counts. The morphology in such instances is erythroid hyperplasia, which looks essentially the same irrespective of the cause. In contrast, information from the bone marrow examination can cinch the diagnosis in a hypoproliferative anemia with a low reticulocyte count.

A hematologist or oncologist performs the bone marrow procedure with the pathologist providing the official interpretation. The clinician should have sufficient knowledge of the procedure to allow proper interpretation of the pathology report. The clinical picture and the diagnostic possibilities associated with it can tilt the interpretation of the bone marrow. The physician overseeing the patient's care should maintain a high vigilance when reviewing the elements of the report.

The two methods of examining the bone marrow can in some instances provide different information. The *bone marrow biopsy* involves the removal of a core that contains cancellous bone as well as the surrounding marrow elements. The bone marrow biopsy is carried out in a fixing solution (usually Zenker's) that preserves cellular architecture during the subsequent slicing and staining process. Hematoxylin and eosin are the standard stains for bone marrow biopsy samples. The fixation requirement means that results of the procedure are not available for 2–3 days at the earliest.

The bone marrow biopsy is the sole way of determining the cellularity of the marrow. Under normal circumstances, "stromal" cells consisting of fat cells and fibroblasts comprise about half of the bone marrow content. The remaining cells are largely hematopoietic in origin. The marrow cellularity varies tremendously with hypoproliferative anemias depending on the etiology of the condition. Aplastic anemia presents the classic picture of absent hematopoietic cells replaced by stroma and fat. Hematopoietic cells often comprise less than 10% of the total cell content in cases of aplastic anemia. In contrast, cases of myelodysplasia can have hematopoietic cellularities in the range of 80%. In the former case, the anemia is due to the absence of hematopoietic cells. In the latter, the hematopoietic cells are present but fail to produce sufficient numbers of mature erythrocytes.

The biopsy provides information about the architecture of the bone marrow that otherwise is unattainable. The platelet-producing cells (megakaryocytes) are most abundant near the edges of a cancellous bone. Subtypes of hematopoietic cells tend to form clusters in which individual cells range from early to late stages of maturation. The erythroid lineage contains clusters with cells ranging from proerythroblasts, which are the earliest visually defined red cell precursors, to late normoblasts that are on the verge of extruding their nuclei to become reticulocytes. Disturbance of the organizational pattern occurs with many hypoproliferative anemias.

A *bone marrow aspiration* involves puncturing the cortical bone with a needle and aspirating marrow contents. The aspirate is spread on a coverslip or a microscope slide and allowed to air dry. The sample is ready for examination after staining with Wright-Giemsa pigment. The whole procedure takes less than an hour, making it the preferred approach when information about the bone marrow is needed rapidly.

The overlap in information provided by the bone marrow aspirate and biopsy is substantial but not total. The aspirate only approximates the bone marrow cellularity and provides no information about architecture. The biopsy is superior for the detection of foreign cells such as in metastatic malignancy. Both the biopsy and aspirate highlight abnormal plasma cells in multiple myeloma. However, biopsy best pinpoints the sheets of plasma cells characteristic of the disorder.

The aspirate is superior to the biopsy on other points. The most important area is the evaluation of iron stores. The bone marrow is the gold standard in the assessment of iron deficiency. The presence of the mineral in reticuloendothelial cells is the key to the diagnosis. The fixation of the biopsy sample washes much if not all the iron from these cells, making the diagnosis of iron deficiency difficult when based on biopsy. As discussed in Chapter 7, bone marrow examination is rarely needed for the diagnosis of iron deficiency. In those unusual instances that do require this invasive procedure use of the proper sampling technique is imperative.

The bone marrow aspirate preserves many aspects of subcellular structure more completely than does the biopsy. The changes characteristic of myelodysplasia are more readily detectable, including prominent nucleoli in proerythroblasts and myeloblasts, poor granule accumulation in metamyelocytes, and abnormal normoblast nuclei. Vacuoles in erythroid precursors, such as those seen with ethanol toxicity, often are easier to recognize on aspiration than by biopsy. The clinician should be aware of whether the bone marrow sampling technique adequately addresses the question at hand.

■ OTHER LABORATORY TESTS

Both the general blood chemistry profile and other specialized blood tests can aid in the evaluation of anemia. Table 1-5 briefly lists tests from each category. The routine laboratory tests are particularly important since they are universally available. Review of old laboratory data of a patient with newly diagnosed anemia sometimes gives clues regarding the inception of the disorder. Modest elevations in the blood urea nitrogen (BUN) and creatinine often exist months or years before anemia secondary to chronic renal insufficiency unfolds, for instance. Routine laboratory tests sometimes point to the etiology of a problem before specific diagnostic test results are available. A patient suspected of having a hemolytic transfusion reaction often will have a urinalysis that tests positive for heme in the absence of red cells. This result, due to intravascular red cell destruction with the transfusion reaction, is available almost immediately and can allow early intervention in an urgent clinical setting.

The specialized laboratory tests are not used for general screening but rather to confirm a suspected diagnosis. A small quantity of the protein haptoglobin normally exists in serum, for instance. The protein has a high affinity for hemoglobin but a very low capacity. Hemoglobin released into the plasma with hemolysis quickly binds to haptoglobin with subsequent clearance by hepatic receptors. Serum haptoglobin falls to a low level or vanishes with intravascular hemolysis of any etiology.

TABLE 1-5 | **LABORATORY TESTS USEFUL IN THE EVALUATION OF ANEMIA**

Laboratory Test	*Comment*
Routine Laboratory Tests	
BUN/CREAT	Elevated with anemia secondary to chronic renal insufficiency
LDH	Elevated with hemolysis
Bilirubin	Unconjugated bilirubin increases with hemolysis
Urinalysis	Positive for heme with either bleeding into the urinary tract or intravascular hemolysis. With bleeding, intact RBCs exist. With intravascular hemolysis, there are no intact RBCs despite the positive heme test
Urine hemosiderin	Positive for several weeks *after* an episode of intravascular hemolysis. Provides support for suspected intravascular hemolysis that was missed.
Erythrocyte sedimentation rate	Elevated in anemia secondary to chronic inflammation.
Special Laboratory Tests	
Serum haptoglobin	Low or absent with hemolysis
Serum hemoglobin	Elevated with intravascular hemolysis
Serum erythropoietin level	Low with chronic renal failure. Can be low with myelodysplasia

BUN, blood urea nitrogen; CREAT, creatinine; LDH, lactate dehydrogenase.

The serum erythropoietin level is particularly useful in the evaluation of patients with anemia in the setting of chronic renal insufficiency. The serum BUN and creatinine reflect renal dysfunction but often do not directly correlate with serum erythropoietin levels. Some patients with only modest renal insufficiency as defined by BUN and creatinine values have very low erythropoietin levels. The erythropoietin level can help guide replacement therapy with the hormone in these instances. Erythropoietin also raises the hematocrit of some patients with myelodysplasia. Patients with low erythropoietin levels in association with myelodysplasia respond better to hormone therapy than do those with normal erythropoietin levels, providing a guide to the therapeutic approach.

■ PHYSICAL EXAMINATION

The physical examination of a patient with anemia can uncover clues to the etiology of the condition. The physiognomy of the patient can point to a number of disorders, particularly those of a congenital nature. Classic cases of Fanconi's anemia, for instance, present with a range of physical abnormalities including skin discoloration, short stature, and skeletal problems such as misshapen or missing thumbs. The severity of the condition varies such that some patients escape diagnosis until adolescence or even early adulthood. Formes fruste of Fanconi's anemia and other "childhood disorders" are often uncovered when the physician keeps them in mind. Irrespective of patient age, all clinicians should look for clues such as short stature or odd facies in the anemia work-up.

A careful examination of the quality and quantity of hair is essential to the anemia work-up. Iron deficiency, for instance, produces thinning and loss of hair because hair follicle cells require iron to proliferate. Loss of the lateral aspects of the eyebrows raises the possibility that hypothyroidism might underlie a normochromic, normocytic anemia. Patients on total parenteral nutritional support can develop significant copper deficiency with associated anemia and brittle hair.

Clues to the etiology of an anemia can surface with careful skin examination. Anemia commonly produces pallor. However, the finding often is masked in patients with prominent skin pigmentation. Careful examination of unpigmented regions of epithelium such as mucous membranes and the nail beds can unveil otherwise cryptic pallor. Jaundice can reflect rapid erythrocyte turnover due to a hemolytic anemia. Jaundice due to increased unconjugated bilirubin also occurs with hepatic injury, in which case anemia might be secondary to a problem such as chronic active hepatitis.

Vitiligo can be a part of an autoimmune complex that includes cobalamin deficiency. Immune reaction to the gastric cells that produce intrinsic factor accompanies the immunologic process associated with vitiligo. Prominent macrocytic anemia can develop in such cases. Telangiectasias in the mouth or around the ears raise the possibility of gastrointestinal bleeding from similar lesions in the gut as the cause of anemia. Skin ulcers over the lower extremities sometimes are prominent clinical findings in patients with hemolytic anemias such as sickle cell disease or thalassemia.

Spooning of the fingernails or "koilonychia" occurs with long-standing cases of iron deficiency. The feature often is most prominent in the thumbs where pressure from writing or holding eating utensils produces the concave curvature of the nail. Splinter hemorrhages of the nail beds raise the possibility that anemia is secondary to underlying bacterial endocarditis.

Ocular examination often shows pale retinae in association with severe anemia. Some retinal abnormalities such as the "sea fan" and "salmon patch" defects of sickle cell disease are visible only with indirect ophthalmoscopy. Blue sclerae are common to iron deficiency. Thinning of the scleral membrane highlights the bluish coloration of the underlying epithelium. Icteric sclerae occur with hemolytic anemias of all types.

Angular stomatitis can result from deficits of iron or cobalamin. The lesions often are painful and may be the first symptom that attracts medical attention to a patient with chronic anemia. Glossitis characterized by a smooth, shiny tongue also develops in many instances of iron or cobalamin deficiency. The patient might initially present to an otolaryngologist for evaluation of a sore tongue. The insidious nature of cobalamin deficiency might not force the patient to further medical attention before serious and irreversible neurologic injury develops. The imperative of recognizing the connection between glossitis and anemia is great in this circumstance.

Chronic severe anemias can produce cardiomegaly related to prolonged high cardiac output. Enlarged hearts in patients with disorders such as thalassemia are usually hyperdynamic. Later, high output heart failure can occur. A third heart sound in a patient with long-standing severe anemia bodes ill.

Abdominal examination can be particularly revealing in the evaluation of anemia. Splenomegaly occurs with many types of anemia. The palpable quality of the spleen provides additional information. A soft spleen is typical of hemolytic anemias such as autoimmune hemolytic anemia or pyruvate kinase deficiency. An enlarged firm spleen can develop with infiltrative disorders such as myeloid metaplasia with myelofibrosis or Gaucher's disease. However, in chronic hemolytic states (e.g., hereditary sphero-cytosis, thalassemia major) the enlarged spleen is usually firm.

Splenomegaly exacerbates anemia by exposing erythrocytes to an environment that is relatively hypoxic and acidic. Metabolically compromised cells, such as those deficient in glucose-6-phosphate dehydrogenase (G6PD) can suffer severe splenic sequestration. Hemolysis is magnified in this circumstance. The spleen also has a prominent representation of reticuloendothelial cells. Antibody-coated erythrocytes that linger in the splenic sinusoids neither live long nor prosper.

Hepatomegaly occurs with primary liver disorders such as acute hepatitis. Anemia in this situation can reflect ongoing viral infection. Large firm livers occur with myeloid metaplasia and myelofibrosis. Metastatic cancer also produces this hepatic picture, sometimes in association with a leukoerythroblastic anemia due to coincident bone marrow invasion by malignant cells. Shrunken livers are typical of cirrhosis and end-stage liver disease. Anemia in this circumstance can have multiple contributors in addition to the primary hepatic insult, including gastrointestinal bleeding from varices, hypersplenism due to elevated portal vein pressure, or hemolysis due to spur cell defects of erythrocytes.

Rectal examination is one of the most important aspects of the physical examination of patients with anemia. The examination can show occult gastrointestinal bleeding as the cause of anemia. This is a particular concern in adults where colonic cancer is a major concern. In contrast, rectal hemorrhoids in a patient with iron deficiency anemia can be a cause for relief.

Neurologic abnormalities associated with anemia vary markedly in presentation and setting. In some cases, such as Pearson's syndrome, the neurologic defects develop during childhood. The manifestations in such instances often are extreme. In other cases, the neurologic deficit develops later, as with pernicious anemia (cobalamin deficiency) and the degeneration of the posterior and lateral tracts in the spinal column.

■ FAMILY HISTORY

A careful family history is essential to the work-up of anemia. The primary disorder sometimes is inherited, as with Fanconi's anemia or pyruvate kinase deficiency. In other instances, an inherited defect predisposes to anemia. Hereditary telangiectasia with associated chronic gastrointestinal bleeding exemplifies such a disorder. A good family history gives the clinician a running start in the anemia evaluation.

A few issues potentially complicate the family history when considering anemia. The frequent occurrence of iron deficiency in menstruating women means that many patients will give a family history skewed by iron deficiency anemia. For instance, questions about anemia in male family members that seek a hereditary pattern are sometimes obscured by unrelated instances of iron deficiency anemia involving females.

The family history often is more accurate when the anemia in question produces severe manifestations. A family with β-thalassemia genes often has members affected with thalassemia major or intermedia. These affected people are hard to miss. In contrast, a family with a gene producing mild pyruvate kinase deficiency might report a much less striking history.

Finally, the physician should not assume that the patient knows the meaning of medical terms such as anemia. Some people might refer to anemia as "poor" blood, "thin" blood, or "low" blood. The latter in particular must be distinguished from low blood pressure. Equally important, a positive family history might not reflect a hereditary disorder. An environmental toxin can produce a familial picture if most of the family members live in the contaminated area. For instance, a family history of anemia in a clan that hails from an old mining region in Colorado could represent widespread lead intoxication from contaminated ground water. The physician must carefully tease apart the information so that the boon of a family history does not become a bane.

■ CONTEXT OF ANEMIA

Anemia occurs as a primary defect or a secondary problem. The bone marrow is the erythrocyte production organ. Failure of its cellular machinery causes primary anemia. Aplastic anemia is the sine qua non in this category. With other anemias, the bone marrow functions normally while the red cells are lost prematurely. Peptic ulcer disease with bleeding into the gastrointestinal tract can cause this problem. Classification of the anemia as a primary or secondary problem is a key early step in the evaluation. The reticulocyte count is the test that defines this branch point. Table 1-6 provides an overview of this bifurcation with a small number of specific examples.

The wide range of primary defects that produce anemia creates a potentially difficult process of elimination. Fortunately, some primary disease processes confer ancillary features to the anemia that can narrow the possible etiologies from hundreds

TABLE 1-6	CLASSIFICATION OF ANEMIA

A. Impaired bone marrow activity
    Bone marrow failure syndromes
        Aplastic anemia
        Diamond-Blackfan syndrome
        Myelodysplasia
    Bone marrow replacement
        Metastatic cancer
        Myelofibrosis
        Gaucher's disease
    Nutritional or hormone deficiency
        Iron deficiency
        Cobalamin deficiency
        Erythropoietin deficiency (chronic renal insufficiency)
    Toxicity
        Lead
        Gold
        Chronic inflammation
        Ethanol

B. Early loss of red cells
    Brisk bleeding
        Peptic ulcer disease
        Colonic arteriovenous malformations
    Hemolysis
        Autoimmune hemolytic anemia
        Sickle cell disease
        Hereditary spherocytosis
        Pyruvate kinase deficiency
    Hypersplenism
        Cirrhosis
    Osmotic lysis
        Fresh water drowning
    Malaria

This table provides a conceptual classification of anemia in which causes are grouped by low bone marrow activity or early loss of red cells. Some of the examples, such as chronic ethanol ingestion, apply to more than one classification but are listed in one for the sake of simplicity.

down to fewer than a dozen. Sometimes the supplemental clue involves a property of the red cell such as microcytosis. The important step is to place the anemia in a broad framework that includes variables such as the environment, patient activity, and comorbid conditions.

A single value defines anemia, for instance, a hemoglobin level of 9 g/dL. Consideration of the overall clinical context of the anemia, however, completes the interpretation of the number. A patient presenting with "mild fatigue and weakness" could on evaluation have a hemoglobin value of 4 g/dL. Another patient who complains of marked fatigue and lethargy might have a hemoglobin value of 10 g/dL. These different presentations provide valuable initial clues in the work-up. The first patient has inveterate anemia. Physiological and behavioral adaptations over time mask the gravity of the condition. An anemia of this severity with such mild symptoms might reflect a chronic nutritional deficit, such as iron deficiency due to bleeding from intestinal infestation with helminths. The second patient has developed anemia more rapidly and without time to adapt. An acute problem such as a brisk gastrointestinal bleed could produce such a picture. Blood loss is the ultimate cause of anemia in each case. The pathophysiology of the anemias differs strikingly, however.

Nutritional deficiencies often have associated features involving other organs since cells other than developing erythrocytes could require the nutrient. Glossitis accompanies cobalamin deficiency reflecting the need for the vitamin by the rapidly proliferating cells of the gastrointestinal tract. The tongue is easy to assess, making changes secondary to cobalamin deficiency easy to detect. Aplasia and flattening of the intestinal villi in the jejunum and duodenum are less familiar manifestations of cobalamin deficiency. These changes nonetheless are more significant than the oral irritation produced by glossitis. Malabsorption of other nutrients by the injured duodenum and jejunum can compound the seriousness of cobalamin deficiency.

Symptoms related directly to anemia include fatigue, tachycardia, and dyspnea on exertion. Fatigue reflects insufficient delivery of oxygen to end organs, particularly muscles. Oxygen delivery is a function of the oxygen-carrying capacity of blood and the rate at which blood circulates. The low hemoglobin level of anemia reduces blood's oxygen-carrying capacity. Tachycardia increases the cardiac output. These factors can offset each other to a degree, allowing continued delivery of adequate quantities of oxygen to the tissues. As the hemoglobin level continues to fall, a point occurs at which the augmented cardiac output cannot compensate for the diminished oxygen-carrying capacity of the blood. This crisis point varies greatly between individuals. Factors such as activity level and coincident disease greatly influence the clinical situation. For example, a young woman who runs long distance track for her college team will develop symptoms due to iron deficiency and early anemia much sooner than would a sedentary classmate. The athlete could develop symptoms without formally meeting the criteria of anemia as defined by population cutoffs. The runner likely would recognize a fall in hemoglobin from 14 to 12.5 g/dL as she fights for maximum energy output. The sedentary classmate likely would notice nothing as she sits and fights her way through Dreiser's *An American Tragedy*.

Vascular integrity also modulates blood flow to tissues. Angina pectoris due to partial occlusion of coronary arteries is a well-recognized clinical problem. An atheromatous plaque in a coronary artery caps blood flow to regions of cardiac muscle. Exercise or other factors can create an oxygen demand that outstrips the blood's delivery capacity. Anemia can reduce the oxygen-carrying capacity of blood to the point that a patient with coronary artery disease suffers angina pectoris with minimal or no exertion. In the absence of coronary artery disease, the patient might tolerate the anemia without problem.

Any definition of anemia that uses the "normal" population under "normal" circumstances does not apply to everyone. Chronic obstructive pulmonary disease impedes oxygenation of blood as it passes through the lungs so that the arterial oxygen saturation often falls to levels substantially below normal. Tissue oxygen demand can be met in this circumstance by a higher blood-oxygen-carrying capacity. In other words, patients with severe chronic obstructive pulmonary disease require unusually high hemoglobin levels. A hemoglobin value of 14 g/dL might produce significant symptoms in such a patient despite being in the "normal" range.

Disease is not the only reason to adjust the definition of anemia. Sherpas in the mountains of Nepal have higher baseline hemoglobin values than do shepherds in New Zealand. Although other physiologic changes contribute to high altitude conditioning, a high baseline hemoglobin is a key factor. Anyone who has flown from sea level to a vacation ski trip in the mountains can attest to this fact. For people who live and work at very high altitude, however, a supernormal baseline hemoglobin level is essential. A Sherpa with a hemoglobin level of 14 g/dL could have problems on the road to Everest.

■ TREATING ANEMIA

The range of possible anemia treatments is limited only by the range of causes of the condition. A direct treatment exists for some forms of anemia, as with cobalamin replacement for pernicious anemia. Other types of anemia such as Fanconi's anemia have no specific remedy. Transfusion provides additional red cells and temporarily corrects most anemias. The benefit is ephemeral since the transfused cells become senescent and are destroyed over intervals ranging from days to weeks. Several general principles underlie the basic guidelines to correction of anemia, however.

Whenever possible, the treatment should be specific to the cause of the condition. When the anemia results from a fault involving the bone marrow, correcting the defect should be the goal. Replacement of iron is the ideal treatment for iron deficiency anemia. For anemias linked to a more generalized underlying disorder, the goal should be to correct the disease process. Kidney transplantation is the best treatment for the anemia of end-stage renal disease. If the disease process cannot be reversed, interventions to relieve the impact of the disorder should be undertaken. Erythropoietin replacement is the treatment of choice for people with end-stage renal disease who cannot receive a kidney transplant. Transfusion is the intervention of last resort for anemia. Transfusions should be used to correct anemia in people with end-stage renal disease only when erythropoietin is unavailable.

The evanescence of the transfusion effect makes the procedure the "band aid" of anemia therapy. Transfusions benefit most profoundly those people with a temporary anemia. A postsurgical patient who requires transfusion immediately following the procedure is a perfect example of the procedure used to tide over an anemia. The patient's endogenous erythrocyte production system quickly takes control of the situation obviating requirements for further transfusion.

Transfusions can also correct chronic anemias. The ongoing need for blood replacement creates its own problems, of which the most important is iron overload. Each unit of blood delivers more than 200 mg of iron, which is an intrinsic component of heme. As discussed in Chapter 7, no physiologic iron excretion mechanism exists, meaning that chronic transfusion can produce astronomical body loads of the mineral.

Untreated transfusional iron overload is invariably fatal. Effective interventions for transfusional iron overload exist, but are difficult to undertake. The specter of iron overload must be balanced against the morbidity of the anemia. Transfusion often is the only option for life-threatening chronic anemia, such as that produced by thalassemia major. For patients with severe anemia where the threat to life is not measured in months or a few years, such as severe hereditary spherocytosis, the risk of morbidity from the primary disorder must be weighed against the perils of transfusion.

Patients with severe anemia from chronic nutritional deficiency are a particular challenge to clinicians. In a person discovered to have a hemoglobin value of 4 g/dL, a great temptation exists to transfuse blood rapidly and bring the hemoglobin up toward the normal range. This can be a disaster. A variety of physiological adjustments allow the person in question to function despite the profound hemoglobin deficit. Expansion of the plasma volume is one of those adaptations. Transfusion of three units of blood aimed at correcting the hemoglobin value can push the patient into major fluid overload with the risk of morbidity and even death.[12]

Slow is the way to go in this circumstance. A person with severe anemia due to cobalamin deficiency usually does not require transfusion because the hemoglobin rises extremely rapidly with vitamin replacement. This approach avoids the risk of fluid overload and the other potential problems of transfusion, such as viruses transmitted by transfusion. The same holds for patients with severe iron deficiency anemia. The most important aspects to the treatment of anemia are gauging the overall clinical context and weighing immediate and long-term needs. Errors are less likely with a measured approach to anemia.

References

1   Fairbanks VF, Klee GG, Wiseman GA, et al. 1996. Measurement of blood volume and red cell mass: Re-examination of ^{51}Cr and ^{125}I methods. Blood Cells Mol Dis 22:169–186.

2   Greendyke RM. 1963. Revised normal values for hemoglobin, hematocrit and erythrocyte count in adult males. Postgrad Med 33:A44–A50.

3   Lovric VA. 1970. Normal haematological values in children aged 6 to 36 months and socio-medical implications. Med J Aust 2:366–370.

4   Dien K, Lentner C, eds. 1973. Documenta Geigy, Scientific Tables, 7th edn. Basle, Switzerland: CIBA-Geigy Limited, p. 617.

5   Stewart JW. 1966. A comparison of different methods of determinating the haematocrit. Bibl Haematol 24:101–108.

6   Windholz M, ed. 1983. The Merck Index, 10th edn. Rahway, NJ: Merck & Co., Inc, p. 672.

7   NCLLS. 2000. Reference and selected procedures for the quantitative determination of hemoglobin in blood; approved standard-third edition. NCCLS document H15-A3 (ISBN 1-56238-425-2). Wayne, PA: NCCLS

8   Kim YR, Ornstein L. 1983. Isovolumetric sphering of erythrocytes for more accurate and precise cell volume measurement by flow cytometry. Cytometry 3:419–427.

9   Dallman PR, Yip R, Johnson C. 1984. Prevalence and causes of anemia in the United States, 1976 to 1980. Am J Clin Nutr 39:437–445.

10   Tsang CW, Lazarus R, Smith W, Mitchell P, Koutts J, Burnett L. 1998. Hematological indices in an older population sample: Derivation of healthy reference values. Clin Chem 44:96–101.

11   Anià B, Suman V, Fairbanks V, Rademacher D, Melton 3rd L. Incidence of anemia in older people: An epidemilogic study in a well defined population. J Am Geviatr Soc 45:825–831.

12   Duke M, Herbert VD, Abelmann WH. 1964. Hemodynamic effects of blood transfusion in chronic anemia. N Engl J Med 271:975–980.

ANEMIA AND AGE

A remarkable set of surveillance and regulatory mechanisms maintain hemoglobin values within a narrow set of parameters for most of a person's life. The renal oxygen sensing mechanism that is part of the erythropoietin feedback system is the primary hemoglobin rheostat. In the absence of pathological processes such as temporary erythroid shutdown due to parvovirus B19 infection, remarkably little fluctuation occurs in the hemoglobin value of an individual. Pregnancy is the one physiological state that substantially, although temporarily, resets the baseline hemoglobin value.

The picture with respect to hemoglobin is not so equitable very early in life or very late in life. The change in status from fetus to neonate is the most profound in life. The physical change required to move from total dependence on the mother to a life as a truly independent being is one of the most dramatic events in nature. Equally profound are the changes in physiology that make possible a solitary survival by the neonate. With this backdrop of events, the changes in hemoglobin values during infancy and childhood along with the parameters that define anemia come as little surprise. Pediatricians face the challenge of defining a "normal" hemoglobin value in what may appear to be a turbulent sea.

Adult providers who care for people whose age begins to press the envelope of human endurance face similar challenges. What is a "normal" hemoglobin value when one has seen four score and seven years go by? Does the fatigue and wear that take a toll on so many organ systems also grind down the erythron and dampen hemoglobin production? Answers to these questions profoundly influence medical management. Reasoned medical care requires insight into the intricacies of such issues.

■ PHYSIOLOGICAL ANEMIA OF INFANCY

At birth, the concentration of hemoglobin averages 16.5 gm/dL. The relative polycythemia of the newborn is attributable to the low arterial Pao_2 in utero that stimulates erythropoietin (EPO) production with a consequent high rate of erythropoiesis. In the fetus and neonate, most EPO production occurs in the liver, rather than the kidney. After birth and the establishment of respiration, the arterial Pao_2 rises, triggering sharp declines both in EPO production and the rate of erythropoiesis. The dampened red cell production is reflected in the disappearance of nucleated red cells and a fall in the reticulocyte count that continues for 6–8 weeks. During this period, the red cell life span is only about 90 days, compared with the 120 days in adults. Hemoglobin levels in the term baby fall from steadily from about 16.5 gm/dL to about 11.0 gm/dL at 6–8 weeks of age due to decreased red cell production and increased destruction. This fall, which reflects the physiologic transition from the relatively hypoxic intrauterine environment to the oxygen-replete extrauterine state, is called the *physiological anemia of infancy.* After 6–8 weeks, red cell production resumes as indicated by a rise in reticulocyte count, stabilization of the hemoglobin level, followed by an increase in hemoglobin level that plateaus at an average of 12.5 gm/dL for the first 5–6 years of life. The rate of RBC production is sufficient to maintain a stable hemoglobin level despite the threefold increase in blood volume that occurs in the first years of life unless there is inadequate iron in the diet.

In the preterm infant, the postnatal fall in hemoglobin concentration is more marked and occurs sooner than in the full-term infant—the smallest infants having the greatest decline in hemoglobin concentration. This is called the early anemia of prematurity, which is an exaggerated physiological anemia. Premature infants have inappropriately low EPO levels for the severity of the anemia, perhaps because hepatic EPO production is less sensitive to reduced oxygen concentrations relative to the renal production mechanism. However, the clinical benefit of EPO therapy is controversial and today the drug is not standardly administered to small premature infants. Other factors that contribute to the early anemia of prematurity include a very large expansion of blood volume (so called "bleeding into the circulation!"), a red cell life span that is even shorter than is typical for this age, and especially the relatively large amounts of blood removed for laboratory studies in sick premature infants. The average 12.5 gm/dL of hemoglobin during childhood is considerably lower than that of adults. It has been hypothesized that this is because the relative hyperphosphatemia of children may result in increased levels of organic phosphate compounds, especially 2,3-DPG within the RBC, which shift the oxygen dissociation curve resulting in more effective delivery of oxygen to the tissues.

Average hemoglobin levels of African American children are about 0.5 gm/dL lower than those of Caucasian children and the difference cannot be ascribed to thalassemia or iron deficiency.

■ ADVANCING AGE AND ANEMIA

Erythrocyte production in adults is remarkably constant. Normal hemoglobin values used in clinical practice are based on determinations from healthy adults of all ages.[1] The baseline hemoglobin value changes little over the course of years in the absence of disturbances such as nutritional deficiencies or major illnesses. The high prevalence of anemia in older adults begs the question of whether the general norms apply to older people. Separating the relationship between hemoglobin and age from perturbations due to pathological disturbances to hematopoiesis that accumulate with age is not straightforward. Anemia is particularly problematic in older people since it lowers the quality of life and can rob people of their independent status. As such, an understanding of anemia and age is vital to proper patient management.

The frequency of anemia in adults rises with advancing age.[2,3] This pattern mirrors the evolution of many disorders that begin in adulthood, ranging from hypertension to cancer. Anemia is a secondary phenomenon to many medical conditions that arise in adults. In some instances, such as the anemia of chronic renal insufficiency caused by a dearth of erythropoietin, the effect is relatively direct and easy to comprehend. Other cases of anemia reflect a complex interplay between the disease process and the erythropoietic machinery. The anemia of chronic inflammation exemplifies this category of disorder.[4] The fact that so many disorders common in older people produce concurrent anemia makes inevitable the rise in the incidence of anemia with age.

The key question with respect to age and anemia is whether advancing age per se produces anemia. If the answer is "no" then anemia in an older person reflects a concomitant and perhaps cryptic disorder whose nature should be uncovered. A low hemoglobin value in an 80-year-old person therefore could not be dismissed simply as an effect of "old age." On the other hand, should aging alone produce anemia, a less vigorous pursuit of etiology might be reasonable in such a patient.

The idea of a body component "wearing out" with age is intuitive in some circumstances. Joints are a fine example of a body part, articular cartilage, which is lost over time due to wear. Osteoarthritis, a common problem for older people, results from years of wear and tear on the joints. The body's repair mechanism for articular cartilage does not correct joint injury with complete fidelity. The result is slow loss of joint substance. Repetitive trauma, such as that occurs with years of long-distance running, accelerates joint degeneration and produces osteoarthritis in some relatively young people. On the whole, however, the condition is confined to older adults.

Could erythropoiesis also suffer "wear" leading to anemia with aging? The bone marrow machinery is not a structural entity like the knee, and therefore does not undergo physical stress. Rather, erythropoiesis is a repetitive process of cell generation beginning with the hematopoietic stem cell. Could the precision of the erythropoietic process decline over time due to acquired defects in the erythropoietic machinery?

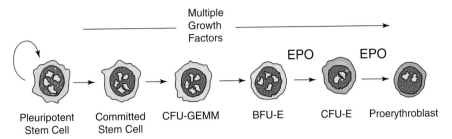

Multiple
Growth
Factors

EPO   EPO

Pleuripotent   Committed   CFU-GEMM   BFU-E   CFU-E   Proerythroblast
Stem Cell   Stem Cell

FIGURE 2–1 *Self-renewal of a hematopoietic stem cell. The hematopoietic stem cell produces mature red cells after multiple steps that involve multiplication, maturation, and differentiation. The stem cell divides and starts down this path infrequently. Even less frequently, the hematopoietic stem cell undergoes a self-renewal process, indicated by the looped line. The loss of stem cells due to direct injury or failure to self-renew can ultimately reduce red cell production.*

The idea is plausible, in particular given the slow accumulation of DNA damage over the years due to background radiation, environmental mutagens, and the like.

The pluripotent hematopoietic stem cell divides rarely, reproducing itself while generating a daughter cell that moves into the pathway of hematopoietic cell production (Figure 2-1). Could some of these self-replications fail to produce a new stem cell, leading to a decline over time in their number? Stem cells comprise a tiny fraction of the hematopoietic cells in the bone marrow. Consequently, the production capacity of the hematopoietic machinery could suffer significantly from the loss of a small number of these cells.

Surprisingly few studies have directly addressed this issue. One investigation examined the number of erythropoietic precursor cells in three cohorts of people.[5] One was a group of elderly people with unexplained anemia. Another was a group of elderly people without anemia. Finally there was a group of young people without anemia who served as controls. The investigators assessed the number of burst-forming units-erythroid (BFU-E), which are red cell precursors that are fairly far along in the erythroid maturation process. No difference existed in the number of BFU-Es in the elderly subjects with or without anemia. Both groups had significantly fewer BFU-Es than did the younger, nonanemic subjects. This suggested that although elderly people have fewer BFU-Es than do their younger counterparts, that fact does not per se portend anemia. The cultured cells responded appropriately to externally added erythropoietin and other growth-promoting factors. The investigators concluded that erythroid precursor cells in older people are functionally normal despite their lower number relative to precursor cells in younger people. The crux of the paper, however, was that advancing age does not produce anemia.

An important point in this context is that BFU-Es are not hematopoietic stem cells. The study does not rule out the possibility that the number of true hematopoietic stem cells is equivalent in younger and older adults. A host of steps that require cytokines and other growth factors exist between stem cells and BFU-Es. Diminished production of one of these factors or aberrant response to a cytokine could account for the difference between older and younger subjects with respect to the number of BFU-Es seen in bone marrow cultures. The conclusion of the work is best framed by saying that relative to younger counterparts the functional reserve of the erythron is lower in elderly adults. Nonetheless the lower functional reserve does not necessarily entail anemia.

Other investigators examined bone marrow from a group of healthy people who were 88 years of age.[6] The hemoglobin values in these people ranged from normal to the level of mild anemia. In vitro assays showed fewer erythroid precursor cells in this group than in a control group of younger people (ages 21–57 years). Marrow precursor cells from the older and younger age groups responded similarly to externally added growth factors. Generally speaking, cytogenetic abnormalities of erythroid precursor cells are more common in older people than in younger counterparts. These changes likely represent low-grade injury to the erythron that accumulates over time. Some cytogenetic changes, such as the loss of the long arm of chromosomes 5 or 7 ($5q^-$ or $7q^-$), are markers for bone marrow failure syndromes. The investigators found no consistent pattern of cytogenetic abnormalities in subjects from the older age group.

Overall, these data point to a decline in the functional capacity of the erythron without anemia as a necessary correlate. The lower functional erythroid reserve in older people does however increase the chance that outside stresses on the erythron will produce anemia. Hemolysis due to a leak around an artificial aortic value would more likely produce anemia in a person 80 years of age than in one of age 40. The key conclusion, however, is that anemia in older people is not the norm.

The cause of anemia in otherwise healthy older subjects often remains a mystery, even with careful examination.[7,8] In an effort to determine whether anemia in older people is pathological or merely the result of physiological changes with aging, investigators assessed the level of 2,3-diphospho glycerate (2,3-DPG) in three cohorts consisting of otherwise healthy elderly subjects with anemia, elderly subjects without anemia, and younger adults also without anemia.[9] 2,3-DPG is a small molecule in red cells that binds to hemoglobin and promotes oxygen release from the protein. Red cell levels of 2,3-DPG are higher in pathological conditions that produce relative tissue hypoxia. The older subjects with anemia had significantly higher erythrocyte 2,3-DPG levels than did the elderly subjects without anemia. This suggested that the anemia in these subjects was pathological and produced relative tissue hypoxia with associated compensatory production of 2,3-DPG. As with the studies cited earlier, these observations support the conclusion that anemia in otherwise healthy older people is pathological and not a normal condition.

Investigations involving cohorts of healthy older people support the conclusions of these smaller studies. A retrospective analysis of over 1000 people showed no decline in mean hemoglobin values in people up to the age of 85 years.[10] Other analyses have shown that healthy older people who live at home and who are not deficient in micronutrients such as iron maintain steady hemoglobin values.[11] The prevalence of anemia does rise with age, reflecting the higher incidence of conditions that produce anemia as a side effect, such as gastrointestinal disease, chronic inflammatory disorders, and renal insufficiency.[12,13] Nutritional deficiency, however, is the leading cause of anemia in older people.[8]

TABLE 2-1	CAUSES OF ANEMIA IN OLDER PEOPLE
Condition	*Example*
Chronic inflammatory conditions	Rheumatoid arthritis, chronic infection
Iron deficiency	Gastrointestinal bleeding
Renal dysfunction	Hypertension, diabetes mellitus, drugs
Cobalamin or folate deficiency	Nontropical sprue
Myelodysplasia	"Preleukemic" syndromes
Drugs	Ceftriaxone (hemolytic anemia)
Unexplained	

■ ETIOLOGY OF ANEMIA IN OLDER PEOPLE

A plethora of reports broadly address the prevalence of anemia in older people. The criteria used to define anemia varies in these studies, but most use the WHO designation that defines anemia as hemoglobin values below 13 g/dL in men or 12 g/dL in women.[14] Not surprisingly, anemia is most common among people in nursing homes or in hospitals.[15,16] The medical conditions that create the need for such facilities often produce anemia as a by-product of their pathology.[17] Chronic renal insufficiency and inflammatory conditions such as rheumatoid arthritis often underlie the anemia seen in these circumstances (Table 2-1).[18,19] Nutritional deficiencies such as iron and cobalamin deficit also commonly produce anemia in older people.[8,20,21] The former most often reflects low-grade gastrointestinal bleeding while the latter frequently results from poor cobalamin absorption.[22]

The high incidence of iron deficiency as a cause of anemia in older people is a cause for both hope and concern.[23] The hope derives from the fact that iron deficiency is readily corrected by either oral or parenteral supplementation of the mineral (Chapter 7). Concern derives from the fact that health-care providers often fail to diagnose iron deficiency even in hospitalized patients.[24] Early diagnosis of an underlying pathology prompted by the appropriate work-up of iron deficiency can be a life or death proposition. In some cases, iron deficiency heralds deadly conditions such as colonic adenocarcinoma.[25] Even without a surgical cure, treatment or palliation of malignancy is more effective with earlier diagnosis. Often, however, the iron deficiency results from benign conditions such as gastritis or peptic ulcer disease.[15,26,27] The underlying conditions often can be corrected with simple measures, such as thorough treatment with antibiotics and histamine H_2 receptor blockers. The benefit to patients is enormous in such circumstances (Table 2-2).

TABLE 2-2 | **KEY DIAGNOSTIC POINTS**

Issue	*Manifestation*	*Approach*
Anemia in the infant	Hemoglobin of 16.5 g/dL at birth falling to <11 g/dL at 8 weeks	• Check micronutrients such as iron and folate. • Observe clinical state. • Transfusion only if clinically indicated.
Anemia in elderly	• Hb <12 g/dL in women • Hb <13 g/dL in men	• Check micronutrients, including iron, folate, and cobalamin. • Rule out occult blood loss. • Rule out occult malignancy or inflammatory process. • Assess clinical state. • Transfuse only for clinical compromise.

■ RAMIFICATIONS OF ANEMIA IN OLDER PEOPLE

Anemia adversely affects the lives of older people to a substantially greater degree than it does to those who are relatively young. Fatigue is the most common symptom, and objective measures of physical performance bear out the negative impact on people's lives.[28] Diminished strength and lower exercise tolerance are the most profound objective findings and the most disturbing abnormalities for many anemic older people.[29] Inability to work or perform household chores clearly has a negative impact on a person's lifestyle. Equally important is the creeping inertia of a sedentary existence that robs a person of many simple pleasures in life.

Weakness due to anemia also increases the risk of falls. While a bruise is one possible outcome of a fall of an older person, the result too often is a bone fracture. Slowed reflexes mean that a person is more likely to strike the surface at an awkward or infelicitous angle. Osteoporosis heightens the chance that the impact will shatter a bone. Hip fractures are a key cause of morbidity in older people.[30] As many as one-quarter of people with hip fractures in assisted care settings die within three months of their accident.[31] While the prospects are better for people who have hip fractures at home, the death rate at three months is still a frightening one-in-ten. Hip fractures have potentially deadly side effects such as deep venous thrombosis and pulmonary embolism. The higher mortality in older people who have a greater than average number of medical problems at the time of their injury is no surprise.[32]

Many older people require prolonged stays in rehabilitation facilities after surgical repair of the injured joint. Decubitus ulcers, infections, and cellulitis are debilitating complications of hip fractures that frequently result from poor care and assistance during the recovery phase from the injury. For many people, diminished muscle tone due to immobility adds another challenge to the goal of reestablishing an independent lifestyle following the injury. Too often, a hip fracture is the first step of a slow downward spiral in health quality.

The overall risk of death is higher in older people who are anemic than is the case for those who are not.[33] Since anemia sometimes presages underlying malignancy or other medical problems that eventually become life-threatening, death related to anemia often is due to the blossoming of these afflictions.[34]

■ EVALUATION AND TREATMENT OF ANEMIA IN OLDER PEOPLE

The approach to anemia in older people should not differ from that applied to younger adults (See Chapter 1). The potential impact of the anemia should be weighed against the overall well-being and life expectancy of the patient. Evaluation and treatment must reflect the most ethical and humane approach to the problem. This principle underlies the art of medicine and is universally applicable (Table 2-3).

One issue that remains a point of debate is the appropriate target hemoglobin for older people. Data from a longitudinal study of older people in Sweden showed a decline in the mean hemoglobin values of both women and men between the ages of 70 and 88 years.[35] The investigators suggested that the "normal" hemoglobin ranges in older adults should be reduced from the WHO standards of 12 mg/dL

TABLE 2-3 | KEY MANAGEMENT POINTS

Issue	Comment
Anemia in infancy and childhood	The hemoglobin decline from 16.5 to 11 g/dL over the first 8 weeks of life is a physiological reset from relative hypoxia in utero to atmospheric oxygen tensions. Occasional infants, especially premature infants, dip below the trough, but almost all rebound without intervention.
	Iron deficiency is frequent in 9-month to 3-year-old infants because of poor intake and rapid growth. This can be prevented by use of iron-supplemented formula and cereals.
	The prevalence of iron deficiency anemia rises sharply in adolescent girls.
Anemia in elderly	No "anemia of old age" exists. The higher frequency of anemia in older people reflects comorbid and sometimes cryptic problems. Anemia per se can produce substantial morbidity. The basis of the anemia should be ascertained and the problem corrected when possible.

for women and 13 mg/dL in men to account for this decline. Other investigations suggest that the WHO hemoglobin standards in fact are too low.[36] Assessment of the relationship between hemoglobin level and mobility in older women showed better performance at hemoglobin levels higher than the WHO "normal" values.[37] The investigators who conducted the study suggested that target hemoglobin levels in elderly women (and presumably men) should be higher than the WHO standards. No trial has been performed to determine whether raising hemoglobin levels to beyond the WHO standard *improves* performance levels in healthy subjects.

The final word, however, is that anemia in older people should not be ignored.

References

1 NCLLS. Reference and selected procedures for the quantitative determination of hemoglobin in blood; approved standard-third edition. NCCLS document H15-A3 (ISBN 1-56238-425-2). Wayne, PA: NCLLS.

2 Balducci L. 2003. Epidemiology of anemia in the elderly: Information on diagnostic evaluation. J Am Geriatr Soc 51:S2–S9.

3 Anià B, Suman V, Fairbanks V, Rademacher D, Melton, 3rd, L. 1997. Incidence of anemia in older people: An epidemiologic study in a well defined population. J Am Geriatr Soc 45:825–831.

4 Andrews N. 2004. Anemia of inflammation: The cytokine-hepcidin link. J Clin Invest 113:1251–1253.

5 Hirota Y, Okamura S, Kimura N, Shibuya T, Niho Y. 1988. Haematopoiesis in the aged as studied by in vitro colony assay. Eur J Haematol 40:83–90.

6 Nilsson-Ehle H, Swolin B, Westin J. 1995. Bone marrow progenitor cell growth and karyotype changes in healthy 88-year-old subjects. Eur J Haematol 55:14–18.

7 Lipschitz D, Mitchell C, Thompson C. 1981. The anemia of senescence. Am J Hematol 11:47–54.

8 Guralnik J, Eisenstaedt R, Ferrucci L, Klein H, Woodman R. 2004. The prevalence of anemia in persons age 65 and older in the United States: evidence for a high rate of unexplained anemia. Blood 104:2263–2268.

9 Lipschitz D, Udupa K, Milton K, Thompson C. 1984. Effect of age on hematopoiesis in man. Blood 63:502–509.

10 Timiras M, Brownstein H. 1987. Prevalence of anemia and correlation of hemoglobin with age in a geriatric screening clinic population. J Am Geriatr Soc 35:639–643.

11 Olivares M, Hertrampf E, Capurro M, Wegner D. 2000. Prevalence of anemia in elderly subjects living at home: Role of micronutrient deficiency and inflammation. Eur J Clin Nutr 54:834–839.

12 Bird T, Hall MR, Schade RO. 1977. Gastric histology and its relation to anaemia in the elderly. Gerontology 23:309–321.

13 O'Neal RM, Abrahams OG, Kohrs MB, Eklund DL. 1976. The incidence of anemia in residents of Missouri. Am J Clin Nutr 29:1158–1166.

14 World Health Organization. Nutritional Anaemias: Report of a WHO Scientific Group. Geneva, Switzerland: World Health Organization; 1968.

15 Kalchthaler T, Tan M. 1980. Anemia in institutionalized elderly patients. J Am Geriatr Soc 28:108–113.

[16] Artz A, Fergusson D, Drinka P, et al. 2004. Mechanisms of unexplained anemia in the nursing home. J Am Geriatr Soc 52:423–427.

[17] Dunn A, Carter J, Carter H. 2003. Anemia at the end of life: Prevalence, significance, and causes in patients receiving palliative care. J Pain Symptom Manage 26:1132–1139.

[18] Beghe C, Wilson A, Ershler W. 2004. Prevalence and outcomes of anemia in geriatrics: A systematic review of the literature. Am J Med 116:3S–10S.

[19] Joosten E, Pelemans W, Hiele M, Noyen J, Verhaeghe R, Boogaerts M. 1992. Prevalence and causes of anaemia in a geriatric hospitalized population. Gerontology 38:111–117.

[20] Joosten E, Ghesquiere B, Linthoudt H, et al. 1999. Upper and lower gastrointestinal evaluation of elderly inpatients who are iron deficient. Am J Med 107:24–29.

[21] Chui C, Lau F, Wong R, et al. 2001. Vitamin B12 deficiency—need for a new guideline. Nutrition 17:917–920.

[22] Bird T, Hall MR, Schade RO. 1977. Gastric histology and its relation to anaemia in the elderly. Gerontology 23:309–321.

[23] Dallman P, Yip R, Johnson C. 1984. Prevalence and causes of anemia in the United States, 1976 to 1980. Am J Clin Nutr 39:437–445.

[24] Smieja M, Cook D, Hunt D, Ali M, Guyatt G. 1996. Recognizing and investigating iron-deficiency anemia in hospitalized elderly people. CMAJ 155:691–696.

[25] Annibale B, Capurso G, Chistolini A, et al. 2001. Gastrointestinal causes of refractory iron deficiency anemia in patients without gastrointestinal symptoms. Am J Med 111:439–445.

[26] Gordon S, Smith R, Power G. 1994. The role of endoscopy in the evaluation of iron deficiency anemia in patients over the age of 50. Am J Gastroenterol 89:1963–1967.

[27] Annibale B, Capurso G, Delle Fave G. 2003. The stomach and iron deficiency anaemia: A forgotten link. Dig Liver Dis 35:288–295.

[28] Penninx B, Pahor M, Cesari M, et al. 2004. Anemia is associated with disability and decreased physical performance and muscle strength in the elderly. J Am Geriatr Soc 52:719–724.

[29] Penninx B, Guralnik J, Onder G, Ferrucci L, Wallace R, Pahor M. 2003. Anemia and decline in physical performance among older persons. Am J Med 115:104–110.

[30] Lu-Yao GL, Baron JA, Barrett JA, Fisher ES. 1994. Treatment and survival among elderly Americans with hip fractures: A population-based study. Am J Public Health 84:1287–1291.

[31] Levi N. 1996. Early mortality after cervical hip fractures. Injury 27:565–567.

[32] Kenzora JE, McCarthy RE, Lowell JD, Sledge CB. 1984. Hip fracture mortality. Relation to age, treatment, preoperative illness, time of surgery, and complications. Clin Orthop 186:45–56.

[33] Izaks G, Westendorp R, Knook D. 1999. The definition of anemia in older persons. JAMA 281:1714–1717.

[34] Kikuchi M, Inagaki T, Shinagawa N. 2001. Five-year survival of older people with anemia: Variation with hemoglobin concentration. J Am Geriatr Soc 49:1226–1228.

[35] Nilsson-Ehle H, Jagenburg R, Landahl S, Svanborg A. 2000. Blood haemoglobin declines in the elderly: Implications for reference intervals from age 70 to 88. Eur J Haematol 65:297–305.

[36] Zauber N, Zauber A. 1987. Hematologic data of healthy very old people. JAMA 257:2181–2184.

[37] Chaves P, Ashar B, Guralnik J, Fried L. 2002. Looking at the relationship between hemoglobin concentration and prevalent mobility difficulty in older women. Should the criteria currently used to define anemia in older people be reevaluated? J Am Geriatr Soc 50:1257–1264.

The human family is marvelous both in its uniformity and its diversity. The human clan began on the plains of East Africa and rapidly spread to occupy every continent on the planet with the exception of Antarctica. Using its most valuable tool, a quick and nimble mind, mankind developed the technology to plant a permanent presence on even the most forbidding soil. The same cleverness opened the road leading off the Earth, placing human footprints on a heavenly body that was formerly confined to the realm of poetry and myth.

The Human Genome Project peered into the very essence of the human organism. The work showed a oneness in humanity that persists despite the hundred thousand year Diaspora from the plains surrounding Olduvai. Over time, however, the human family has acquired a rainbow of different external features. Variety in hair texture, skin tone, and eye shape are among the most obvious of these visible adornments. These and other aspects of human diversity distribute unevenly across the family, with dark skin and dark hair common to people in some regions while light skin and hair are seen frequently among people in other areas of the globe.

Some of these features clearly have regional survival value. The high melanin content common to the skin of people who live in the Earth's circumequatorial belt protects against injury from intense sunlight whose effects range from skin blistering to skin cancer. In contrast, other characteristics such as the oval eye features common to people of Asian background lack a clear selective attribute.

Beneath these superficial alterations are other genetic characteristics that in the past have aided human survival. The threat of disease selected for some of these characteristics. Malaria provided the selective pressure for a number of traits. Glucose-6-phosphate dehydrogenase deficiency, the sickle hemoglobin gene, and the variety of alterations that produce thalassemias all trace their high prevalence to this disease. The alteration in gut uptake of iron that sometimes causes iron overload in people with hereditary hemochromatosis likely was an adaptation to the low availability of dietary iron in regions of northern Europe.

Hemoglobin levels change dramatically throughout the course of a person's life. The very high hemoglobin values at birth quickly decline and then slowly rise during childhood (Chapter 2). Consequently, hemoglobin determinations in children must be assessed using age-specific scales. After puberty, hemoglobin levels consistently differ between men and women, with men showing higher values even when the two groups have adequate iron stores. The physiology of the sexes differs in a number of ways that produce inequities in hemoglobin values.

Differences also exist in the mean hemoglobin values seen in people of predominately African heritage compared to people whose genetic roots ply more deeply into European soil. In the United States, these differences have triggered debate that is both scientific and political. The place of "race" as a meaningful term in the scientific lexicon is a point of great contention. The history of using characteristics such as skin color to justify political or economic hegemony by one group of people over another has imbued the word "race" with a negative subtext. The attempts to link "race" with nebulous characteristics such as intelligence, industriousness, and moral rectitude have largely disappeared into the dustbin of history. Unfortunately, the echoes of the past reverberate into the present, often making impossible rational discussions of any characteristic in which "race" is a point of reference.

And yet, medical differences clearly exist between the races loosely defined in the United States as "black" and "white." African Americans or black Americans start life at a disadvantage with respect to their white counterparts. The infant mortality rate is more than twofold higher in blacks than in whites in America. The drumbeat of disadvantage continues with higher rates of morbidity and mortality for conditions ranging from childhood asthma to breast cancer. Many of the problems derive from socioeconomic differences between the races in the United States. The task of untangling the web of social ills from aspects of biology or medicine, however, is often devilishly difficult.

Should medical characteristics that differ between races affect medical, social, and governmental policy, assuming that such differences exist? The history of mendacious social and legal policy based on racial stereotyping gives pause to any fair-minded person. The enormity of some "medical investigation" focused on black Americans, embodied most starkly by the infamous Tuskegee Experiment, left a persistent cloud over the integrity of the biomedical community in the minds of minorities and many others in the United States. Nonetheless, lifesaving interventions can result from the identification of a clustering of medical conditions. Newborn screening for sickle cell disease, which initially targeted black neonates, has saved the lives of untold thousands of infants over the past two decades by allowing timely treatment with prophylactic penicillin and appropriate immunization. Prenatal diagnosis of Tay-Sachs disease in people of Ashkenazi Jewish background has allowed thousands of couples to make informed decisions about their families.

The "normal" values for many laboratory tests derive from samples drawn from a large group of people in a population. The result in most cases is a range of values that approximate a Poisson distribution. The range of "normal" usually entails those values within two standard deviations of the mean. The samples upon which the standard is based should come from a valid representation of the people to whom it will be applied. The values for normal height determined for people in Sweden clearly are inappropriate for people in Thailand.

The question that bedevils medicine is whether normal hemoglobin values determined for people of European background are appropriate for people of African heritage. The first task is to settle the issue of whether a significant difference actually exists between the hemoglobin values of black and white people. The next item is to determine what such a difference means. And finally, there is the question of how the health-care community should approach the point.

■ HEMOGLOBIN VALUES IN BLACK AND WHITE

The possibility that mean hemoglobin values might differ between blacks and whites crept into the medical consciousness somewhat slowly.[1] Nutritional deficiency, particularly low iron stores, is a common problem for many Americans that complicates the assessment of baseline hemoglobin values.[2] Iron deficiency is particularly prevalent in poor women and children.[3] Nearly 20% of children between the ages of 10 months and 3 years were anemic in some studies of inner-city communities.[4] Another limitation of the earlier studies was the relatively small number of subjects who were evaluated. The degree to which the conclusions of these investigations could be generalized to larger groups was a legitimate concern.

The National Health and Nutrition Examination Survey (NHANES) provided a new base of information that touched on the question of anemia in black Americans.[5] The Centers for Disease Control (CDC) conducted the survey between 1971 and 1974 with the broad aim of assessing the health and nutritional status in the noninstitutionalized US civilian population. The data were widely available to investigators who could examine subsets for trends in their particular fields of expertise and interest.

One group of investigators dissected the data to assess the hemoglobin levels in two cohorts of subjects, one consisting of nonpregnant white women and the other of nonpregnant black women.[6] The frequency distribution for hemoglobin levels in black women was shifted smoothly to lower values vis-à-vis those seen in white women. By stratifying hemoglobin values from the two groups across a range of transferrin saturation, the investigators could better assess the relationship between iron status and hemoglobin level. Black women had lower hemoglobin levels for any degree of transferrin saturation, meaning that the hemoglobin values did not reflect the effect of iron deficiency. The intrinsic hemoglobin level appeared to be lower in black women relative to their white counterparts.

Using the WHO standard that defines hemoglobin levels of 12 g/dL as the lower limit of normal for women,[7] the incidence of anemia approached 20% among black subjects compared to a 4% incidence in whites.[8] When the definition of anemia was derived from the Gaussian distribution of hemoglobin values in each group, only 1% of white women and 3% of black women were designated as anemic. The results indicated that the standard for anemia derived from whites inappropriately designates too many black subjects as "anemic" and therefore is inappropriate for this group.

Another analysis of NHANES hemoglobin data from black and white subjects excluded people with low transferrin saturation values in an effort to reduce or eliminate the impact of iron deficiency on the results.[9] The investigators also matched age and income of subjects in each group to reduce the effect of socioeconomic status on the outcome. A 0.7-g/dL difference in hemoglobin values persisted between black and whites nonetheless. Another analysis using different transformations of the data showed a mean hemoglobin value that was lower in blacks than in whites by

0.6 g/dL.[10] The latter difference existed even in a range of transferrin saturation that eliminated iron deficiency as a factor. The implication was that black Americans have an intrinsically lower mean hemoglobin level than do their white counterparts.

The military is another possible source of information on medical parameters derived from a large group of healthy people. Military records provide data on a selected population, but the information is collected in a relatively uniform fashion. Hemoglobin levels in over 300 black men were about 0.3 g/dL lower than those determined for over 2000 white men.[11] While significant, the difference was smaller than those reported in earlier studies. Furthermore, the degree of difference declined when the subject set was limited to men who reported an iron intake consistent with recommended daily allowances. The report concluded that relatively lower iron stores in black recruits contributed significantly to the baseline discrepancy between hemoglobin levels in black and white enlisted men.

In contrast, another study of nearly 500 military personnel found mean hemoglobin values that were lower in black men and women relative to their white counterparts by 1.8 g/dL and 2.2 g/dL, respectively.[12] The differences reflected a net shift toward lower values of the entire hemoglobin distribution curve for blacks versus that seen for whites. The symmetrical nature of the curve argued against iron deficiency as the cause of the shift. A subgroup of iron-deficient people in a population with an otherwise normal distribution would produce a bimodal distribution curve.

Some investigators continued to explore the issue of anemia in blacks and whites in small groups of subjects. The smaller number of people involved in these studies was partially offset by the prospect of more detailed evaluation of factors that could alter hemoglobin values. In one study of healthy people, the mean hemoglobin values were lower in black men and women relative to white counterparts by 0.9 g/dL and 0.5 g/dL, respectively.[13] Careful analysis of iron status as assessed by transferrin saturation and ferritin levels argued against a contribution of iron deficit to the lower hemoglobin values in blacks.

The Second NHANES (NHANES II) conducted during the 1970s and 1980s provided a new and larger data set that could be analyzed for differences in hemoglobin values between blacks and whites. In addition to information on transferrin saturation and ferritin levels, the survey included data on erythrocyte protoporphyrin measures as well as nutrition history. Erythrocyte protoporphyrin values are a sensitive screen for iron deficits that alter hemoglobin production.[14,15] In subjects with no apparent iron deficiency, the mean hemoglobin values in black men and women were lower than those of their white counterparts by 0.8 and 0.6 g/dL, respectively.[16] Interestingly, ferritin levels in blacks were systematically higher than the values seen in whites. Black children between the ages of 3 and 12 years had mean hemoglobin values that were 0.6 g/dL lower than those of white children.

The data for children in this study were consistent with those found in earlier investigations.[17] Although black neonates also have lower hemoglobin values than do white newborns, a 3-month period of iron replacement for all anemic infants nearly eliminates the differential in hemoglobin values between the two groups.[18] The implication is that at birth hemoglobin values in blacks and whites are nearly identical. The values diverge over time, producing a statistically significant difference between the two groups by 3 years of age. Interestingly, a switch occurs during this time from red cells with predominately fetal hemoglobin to erythrocytes containing only adult hemoglobin. A contribution of hemoglobin switching to the difference in hemoglobin levels seen in blacks and whites is a tantalizing thought. Interestingly, children of Asian background had hemoglobin values that were equal to those of whites.[17] Other data on Asian peoples outside the United States also show values that closely approximate those of white Americans.[19] American Indian children likewise have hemoglobin values that are indistinguishable from those of white children.[20]

A lower hemoglobin value is not the only difference in the hemograms of black and white people. The neutrophil count also tends to be consistently lower in blacks than in whites.[21–23] The most important point in all the studies, however, is the functional insignificance of these numeric differentials in the levels of circulating neutrophils. No difference exists in the frequency of infectious problems between whites and the subset of blacks with lower neutrophil counts. Indirect data suggest that the lower neutrophil level in blacks reflects a lower granulocyte reserve.[24,25] Nonetheless, the most apt interpretation of the data as a whole is that lower neutrophil counts reflect a difference in the "set point" for circulating neutrophils in the two groups. Blacks have normal neutrophil function, broadly defined as the capacity to prevent bacterial infection. The lower mean neutrophil level in blacks is a quiddity without clinical significance.

The same can be said for the lower hemoglobin value seen in blacks. The consensus from 30 years of investigation is that blacks have a mean hemoglobin level that is about 0.7 g/dL lower than that of whites. The key confounding factor, iron deficiency anemia, has been virtually eliminated in high risk groups by the introduction of iron-fortified infant formulas.[28] Although some investigators still maintain that the difference is an artifact reflecting environmental or other factors,[26,27] most experts feel that the differential is real. The crucial fact is that, real or not, no one considers the difference in mean hemoglobin values between blacks and whites to be physiologically important. Oxygen delivery to peripheral tissues is perfectly adequate in blacks. Furthermore, the ability to respond to hypoxic stress is not compromised by the *statistically* lower hemoglobin values.

The question of whether the lower mean hemoglobin value in blacks is *clinically* significant is a different issue. A laboratory parameter is clinically significant if it produces a physiological problem *or* if it triggers an intervention by the health-care system. Anemia in the absence of a clear cause should be evaluated and treated. Since the standard by which a hemoglobin level will be designated as "anemia" is based on values determined largely from white Americans, a number of black Americans will be inappropriately designated as "anemic." The discrepancy is not as great as that which would result if Swedish standards for height were used in Thailand, but there will be some effect. If the mean hemoglobin value in blacks is 0.5 g/dL lower than that in whites, then perhaps as many as 10% of black people will be erroneously designated as anemic. The key issue is how such a designation might affect the health status of black people in the United States. This point is an issue of medical policy and procedure.

With respect to actual (as opposed to theoretical) medical procedure, black Americans routinely receive substandard medical care relative to their white compatriots.[28] The effect is greater morbidity and mortality in blacks for diseases almost across the board.[29] The problem for black Americans with respect to medical care is that they too often come in below the metaphorical radar screen. The overdiagnosis of anemia would, in a sense, somewhat counterbalance the tendency of the US medical establishment to overlook the health and welfare of black citizens. The chance exists that a spurious diagnosis of anemia in a black person will trigger a well-deserved closer look at health issues that might not otherwise occur. This justification for using the existing anemia standards for black Americans is a far from ideal rationale applied to a far from ideal world.[30]

References

1   Garn S, Smith N, Clark D. 1975. Lifelong differences in hemoglobin levels between blacks and whites. J Natl Med Assoc 67:91–96.
2   O'Neal R, Abrahams O, Kohrs M, Eklund D. 1976. The incidence of anemia in residents of Missouri. Am J Clin Nutr 29:1158–1166.
3   Zee P, Walters T, Mitchell C. 1970. Nutrition and poverty in preschool children. A nutritional survey of preschool children from impoverished black families, Memphis. JAMA 213:739–742.
4   Katzman R, Novack A, Pearson H. 1972. Nutritional anemia in an inner-city community. Relationship to age and ethnic group. JAMA 222:670–673.
5   Simopoulos A. 1981. Overview of nutritional status in the United States. Prog Clin Biol Res 67:237–427.
6   Meyers L, Habicht J, Johnson C. 1979. Components of the difference in hemoglobin concentrations in blood between black and white women in the United States. Am J Epidemiol 109:539–549.
7   World Health Organization. 1968. Nutritional Anaemias: Report of a WHO Scientific Group. Geneva, Switzerland: World Health Organization.
8   Meyers L, Habicht J, Johnson C, Brownie C. 1983. Prevalences of anemia and iron deficiency anemia in Black and White women in the United States estimated by two methods. Am J Public Health 73:1042–1049.
9   Garn S, Ryan A, Owen G, Abraham S. 1981. Income matched black-white hemoglobin differences after correction for low transferrin saturations. Am J Clin Nutr 34:1645–1647.
10 Pan W, Habicht J. 1991. The non-iron-deficiency-related difference in hemoglobin concentration distribution between blacks and whites and between men and women. Am J Epidemiol 134:1410–1416.
11 Jackson R, Sauberlich H, Skala J, Kretsch M, Nelson R. 1983. Comparison of hemoglobin values in black and white male U.S. military personnel. J Nutr 113:165–171.
12 Reed W, Diehl L. 1991. Leukopenia, neutropenia, and reduced hemoglobin levels in healthy American blacks. Arch Intern Med 151:501–505.
13 Williams D. 1981. Racial differences of hemoglobin concentration: Measurements of iron, copper, and zinc. Am J Clin Nutr 34:1694–1700.
14 Paton T, Lembroski G. 1982. Fluorometric assay of erythrocyte protoporphyrins: Simple screening test for lead poisoning and iron deficiency. Can Med Assoc J 127:860–862.
15 Mei Z, Parvanta I, Cogswell M, Gunter E, Grummer-Strawn L. 2003. Erythrocyte protoporphyrin or hemoglobin: Which is a better screening test for iron deficiency in children and women? Am J Clin Nutr 77:1229–1233.

[16] Perry G, Byers T, Yip R, Margen S. 1992. Iron nutrition does not account for the hemoglobin differences between blacks and whites. J Nutr 122:1417–1424.

[17] Dallman P, Barr G, Allen C, Shinefield H. 1978. Hemoglobin concentration in white, black, and Oriental children: Is there a need for separate criteria in screening for anemia? Am J Clin Nutr 31:377–380.

[18] Reeves J, Driggers D, Lo E, Dallman P. 1981. Screening for anemia in infants: Evidence in favor of using identical hemoglobin criteria for blacks and Caucasians. Am J Clin Nutr 34:2154–2157.

[19] Khusun H, Yip R, Schultink W, Dillon D. 1999. World Health Organization hemoglobin cut-off points for the detection of anemia are valid for an Indonesian population. J Nutr 129:1669–1674.

[20] Yip R, Schwartz S, Deinard A. 1984. Hematocrit values in white, black, and American Indian children with comparable iron status. Evidence to support uniform diagnostic criteria for anemia among all races. Am J Dis Child 138:824–827.

[21] Bain B. 1996. Ethnic and sex differences in the total and differential white cell count and platelet count. J Clin Pathol 49:664–666.

[22] Freedman D, Gates L, Flanders W, et al. 1997. Black/white differences in leukocyte sub-populations in men. Int J Epidemiol 26:757–764.

[23] Zezulka A, Gill J, Beevers D. 1987. 'Neutropenia' in black west Indians. Postgrad Med J 63:257–261.

[24] Mason B, Lessin L, Schechter G. 1979. Marrow granulocyte reserves in Black Americans. Hydrocortisone-induced granulocytosis in the "benign" neutropenia of the Black. Am J Med 67:201–206.

[25] Bain B, Seed M, Godsland I. 1984. Normal values for peripheral blood white cell counts in women of four different ethnic origins. J Clin Pathol 37:188–193.

[26] Jackson R. 1990. Separate hemoglobin standards for blacks and whites: A critical review of the case for separate and unequal hemoglobin standards. Med Hypotheses 32:181–189.

[27] Kent S. 1997. Interpretations of differences in population hemoglobin means: A critical review of the literature. Ethn Dis 7:79–90.

[28] Yip R, Binkin NJ, Fleshood L, Trowbridge FL. 1987. Declining prevalence of anemia among low-income children in the United States. JAMA 258:1619–1623.

[29] Weissman JS, Stern R, Fielding SL, Epstein AM. 1991. Delayed access to health care: Risk factors, reasons, and consequences. Ann Intern Med 114:325–331.

[30] Gornick ME, Eggers PW, Reilly TW, et al. 1996. Effects of race and income on mortality and use of services among Medicare beneficiaries. N Engl J Med 335:791–799.

[31] Bach PB, Pham HH, Schrag D, Tate RC, Hargraves JL. 2004. Primary care physicians who treat Blacks and Whites. N Engl J Med 351:575–584.

ANEMIA AND PREGNANCY

Pregnancy is the most important physiological state for humankind since it assures the continuation of the species. Pregnancy produces major physical alterations in the mother, supports the fetus as it develops the capability of independent existence, and introduces a new organ in the form of the placenta that provides the link between the two. The placenta places the maternal and fetal circulatory systems into close juxtaposition, facilitating the delivery of vital nutrients from mother to fetus as well as retrograde transit of waste products from the fetus to the mother for subsequent disposal. The placenta is not, however, a disinterested arbiter in the relationship between mother and fetus. In every interaction between the two, the placenta is the fetal proxy with the role of safeguarding the health and welfare of its young charge. At times, maternal physiology must accept and adjust to this separate and unequal treatment.

The alterations in the hematological status of pregnant women are profound. Modifications in the production of red cells and changes in plasma volume shift fundamental parameters such as the hematocrit. The nutritional demands of the fetus, particularly as they relate to iron and micronutrients, place an additional burden on the mother. Understanding the basic features of the hematological program during pregnancy is vital to the proper care of pregnant women and the fetuses they carry.

■ HEMATOLOGICAL BASELINE IN PREGNANCY

The two most pronounced hematological changes during pregnancy involve increases in plasma volume and total red cell mass. The plasma volume rises by about 30%

while the total red cell mass (and number of red cells) increases by only about 20%. The result is a fall in hematocrit, since this variable is defined as the volume of packed red cells in a given volume of plasma. This decline in hematocrit is called the "physiological anemia" or "dilutional anemia" of pregnancy. While these terms seem reasonable at first blush, both are inaccurate.

True anemia represents a fall in the oxygen transport capacity of blood relative to the normal physiological state. This is not the case during pregnancy where the oxygen-carrying capacity is higher than in the nonpregnant state. Also, the term "anemia" implies pathology. The word is properly applied to a host of conditions such as sideroblastic anemia, Diamond-Blackfan anemia, and Cooley's anemia where a pathological process reduces the hemoglobin value from the baseline seen in normal people. "Anemia" is not a correct designation for the hemoglobin status during pregnancy. The shift in the relationship between plasma volume and red cell mass is an adjustment toward the proper physiological norm of the pregnant state. The hematocrit *corrects* with the onset of pregnancy rather than declines. Terms such as "dilutional anemia" are well ensconced in the medical argot and will not soon change. The critical observer must be aware of this nosological inconsistency and avoid being mislead by the term "physiological anemia" when looking at a pregnant patient.

The rise in plasma volume begins at about 6 weeks into the pregnancy. The rise is initially rapid but the pace slows after about week 30. The plasma volume at term is about 1200 mL greater than that in the nonpregnant baseline, which translates into an increase of nearly 50%. The red cell mass also increases over this time, with a net rise that by term ranges between 250 and 400 mL.[1] This renders an increase of between 20% and 30% over the nonpregnant value. The relative difference between the degree to which the plasma volume expands and the red cell mass increases accounts for the fall in hematocrit. The oxygen delivery capacity of blood is greater during pregnancy as reflected by higher venous oxygen saturation relative to the nonpregnant state. The higher oxygen-carrying capacity associated with the greater red cell mass means that less oxygen must be extracted per volume of blood to meet tissue requirements.

The hematocrit normally declines into the second trimester, but rises slowly thereafter (Figure 4-1). Consequently, the hemoglobin value that is the gauge of true anemia is not static, but shifts over the course of the pregnancy. Keeping track of a moving target can sow confusion. The most equitable means of approaching the problem is to assign 11 g/dL as the lower limit of normal hemoglobin values during pregnancy.[2] Interestingly, "high" hemoglobin values during pregnancy are not felicitous findings. Unexplained values above 13 g/dL are associated with poor fetal outcome, including intrauterine growth retardation, low birth weight, and preterm birth.[3]

Speculation exists that the lower hemoglobin values associated with pregnancy in some way improve the fetal environment. The reduced blood viscosity associated with the lower hematocrit might, for instance, facilitate blood flow through the placental sinusoids. In any event, the window of maternal hemoglobin values beneficent for the fetus is lower than that typical of the nonpregnant state.

Not surprisingly, a rise in serum erythropoietin values appears to be a key factor in red cell mass expansion during pregnancy.[4] Erythropoietin levels rise to 50%

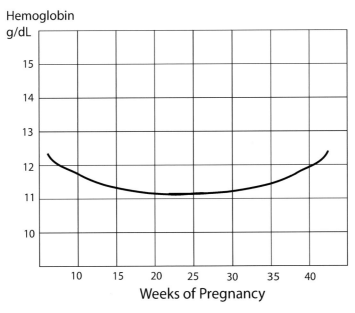

FIGURE 4–1 *Hemoglobin profile during pregnancy. The hemoglobin value declines from the onset of pregnancy into the second trimester. Thereafter, the hemoglobin gradually rises to attain a value close to that seen at the outset of the pregnancy.*

above baseline by the second trimester of pregnancy.[5] The basis of the change in erythropoietin set point is a mystery. Hypoxia is not the basis of the shift, however. A more robust rise in serum erythropoietin level occurs in women who are iron deficient.[6] The lower hemoglobin value associated with iron deficiency probably produces relative renal hypoxia with secondarily enhanced erythropoietin production over that associated with pregnancy in the absence of anemia. Pregnancy has a lower hemoglobin set point, but the compensatory response mechanisms to true anemia are intact.

■ FACTORS THAT INFLUENCE MATERNAL HEMOGLOBIN DURING PREGNANCY

A host of factors influence the hematological status of pregnant women. The higher recommended daily allowance for many vitamins and minerals such as zinc, calcium, and vitamin A reflects the greater demand created by the growing fetus. In the case of iron and folate, the higher recommended daily allowance represents both fetal demand for the nutrients and higher maternal need associated with red cell mass expansion. Adequate intake of these two dietary essentials is vital to both maternal and fetal health.

IRON

Optimal iron availability is essential to healthy fetal maturation. The complex physiological machinery that supports delivery of the mineral to the fetus underscores the central importance of iron in pregnancy. The fetus and its surrogate operator, the placenta, tremendously influence maternal iron metabolism during the 9 months of their coexistence with the mother. Nearly 1 g of iron is diverted from the mother to support the growth and maturation of the fetus over the course of a pregnancy. Simultaneously, the maternal red cell mass increases by as much as 30%. To accommodate the vastly greater iron requirement of pregnancy, maternal iron absorption from the gastrointestinal tract more than doubles over the course of gestation.

Pregnancy and Iron Absorption

Many factors influence gastrointestinal iron absorption, with the plasma iron turnover (PIT) being one of the most important. In the nonpregnant state, bone marrow erythropoiesis is the primary determinant of PIT since erythron consumption accounts for nearly 90% of plasma iron use (Figure 4-2). Pregnancy adds a new dimension to the equation. The cells that line the maternal interface of the placental sinusoids are rich in transferrin receptors and efficient in the removal of iron from its circulating carrier protein.[7,8] The placenta strips as much as 30% of the iron from transferrin during a single pass of blood through the organ. The dramatic rise in PIT enhances gut absorption of maternally consumed oral iron.

The bioavailability of iron in the GI tract is a key determinant of whether the increase in maternal gastrointestinal iron absorption is sufficient to satisfy the needs of the placenta and fetus.[9] Gastrointestinal uptake of heme iron from animal sources far exceeds that seen with the iron salts common to cereals and other plant sources of the mineral. Many women in the world have diets that are low in bioavailable iron and consequently fall into a deficit with respect to iron balance. The needs of the fetus are physiologically paramount, meaning the placenta will remove iron from the maternal plasma to whatever extent necessary to meet fetal demand.[10] Mobilization of maternal iron reserves helps meet that demand when GI iron absorption proves insufficient. On average, mobilization of 8% of maternal iron stores occurs over the 280 days of gestation. The result is depletion of maternal iron stores often to the point of frank maternal iron deficiency.

The placenta is a powerful ally to the fetus and defends fetal welfare against all other interests, including those of the mother. Mothers reduced to frank iron deficiency during pregnancy can become severely anemic. In contrast, iron deficiency anemia is rare among the infants born to these women.[11] The highly efficient placental iron extraction machinery provides a safety umbrella for the fetus during its growth in an iron-deficient environment, namely the mother. Problems arise after birth, however, when placental protection from iron deficit no longer exists for the neonate. Maternal iron deficiency during pregnancy commonly is a socioeconomic problem. The neonate enters the same iron-deficient environment in which the mother dwells and faces the same obstacles to adequate iron intake. Often the barriers reflect poverty, although other social ills such as drug abuse or mental illness can be equally mendacious.

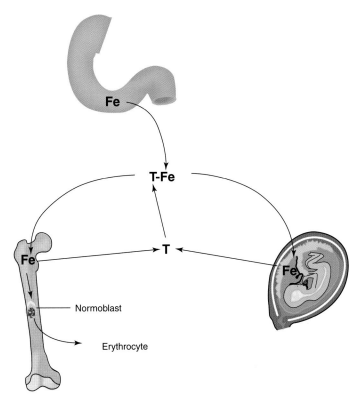

FIGURE 4–2 *Iron uptake and metabolism during pregnancy. Iron (Fe) absorption occurs in the small intestine, primarily the duodenum. Transferrin in the circulation binds the mineral and transports it to all the cells in the body. Normally, the bone marrow is the destination of nearly 90% of absorbed iron thus permitting the production of heme by the developing normoblasts. In this circumstance, marrow erythropoietic activity is the primary determinant of plasma iron turnover (PIT). Pregnancy introduces a second major site of iron removal from the plasma, namely the placenta. The fraction of iron shunted to the placenta increases as gestation progresses with a consequent rise in the PIT. The augmented PIT prompts the increase in iron absorption that characterizes normal pregnancies.*

Without the placenta as a physiological guardian, the neonate often falls victim to the malevolent consequences of iron deficit.

Significant iron deficiency during the neonatal and early childhood periods causes developmental delay.[12,13] Even modest iron deficiency in young children produces neurocognitive problems, the ramifications of which persist for years if not indefinitely.[14] Maternal iron deficiency does not produce neonatal anemia unless the deficit is desperately severe. The primary problem that confronts a neonate born to an iron-deficient mother is both insidious and profound. Neonatal iron stores commonly are low or nonexistent. The low GI iron absorption characteristic of the immature infant gut further magnifies the problem of iron deficit in the newborn.

Iron Supplementation During Pregnancy

Maternal iron supplementation during pregnancy reduces the impact of the imbalance between fetal needs and iron availability.[15] Only a fraction of consumed elemental iron is absorbed on a daily basis, meaning that mild erosion of maternal stores can occur despite supplementation. The average daily iron requirement during pregnancy slightly exceeds 4 mg. This value is close to the upper limit of GI absorptive capacity for iron under optimal conditions. Continuation of iron supplements after pregnancy lessens the impact of depleted maternal iron stores. Supplementation for 8 weeks postpartum is a reasonable practice. This approach is particularly important in multiparous women in whom repletion of iron stores between pregnancies often is incomplete.

Variable reports exist of incidence of iron deficiency anemia at term in women who take no iron supplements during pregnancy. Figures from industrialized countries commonly range between 8% and 14%.[16] In the absence of supplements, half of all women have latent iron deficiency. This is a condition without frank anemia that is characterized by low values for serum ferritin and transferrin saturation along with elevated serum values for the soluble transferrin receptor. Adequate iron supplementation, sometimes as little as 50 mg of elemental iron per day, largely eliminates iron deficiency anemia during pregnancy. Even with this intervention, depletion of iron stores and latent iron deficiency continue to be significant issues.[17]

Iron deficiency during pregnancy takes a particularly heavy toll on many women in the developing world. Nearly every aspect of the iron metabolism equation plays against this unfortunate cohort of women. Iron salts with poor bioavailability of the mineral are the chief sources of the element in the diet. Animal proteins in the diet are scarce along with the valuable heme iron they contain. A high baseline incidence of iron deficiency holds for the general population in many developing nations. The underlying problem commonly is helminthic infestation with organisms such as hookworm. Finally, a significantly larger fraction of women are multiparous relative to their counterparts in developed nations.

Socioeconomic realities impose additional constraints on adequate iron supplementation. The cost of iron supplement tablets places them beyond the economic reach of many women. Remembering a medication that is required daily can be a challenge to anyone. Iron replacement has no external manifestation to show that it is doing any "good," making the supplement easier to overlook. By way of contrast, pain and swelling from an infection are constant reminders of the need for continued antibiotic use. Furthermore, women often come to medical attention later in course of pregnancy, leaving a very narrow treatment window.

Oral supplementation is always the preferred route for iron replacement (see Table 4-1). Parenteral supplementation is however the sole means of rapidly building maternal stores during this critical time. Iron dextran, used clinically now for more than 40 years, allows the rapid repletion of a large fraction of the body iron deficit. An approach called "total dose infusion" at times permits complete replacement of body iron stores.[18] The rare but real cases of anaphylaxis with iron dextran lower the attractiveness of the drug as a replacement vehicle for iron.

TABLE 4-1	**IRON SUPPLEMENTATION IN PREGNANCY**		
Formulation	*Route*	*Benefits*	*Shortcomings*
Iron sulfate	Oral	• Inexpensive	Frequent GI side effects, including cramping, bloating, constipation, and abdominal pain
Iron gluconate	Oral	• Inexpensive • Well tolerated	
Carbonyl iron	Oral	• Inexpensive • Well tolerated • High bioavailability	
Iron polymaltose	Oral	• Well tolerated	Relatively expensive
Iron dextran	Parenteral	• Inexpensive • Rapid administration • Large replacement dose is possible	20% incidence of arthralgias and myalgias Rare anaphylaxis (<1%)
Iron saccharides	Parenteral	• Well tolerated • No anaphylaxis	Limited maximum dose for a single infusion

Fortunately, anaphylaxis is virtually unknown among the host of iron saccharides now available for parenteral use. These agents lack FDA approval for use during pregnancy in the United States, however. This lapse has less to do with intrinsic properties of the drugs than it does with the timorous approach taken by pharmaceutical companies toward medications in pregnancy. Physicians must be aware of the risks and benefits of each mode of iron replacement in this delicate situation.

Assessment of Iron Deficiency During Pregnancy

Just as pregnancy alters red cell mass and plasma volume, important changes occur in parameters central to the assessment of iron stores (Tables 4-2 and 4-3). Pregnancy raises the serum ferritin value, which lowers its diagnostic value as a surrogate marker of iron stores. Simultaneously, serum transferrin values rise while the serum iron level falls. The decline in the iron content of serum reflects in part its incorporation into heme as part of maternal red cell mass expansion. The net result is a transferrin saturation value that on average is lower than that seen in the nongravid state. The resetting of normal physiology during pregnancy lessens the utility of two of the key laboratory parameters in the analysis of iron deficiency.

TABLE 4-2	KEY DIAGNOSTIC POINTS WITH PREGNANCY AND ANEMIA	
Issue	*Manifestation*	*Approach*
Iron deficiency	• True anemia, not "dilutional" • Depleted maternal iron stores • Suboptimal fetal iron stores • Low serum iron level	• Soluble transferrin receptor level • Mean reticulocyte hemoglobin concentration
Folate deficiency	• True anemia, not "dilutional" • Depleted maternal folate stores • Low serum folate level	• Serum folate assay • Serum homocysteine level
Cobalamin deficiency	• Depleted maternal cobalamin stores • Low serum cobalamin level	• Serum cobalamin assay • Serum methyl malonic acid level

The soluble transferrin receptor level is an important diagnostic tool that improves the analysis of iron status during pregnancy.[19] The transferrin receptor is a membrane-bound protein that mediates cellular iron uptake from circulating transferrin. Erythroid precursor cells account for most transferrin receptors in the body. A small fraction of these receptors normally are clipped from the cell membrane and circulate in the plasma in a soluble form, allowing detection by enzyme-linked immunoabsorbent assay.

Expansion of the total mass of erythroid precursors increases the total number of transferrin receptors in the body and with it the number of soluble transferrin receptors in the circulation. The serum level of soluble transferrin receptors in people

TABLE 4-3	KEY MANAGEMENT ISSUES WITH PREGNANCY AND ANEMIA
Issue	*Comment*
Iron deficiency	• Oral iron supplementation should be used whenever possible • Avoid ferrous sulfate because of GI side effects and intolerance. • Parenteral iron replacement only when absolutely necessary.
Iron overload	• No chelation therapy during pregnancy.
Folate deficiency	• Women who might become pregnant should take folate supplements. Higher folate supplementation is needed when actual pregnancy is established.
Cobalamin deficiency	• Most commonly an issue in women with mild pernicious anemia. • Significant cobalamin deficiency can exist without frank anemia. • Replacement entails parenteral cobalamin injection.

with severe thalassemia, for instance, is far higher than normal due to the tremendous expansion of red cell mass associated with the condition. In contrast, iron deficiency dramatically increases the number of transferrin receptors on individual erythroid precursor cells. As a consequence, the total number of transferrin receptors increases as does the content of soluble transferrin receptors in the serum.[20] Pregnancy per se only slightly perturbs the serum level of soluble transferrin receptors, making this marker a valuable index of iron deficiency.[21]

Iron deficiency constrains hemoglobin synthesis by erythroid precursors with a consequent lowering of the mean corpuscular hemoglobin concentration (MCHC) and mean corpuscular volume. Assessment of the fall in MCHC during pregnancy works poorly as an index of iron deficiency, however. The difficulty lies in the long half-life of red cells in circulation. As iron deficiency develops, red cells with low MCHC values mix with older cells already in the circulation with normal MCHC values. This admixture minimizes the impact of the recently formed red cells since the older cells swamp their contribution to the mean MCHC signal determined by electronic blood analyzers. The 40-day red cell half-life means that the "archival" MCHC data of the older red cells persists as the dominant determinant of mean MCHC values long after the onset of iron-deficient erythropoiesis.

Assessment of the reticulocyte hemoglobin content (CHr) eliminates the problem of archival data. Reticulocytes exist in the circulation for 2–3 days before becoming mature erythrocytes that are essentially identical to the older cells in the blood. Having just emerged from the bone marrow, reticulocytes are a window to the current status of erythropoiesis. Iron-deficient erythropoiesis produces reticulocytes whose hemoglobin content is low (low CHr). The CHr therefore provides a dynamic, real-time index of iron availability to red cell precursors. The combination of CHr with soluble transferrin receptor analysis gives the most accurate index of iron status and erythropoiesis during pregnancy.[22]

IRON OVERLOAD IN PREGNANCY

Until recently, the issues of iron overload and pregnancy were largely mutually exclusive. Women with hereditary hemochromatosis do not develop iron overload until after menarche. The physiological iron loss during menses provides protection and delays the onset of clinically apparent hemochromatosis by nearly 10 years relative to men. The childbearing age is past when most women with hereditary hemochromatosis develop iron overload. In women with transfusion-dependent anemias such as thalassemia, transfusional iron overload was severe to the point that endocrine dysfunction was typical and gonadal failure was the norm.[23] Pregnancy was not an issue.

The picture changed with the institution of effective iron chelation strategies, primarily using the chelator deferoxamine (Desferal).[24] The chelation regimen with this agent is both tedious and taxing. However, adherence to the protocol spares end organs from iron-mediated injury allowing near normal function in some instances. Pharmacological hormone manipulations aid conception in many such women. Pregnancies in women with transfusional iron overload are no longer the rare exceptions of the past.[25]

Desferal crosses the placenta and is potentially harmful to the fetus. Consequently, pregnant women suspend their infusion regimens until they give birth. Many if not most of these patients have substantially high iron stores despite good adherence to the chelation program. The transferrin saturation quickly rises to 80% or beyond due to the large body iron stores. An initial concern was that this circumstance would produce excessive iron delivery to the fetus.

Not surprisingly, the fetal ally and champion, the placenta, stepped to the fore again. The organ protects the fetus and prevents gestational iron loading. This clinical observation mirrored the experimental results in a rat model.[26] Laboratory dams loaded with iron by repeated injections develop marked elevations in serum iron levels and transferrin saturation. Nonetheless, these animals produce fetuses whose iron content is no higher than that of the control group without iron loading. In contrast, the iron content of the placenta was much higher in the experimental animals relative to the controls. The placenta is not a passive conduit for iron. The organ actively acquires iron for the fetus in an environment deficient of the mineral and defends the fetus against a surfeit.

FOLATE

Folate is an essential nutrient from the B complex group of vitamins and serves as a cofactor in numerous intracellular reactions. The vitamin facilitates single-carbon transfer reactions, such as the conversion of homocysteine to methionine, and serves as a source of single-carbon units in different oxidative states. Most folate is bound tightly to enzymes and its cellular availability is both protected and strictly regulated. In animals, the liver controls folate availability through first-pass metabolism, biliary secretion, enterohepatic recirculation, as well as through recycling of senescent erythrocytes.

The causes of folate deficiency are varied and include reduced intake, increased metabolism, and increased requirements secondary to genetic defects. Folate deficiency produces high circulating levels of plasma homocysteine, megaloblastic anemia, and mood disorders. Folate deficiency is also implicated in disorders associated with neural tube defects. Several countries use folate supplementation of grain products such as cereals as a cost-effective means of reducing the prevalence of neural tube defects.

Only iron deficit exceeds folate deficiency as a discreet cause of anemia during pregnancy. The vitamin is key to the synthesis of new red cells. The demands of fetal growth and a higher rate of maternal erythropoiesis both contribute to the greater need for folate during pregnancy. In recognition of this fact, the recommended daily allowance for folate during pregnancy is 600 μg rather than the 400 μg assigned to nonpregnant women. Folate stores in adults range between 5 and 10 mg, which suffice for only 2–4 months in the absence of vitamin intake. Paradoxically, the higher estrogen and progesterone levels associated with pregnancy appear to dampen folate absorption from the gastrointestinal tract.

Folate depletion develops in as many as 75% of women during pregnancy in the absence of vitamin supplements. Despite a substantial fall in maternal folate stores, the fetal folate supply remains sufficiently high to avoid anemia. This phenomenon reflects intercession of the placenta. The organ selectively transfers the vitamin to the fetus, thereby avoiding frank fetal folate deficiency. The ability of the placenta to shield the fetus from some of the effects of folate deficiency does not however obviate the need to provide supplemental folate during pregnancy.

Folate deficiency of sufficient magnitude to produce megaloblastic anemia is rare. Mild macrocytosis occurs commonly during normal pregnancy and does not necessarily indicate a vitamin deficit.[27,28] Detrimental obstetrical conditions and poor pregnancy outcomes possibly related to folate deficiency include toxemia of pregnancy, neuropsychiatric symptoms, prematurity and low birth weight, abruptio placenta, spontaneous abortion and stillbirth, and congenital anomalies.[29] The most detailed studies of these deleterious consequences of folate deficit involve nonhuman primates. The degree to which such results reflect the human condition is unclear.

Randomized control trials indicate that women of childbearing age who consume folic acid supplements, in addition to naturally occurring food folate, have a much lower chance of giving birth to infants affected by spina bifida and anencephaly, as predicted by odds outcome measures.[30–32] Most women do not suspect that they are pregnant until weeks or months of gestation have passed. Folate supplementation triggered by the suspicion of pregnancy therefore misses the window crucial to fetal neurotubular development. These and other considerations are the basis for the 1992 recommendation by the US Public Health Service that all women with the potential of becoming pregnant consume at least 0.4 mg of folic acid daily before conception and during the first 6 weeks of pregnancy.

OTHER NUTRITIONAL DEFICIENCIES IN PREGNANCY

While iron and folate are the primary nutrients whose deficiency adversely affects hematological status during pregnancy, deficits of other vitamins and micronutrients occasionally produce problems. For instance, cobalamin levels tend to fall over the course of pregnancy. Despite this pattern, frank cobalamin deficiency with megaloblastic anemia is uncommon. The problem of maternal cobalamin deficiency arises most commonly in women with mild pernicious anemia. Depressed cobalamin absorption due to the pernicious anemia exhausts the normal 2–3 mg vitamin reserves in the liver. Importantly, these women can have substantial cobalamin deficiency without frank anemia. The circulating level of the cobalamin-dependent metabolite, methylmalonic acid, always is high in this circumstance.

The major concern in this circumstance is a deficit in neonatal cobalamin stores. Such infants can develop severe megaloblastic anemia within several months of birth, particularly if breast milk is the primary source of nutrition. This phenomenon reflects the low cobalamin content of breast milk produced by women who themselves are deficient in the vitamin. Rarely, maternal and fetal cobalamin deficiency occurs in women who are strict vegetarians (vegans) due to dietary deficiency of the vitamin.

Maternal vitamin K deficiency does not produce anemia but can cause the newborn to have low vitamin stores. The lack of intestinal bacteria in neonates to generate vitamin K places these infants at risk of bleeding. Intramuscular administration of the vitamin in the perinatal period is common practice and prevents problems in these children.

Zinc is an important mineral that serves as a cofactor for a number of enzymes. The nutrient has prominent history with respect to anemia due to the significant deficiency that develops in some patients with hemolytic anemia, including sickle cell disease and thalassemia. Zinc deficiency is not common in industrialized countries, but is modestly frequent in areas where diets rely heavily on plant sources since these have low intrinsic zinc content. Infants born to mothers who were zinc deficient during pregnancy sometimes develop central nervous system anomalies. The recommended daily allowance of zinc during pregnancy is 20 mg, quadruple the value for women who are not pregnant.

References

[1] Hytten F. 1985. Blood volume changes in normal pregnancy. Clin Haematol 14:601–612.

[2] Milman N, Byg K-E, Agger AO. 2000. Hemoglobin and erythrocyte indices during normal pregnancy and postpartum in 206 women with and without iron supplementation. Acta Obstet Gynecol Scand 79:89–98.

[3] Koller O, Sagen N, Ulstein M, Vaula D. 1979. Fetal growth retardation associated with inadequate hemodilution in otherwise uncomplicated pregnancy. Acta Obstet Gynecol Scand 58:9–13

[4] Milman N, Agger AO, Nielsen OJ. 1994. Iron status markers and serum erythropoietin in 120 mothers and newborn infants. Effect of iron supplementation in normal pregnancy. Acta Obstet Gynecol Scand 73:200–204.

[5] Riikonen S, Saijonmaa O, Jarvenpaa AL, Fyhrquist F. 1994. Serum concentrations of erythropoietin in healthy and anaemic pregnant women. Scand J Clin Lab Invest 54:653–657.

[6] Milman N, Graudal N, Nielsen OJ, Agger AO. 1997. Serum erythropoietin during normal pregnancy: Relationship to hemoglobin and iron status markers and impact of iron supplementation in a longitudinal, placebo-controlled study on 118 women. Int J Hematol 66:159–168.

[7] Seligman PA, Schleicher RB, Allen RH. 1979. Isolation and characterization of the transferrin receptor from human placenta. J Biol Chem 254:9943–9950.

[8] Wada HG, Hass PE, Sussman HH. 1979. Transferrin receptor on human placental brush boarder membranes. J Biol Chem 254:12629–12637.

[9] Hallberg L. 1982. Iron nutrition and food iron fortification. Semin Hematol 19:31–42.

[10] Agrawal RM, Tripathi AM, Agarwal KN. 1983. Cord blood haemoglobin, iron and ferritin status in maternal anaemia. Acta Paediatr Scand 72:545–550.

[11] MacPhail AP, Charlton RW, Bothwell TH, Torrance JD. 1980. The relationship between maternal and infant iron status. Scand J Haematol 25:141–148.

[12] Pollitt E, Saco-Pollitt C, Leibel RL, Viteri FE. 1986. Iron deficiency and behavioral development in infants and preschool children. Am J Clin Nutr 43(4):555–565.

[13] Delinard AS, List A, Lindgren B, Hunt JV, Chang PN. 1986. Cognitive deficits in iron-deficient and iron-deficient anemic children. J Pediatr 108(5 Pt 1):681–689.

[14] Lozoff B, Jimenez E, Wolf AW. 1991. Long-term developmental outcome of infants with iron deficiency. N Engl J Med 325(10):687–694.

[15] Taylor DJ, Mallen C, McDougall N, Lind T. 1982. Effect of iron supplementation of serum ferritin levels during and after pregnancy. Br J Obstet Gynaecol 89:1011–1017.

[16] Bergmann RL, Gravens-Müller L, Hertwig K, et al. 2002. Iron deficiency is prevalent in a sample of pregnant women at delivery in Germany. Eur J Obstet Gynecol Reprod Biol 102:155–160.

[17] Beard JL. 1994. Iron deficiency: Assessment during pregnancy and its importance in pregnant adolescents. Am J Clin Nutr 59(2 Suppl):502S–508S.

[18] Auerbach M, Witt D, Toler W, Fierstein M, Lerner RG, Ballard H. 1988. Clinical use of the total dose intravenous infusion of iron dextran. J Lab Clin Med 111(5):566–570.

[19] Carriaga MT, Skikne BS, Finley B, Cutler B, Cook JD. 1991. Serum transferrin receptor for the detection of iron deficiency in pregnancy. Am J Clin Nutr 54:1077–1081.

[20] Baillie F, Morrison A, Fergus I. 2003. Soluble transferrin receptor: A discriminating assay for iron deficiency. Clin Lab Haematol 25(6):353–357.

[21] Akesson A, Bjellerup P, Berglund M, Bremme K, Vahter M. 1998. Serum transferrin receptor: A specific marker of iron deficiency in pregnancy. Am J Clin Nutr 68(6):1241–1246.

[22] Thomas C, Thomas L. 2002. Biochemical markers and hematologic indices in the diagnosis of functional iron deficiency. Clin Chem 48(7):1066–1076.

[23] Costin G, Kogut M, Hyman C, Ortega J. 1979. Endocrine abnormalities in thalassemia major. Am J Dis Child 133:497–502.

[24] Rund D, Rachmilewitz E. 1995. Thalassemia major 1995: Older patients, new therapies. Blood Rev 9(1):25–32.

[25] Aessopos A, Karabatsos F, Farmakis D, et al. 1999. Pregnancy in patients with well-treated beta-thalassemia: Outcome for mothers and newborn infants. Am J Obstet Gynecol 180(2 Pt 1):360–365.

[26] Finch CA, Huebers HA, Miller LR, Josephson AM, Shepard TH, Mackler R. 1983. Fetal iron balance in the rat. Am J Clin Nutr 37:910–916.

[27] Cauchi MN, Smith MB. 1982. Quantitative aspects of red cell size variation during pregnancy. Clin Lab Haematol 4:149–154.

[28] Chanarin I, McFadyen IR, Kyle R. 1977. The physiological macrocytosis of pregnancy. Br J Obstet Gynaecol 84:504–508.

[29] Blocker DE, Thenen SW. 1989. Experimental maternal and neonatal folate status relationships in nonhuman primates. Am J Clin Nutr 50:120–128.

[30] Czeizel A, Dudas I. 1992. Prevention of the first occurrence of neural-tube defects by periconceptional vitamin supplementation. N Engl J Med 327:1832–1835.

[31] MRC Vitamin Study Research Group. 1991. Prevention of neural tube defects: Results of the Medical Research Council Vitamin Study. Lancet 338:131–137.

[32] Eskes T. 1997. Folates and the fetus. Eur J Obstet Gynecol Reprod Biol 71:105–111.

CANCER AND ANEMIA

Cancer is one of mankind's most dreaded disorders. The very word often is spoken in hushed and mournful tones by families and friends with loved ones stricken by the condition. Cancer is not a single entity, but rather is a collection of disorders whose unifying characteristic is uncontrolled cell proliferation. Although some forms of cancer can be cured, a disappointingly large number cannot. As a group, pediatric cancers tend to respond more favorably to therapeutic interventions than do their adult counterparts. Cancers that defy surgical excision because of anatomic location or extent of spread often are treated with toxic chemotherapy agents or with radiation therapy, which in themselves can be debilitating and sometimes fatal. In 2002, cancer surpassed cardiovascular disease to become the leading cause of death in the United States, with nearly one-half million victims. The incidence of cancer is rising quickly in the developing world as the mean lifespan of people there increases. Most often, the cause of a specific cancer is unknown. Nonetheless, strong associations exist with environmental factors (e.g., smoking and lung cancer), infections (e.g., hepatitis C and hepatocellular carcinoma), and genetic anomalies (e.g., BCRA1 mutations and breast cancer).

Anemia is a common consequence of cancer. The World Health Organization and the National Cancer Institute each has promulgated scoring schemes for anemia (Table 5-1). Substantial anemia (Hb <10.5 g/dL) exists in as many as 50% of patients with multiple myeloma at the time of diagnosis.[1] One-third of patients with

TABLE 5-1	**ANEMIA GRADING SYSTEMS**	
Severity	*WHO*	*NCI*
Grade 0 (WNL)[a]	≥11.0 g/dL	WNL
Grade 1 (mild)	9.5–10.9 g/dL	10.0 g/dL to WNL
Grade 2 (moderate)	8.0—9.4 g/dL	8.0–10.0 g/dL
Grade 3 (serious/severe)	6.5—7.9 g/dL	6.5–7.9 d/dL
Grade 4 (life threatening)	<6.5 g/dL	<6.5 g/dL

WHO, World Health Organization; NCI, National Cancer Institute.
[a] Within normal limits: female 12.0–16.0 g/dL, male 14.0–18.0 g/dL

non-Hodgkin's lymphoma have anemia (Hb <12 g/dL) when they come to medical attention.[2,3] Thirty percent of women with ovarian cancer have significant anemia at presentation.[4] The European Cancer Anaemia Survey evaluated over 15,000 patients and reported anemia (Hb <12 g/dL) in nearly 40% of subjects.[5] The incidence varied according to tumor type, and most of the anemic patients had hemoglobin values in the range of 10.0–11.9 g/dL. However, severe anemia (Hb 8.0–9.9 g/dL) existed in approximately 20% of patients suffering from head and neck cancer, leukemia, or urogenital cancer (Figure 5-1). Over 30% of subjects who were not receiving treatment at the time of survey enrollment were anemic.

Typically, cancer-related anemia is normochromic and normocytic with a depressed reticulocyte count. However, Macrocytosis (MCV 105-110 fL) is typical finding in patients who are actively receiving chemotherapy. The red cell contour in these anemias most often is normal. Schistocytes point to a hemolytic component of the type seen, for instance, with the disseminated intravascular coagulation that can arise in pancreatic cancer. The condition is often called "red cell fragmentation syndrome" in recognition of the extensive erythrocyte damage. Some tumor cells can invade the lumen of veins where they produce red cell shearing and hemolysis through direct contact with erythrocytes. Renal cell carcinoma produces this problem on occasion. Either of these scenarios can engender severe and sometimes life-threatening anemia. Control of the anemia often is difficult, requiring aggressive measures aimed at tumor suppression. The bleeding diathesis produced by thrombocytopenia and deficiency of coagulation factors due to excess consumption renders the situation even more dire.

Histology shows a bone marrow that appears remarkably placid in most instances of cancer-related anemia. The marrow cellularity as well as the distribution of precursor cells in the marrow is normal. One finding that points to disrupted hematopoiesis is the presence of iron-laden macrophages. Trapping of iron in reticuloendothelial (RE) cells is a long-appreciated hallmark of anemia in cancer for which a pathophysiologic explanation has only recently emerged (see below).

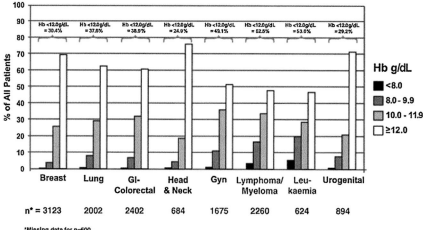

FIGURE 5-1 *Prevalence of anemia in subsets of patients with cancer. The figure shows hemoglobin values at the time of enrollment in the European Cancer Anaemia Survey for patients with various tumor types. Data based on the evaluable population (n = 14,912). Gyn, gynecological; GI, gastrointestinal. (From Ludwig H, Van Belle S, Barrett-Lee P, et al. 2004. The European Cancer Anaemia Survey (ECAS): A large multinational, prospective survey defining the prevalence, incidence, and treatment of anaemia in cancer patients. Eur J Cancer 40:2293–2306. Figure 2. Reproduced with permission of the publisher.)*

Anemia can also result from bone marrow invasion by malignant cells. Among solid tumors, breast carcinoma and prostate cancer are notorious offenders. Tumor cells crowd out the intrinsic marrow elements in a process termed "myelophthisis." Reactive proliferation of bone marrow fibroblasts can further impinge on marrow cavity space normally reserved for hematopoietic precursors. A characteristic finding is a peripheral blood smear containing both nucleated red cell precursors and immature myeloid precursors. Schistocytes are also a prominent part of this "leukoerythroblastic" picture (Figure 5-2). The foreign cells appear to disrupt the barriers that normally confine immature hematopoietic precursors to the marrow. Bone marrow examination shows confluent sheets of dysplastic tumor cells that are visible on aspirate but are best appreciated on biopsy. Interestingly, replacement of normal marrow elements by cells of hematopoietic lineage, such as lymphoma or myeloma cells, produces much less in the way of leukoerythroblastic manifestations.

Malignant cells capable of antibody production, such as those associated with multiple myeloma or chronic lymphocytic leukemia, occasionally generate a paraprotein with specificity for red cell epitopes. The result is an antibody-mediated hemolysis that mirrors the picture seen in autoimmune hemolytic anemia. Brisk hemolytic anemia can be the presenting feature in chronic lymphocytic leukemia or lymphoma. Reticulocytosis is the rule in this setting along with spherocytes and microspherocytes. Rouleaux formation is marked, with long stacks of erythrocytes prominently featured on the peripheral smear.

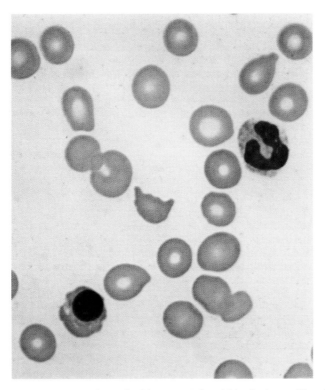

FIGURE 5–2 *Leukoerythroblastic peripheral blood picture. The photomicrograph is from a patient with a mild anemia. The presence of helmet cells and teardrop cells is consistent with erythrocyte destruction by microangiopathic cell shearing in the peripheral circulation. In addition, the orthochromatic erythroblast indicates a breach in the barrier that normally confines immature cells to the bone marrow. (From Kapff CT, Jandl JH. 1981. Blood: Atlas and Sourcebook of Hematology. Boston: Little, Brown and Company. Figure 26-2, p. 69. Reproduced with permission of the publisher.)*

■ ETIOLOGY OF ANEMIA IN CANCER

Table 5-2 lists some of the factors that can contribute to depressed hemoglobin values in cancer patients, including chronic bleeding, hemolysis, and bone marrow invasion by tumor cells. Chemotherapy is a key factor in this setting, reflecting the proliferation arrest and death of erythroid precursor cells that this intervention can produce.

A significant contributor to cancer-related depression of hemoglobin values is a condition interchangeably termed the anemia of chronic disease (ACD) or the anemia of chronic inflammation (ACI). Hemoglobin synthesis depends on a precisely orchestrated pattern of events that includes iron absorption and delivery to the bone marrow as well as hormonally induced maturation of erythroid precursors. Cancer upsets this delicate balance, thereby impairing red cell production. At center stage in

TABLE 5-2	CAUSES OF ANEMIA IN CANCER

Bleeding
Deficiency of folate or cobalamin
Anemia of chronic inflammation
Impaired erythropoietin production
Impaired response to erythropoietin
Tumor infiltration of bone marrow

Chemotherapy
 Hemolysis
Protein/calorie malnutrition

TABLE 5-3	KEY DIAGNOSTIC POINTS WITH CANCER ANEMIA

Issue	Manifestation	Approach
Bone marrow involve with cancer	Leukoerythroblastic peripheral blood smear; nucleated red cells, immature white cells, schistocytes, thrombocytosis Elevated LDH	Aggressive cancer treatment
Antibody-mediated hemolysis	Reticulocytosis, spherocytes, Rouleaux formation Elevated LDH	Aggressive cancer treatment
Red cell fragmentation syndrome	Schistocytes, low platelets Elevated LDH Elevated PTT	Aggressive cancer treatment Replace coagulation factors Replace platelets
Chronic inflammatory response	Depressed serum iron, elevated TIBC, elevated serum ferritin Depressed reticulocyte count Elevated ESR	Aggressive cancer treatment

this picture are iron and the hormone hepcidin, which orchestrates iron uptake from the gastrointestinal tract and modulates its overall distribution in the body.

IRON AND THE ERYTHROCYTE

Iron is a key component of hemoglobin and therefore a key to red cell production. The basic pathways involved in iron metabolism and erythropoiesis are well known (Chapter 7). The mineral is absorbed from the duodenum and subsequently moves throughout the body as a ligand bound to transferrin. About 80% of absorbed iron is delivered to the bone marrow to be used in the production of new red cells. Developing normoblasts incorporate iron into heme, which then is inserted into the heme-binding pocket of globin. Hemoglobin production is impossible without iron, and iron deficiency anemia results from the deficit.

Correction of iron deficiency anemia is a straightforward process. Reticulocytosis begins within 1 or 2 days of intravenous iron replacement in a patient with severe deficiency of the nutrient and peaks at about 10 days. Iron deficiency fosters the generation of reticulocytes with low hemoglobin content due to impaired hemoglobin production.[6] Correction of the iron supply pipeline immediately corrects the problem, allowing production of reticulocytes with normal hemoglobin content. Reticulocytosis persists until the anemia is fully corrected.

ERYTHROPOIETIN AND THE ERYTHROCYTE

Iron is the basic fuel used in red cell production. Erythropoietin, by contrast, is the accelerator that controls the rate of that production.[7] Erythropoietin receptor expression occurs most prominently on early erythroid precursors, primarily the BFU-E and CFU-E (Figure 5-3). In the absence of erythropoietin, these red cell precursors fail to mature into erythrocytes and eventually undergo apoptosis. Anemia due to erythropoietin deficiency can be quite severe. The most clear-cut example of this phenomenon is the anemia associated with chronic kidney disease (CKD). The kidneys are the primary sources of erythropoietin. CKD markedly reduces the levels of the hormone due to loss of erythropoietin-producing renal tissue.

Correction of anemia due solely to erythropoietin deficiency also is a straightforward process. Administration of the hormone to patients, such as those with CKD, where anemia primarily reflects erythropoietin deficiency, produces a prompt and dramatic reticulocytosis.[8] The reticulocyte response continues until the anemia is corrected.

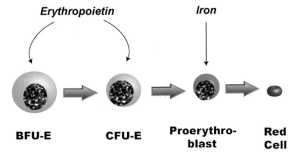

FIGURE 5–3 *Schematic representation of the effect of erythropoietin and iron on the maturation of early erythroid precursors. Iron and erythropoietin operate in concert to promote red cell development. Absence of either factor severely hampers erythropoiesis.*

As shown in Figure 5-3, iron and erythropoietin are complementary factors in red cell development. One does not work without the other. When anemia results from simple deficiency of either factor, exogenous replacement of that factor quickly corrects the red cell deficit.

ANEMIA OF CHRONIC INFLAMMATION

Anemia due to deficiency of either iron or erythropoietin is a simple matter of cause and effect. Consequently, correction of anemia in either scenario is simple. By contrast, anemia in circumstances of chronic inflammation is a complex process reflecting the impact of multiple pathophysiologic disturbances. The ACI occurs in diverse circumstances that include primary inflammatory disorders, such as rheumatoid arthritis, chronic infections, such as tuberculosis, as well as cancers.[9] The discovery of hepcidin provided new insight into an area that previously was poorly understood, at best.

The role of disturbed iron metabolism in ACI has been recognized for decades. Low serum iron, low transferrin saturation, and elevated ferritin levels are the central laboratory features of ACI.[10] Iron supplementation in this setting neither raises the transferrin saturation nor corrects the anemia. Duodenal biopsy in affected patients shows iron accumulation in the enterocytes, leading to the term "mucosal iron block" as a description in ACI. Furthermore, examination of macrophages shows iron accumulation in these cells, again pointing to a disturbance in iron metabolism.

Hepcidin is a liver-derived 25 amino acid polypeptide that blocks iron uptake from the duodenal enterocytes as well as iron release from macrophages.[11,12] Figure 5-4 schematically represents this process. The iron-transport protein ferroportin mediates release of iron both from enterocytes and macrophages and appears to be the target of hepcidin action.[13] Hepcidin blocks ferroportin-mediated iron release, leading to retention of the mineral in enterocytes and macrophages. The overall result is erythropoiesis that is limited by low relative iron availability.[14] Oral iron replacement does not correct the anemia due to the block in iron uptake from the gut. Parenteral iron replacement does not correct the problem due to trapping of iron in RE cells (parenteral iron is composed of microparticles of iron dextran or iron saccharates that must be processed in RE cells before they are bioavailable.) Despite an abundance or even a surfeit of iron in the body, the erythropoietic machinery faces a deficit of the mineral. The scenario is termed "functional iron deficiency."

Hepcidin is a normal polypeptide that modulates iron physiology. The problem in chronic inflammation is hepcidin overproduction, which deranges iron metabolism and ultimately produces anemia. The key question with respect to anemia in chronic inflammatory states is "what is the basis of hepcidin overproduction?" The answer appears to be inflammatory cytokines. IL-6, IL-1α, and IL-1β all enhance hepcidin production by hepatocytes.[15,16] TNF-α is a counter regulatory protein in this context that lowers hepcidin production.

IL-6 is a central factor in many cancers, including multiple myeloma, lymphoma, breast cancer, and non small cell lung cancer.[17–19] In some cases of multiple myeloma, IL-6 appears to derive from direct synthesis by myeloma cells.[20] The source of IL-6 varies in other cancers. Tumor-associated mononuclear cells (lymphocytes and

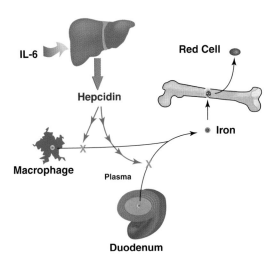

FIGURE 5–4 *Schematic representation of the anemia of chronic inflammation. Interleukin 6 (IL-6) is abundant in cancer, coming from many sources. The IL-6 simulates hepatocytes to secrete hepcidin. Hepcidin in turn blocks iron release from hepatocytes following its uptake from the GI tract as well as iron release from macrophages. The result is iron sequestration that prevents an adequate quantity of the mineral from reaching the bone marrow for red cell production.*

monocytes) from malignant effusions and peripheral blood of patients with ovarian cancer produce high levels of IL-6 and IL-2.[21] This finding suggests that normal cells that are part of the host response to cancer might indirectly foster anemia through the immune response that they mount. In all cases, however, the cancers in question have an associated anemia. In addition to the effect on hematopoiesis, IL-6 expression has negative prognostic significance in some malignancies, such as prostate cancer, multiple myeloma, and ovarian cancer.[22,23]

In contrast to the situations with simple iron or erythropoietin deficiency, no straightforward means exists to correct ACI. Erythropoietin replacement has been used in some conditions. In keeping with the fact that erythropoietin is at least one level removed from the pathophysiologic basis of ACI, correction occurs only with relatively high doses of the hormone. Moreover, this intervention fails in a substantial fraction of patients, perhaps up to 40%.

As shown in Figure 5-4, hepcidin is the lock in ACI, but IL-6 is the key. This inflammatory cytokine is central to hepcidin dysregulation and the consequent disturbances in iron metabolism and erythrocyte production. Interestingly, IL-6 produced by recombinant DNA technology was investigated as a possible therapeutic agent at a time when its role in ACI was not fully elucidated. Marked anemia was a prominent side effect of this intervention.[24] Almost certainly, any agent that blocks IL-6 activity would lessen hepcidin production and increase iron availability for red cell generation. Recombinant DNA technology and "intelligent drug design" are two of the tools used in ongoing efforts to develop countermeasures to ACI.

Inflammatory cytokines disrupt erythropoiesis through effects additional to those on hepcidin and iron metabolism. IL-6 directly suppresses erythropoietin production, creating a state of relative erythropoietin deficiency for a given degree of anemia.[25] Other inflammatory cytokines likely contribute to suppressed erythropoietin production as well.

At the distal end of the erythropoietic pathway, inflammatory cytokines suppress erythropoietin responsiveness of hematopoietic precursor cells. IL-1β, IFN-γ, and TNF-α play very prominent roles in this respect. When added to in vitro cultures of erythropoietic precursors, IFN-γ promotes apoptosis of these cells in direct opposition to erythropoietin activity.[26] Other cytokines including TNF-α directly amplify this detrimental effect on hematopoiesis.[27] This pernicious result of inflammatory cytokines is compounded by a shortening in the half-life of circulating red cells. The anemia induced by inflammatory cells is therefore multifactorial in origin.

Reactive oxygen species (ROS) generated as part of the chronic inflammatory state probably further exacerbate anemia in cancer patients.[28] ROS include a host of injurious compounds such as superoxide, the hydroxyl radical, and nitric oxide. Although nitric oxide is a very important biological second messenger, out of context the molecule is a potent oxidizing agent. These agents can injure cells by promoting production of lipid and protein peroxides as well as DNA cross-links.[29] Heavy oxidant damage leads to cell necrosis. Less severe injury triggers apoptosis with eventual cell death.

Hematopoietic precursor cells are very sensitive to oxidant assault. Erythroid precursors appear to be particularly susceptible to this form of injury, perhaps because of their abundant iron content. Iron is a natural catalyst in the formation of ROS. Cells have a number of defenses against oxidant injury including enzymes such as superoxide dismutase, glutathione peroxidase, and glutathione reductase. Some of these defensive parapets are breached under the assault of cancer and cancer-induced pro-oxidants.[30] These perturbations likely contribute to the hemolysis and ineffective erythropoiesis that frequently characterize cancer-related anemia.

Cancer-related anemia is a complex, multifactorial process. Dysregulation of iron metabolism due to hepcidin overproduction contributes heavily to the phenomenon, but is not the sole factor in the pathogenesis of cancer anemia. Direct suppression of hematopoiesis by inflammatory cytokines is also a key piece of the puzzle. Finally, oxidant compounds of various sorts injure hematopoietic cells, further exacerbating the problem. The complex nature of anemia in cancer means that no single or simple solution to the issue exists.

■ TREATMENT OF ANEMIA IN CANCER

Elimination of the cancer and cure of the patient is the ultimate goal of any cancer treatment. As noted earlier, this goal often is frustratingly elusive, particularly with respect to the most common tumors such as lung, breast, and gastrointestinal malignancies. In these circumstances, problems such as anemia that diminish quality of life (QoL) assume much larger roles in management decisions.

TRANSFUSIONS

For cancer patients not deficient in iron, folate, or cobalamin, blood transfusion is the most clear-cut way to correct an anemia. Transfusion also is relatively straightforward. In the late 1980s in the United States, an estimated one million units of blood were transfused yearly to correct or moderate the severity of anemia in patients with cancer.[31] This figure represented nearly 10% of the nation's blood supply. The end of the 1980s also brought about an unparalleled trial to the practice of blood transfusion.

Blood-borne infection has always been a transfusion risk. Infection with hepatitis viruses, cytomegalovirus, and even malaria were well-known problems within the medical community. However, the entry of the human HIV virus into the blood supply raised concern to the point of crisis. The mysterious nature of the infection struck fear into the hearts of patients and physicians alike. The terror gripped even many blood donors who, for instance, irrationally believed that HIV might be contracted merely by giving blood. The net result was a one of the greatest crises to confront modern medicine. The advent of effective screening procedures virtually eliminated HIV from the nation's blood supply.[32] The psychological damage was done however, leaving blood transfusion under a pall of suspicion that persists to this day.

In addition to infection risk, transfusions pose other problems for cancer patients. Repeated blood transfusions can produce iron overload and a host of consequent problems including heart and liver failure. No transfusion is a perfect antigenic match between donor and recipient. In particular, matching for minor red cell antigens is not routine, in contrast to the case with the major antigens ABO and Rh. Repeated transfusions can generate an immune response to minor antigens called alloimmunization. Alloimmunization complicates crossmatching and can render a patient refractory to transfusion due to the inability to identify compatible units of blood. In addition to these woes, cancer patients face a further burden related to an immune defense system weakened by the cancer itself or the chemotherapy used to treat the cancer. Immune-competent lymphocytes transferred from the blood donor in the transfused blood can trigger an immune attack against the recipient, producing graft-versus-host disease (GVHD). GVHD complicates the management of these already ill patients and at times is fatal. All transfusion products given to cancer patients should be irradiated to kill any lymphocytes and eliminate the risk of GVHD.

These problems gave justifiable pause to the issue of transfusion in cancer patients. One of the few published assessments of transfusion practice in cancer patients showed that although 20% of patients in the late 1980s received a transfusion in the course of their care, the hemoglobin threshold used for those transfusions was quite low, often under 8 g/dL.[33] Concerns about transfusion safety intersected with a reduction in blood supply to impair patient well-being by lowering to a tenuous point the hemoglobin threshold used as a transfusion trigger. The advent of recombinant human erythropoietin (rHuEpo) provided an alternative to blood transfusion for management of anemia in these patients. With the exception of life-threatening or severe anemia (Hb <8 g/dL), rHuEpo products have superseded blood transfusion as the standard of care for these patients.[34]

ERYTHROPOIESIS-STIMULATING AGENTS

The search for alternatives to blood transfusion for the management of anemia intersected with the first great success in the genetic engineering of a drug, namely the production of rHuEpo. Patients with anemia due to renal failure were the first to reap a benefit from this marvel of recombinant DNA technology. Following this initial success, rHuEpo found a niche in the treatment of many other forms of anemia, including that seen in cancer patients.

Cancer itself commonly produces anemia. The addition of chemotherapy raises the proportion from a minority to a large plurality or even a majority, depending on the nature of the drugs used in the particular treatment regimen. Agents in the cisplatin family of drugs are the most likely to produce anemia in cancer patients.[35] These drugs are mainstays in the treatment of many of the most aggressive malignancies, including cancers of the lung and GI tract. That being said, myelosuppressive chemotherapy agents of every class produce some degree of anemia.

The advent of erythropoiesis-stimulating agents (ESAs; so called because some are modifications of natural erythropoietin) provided a new option for the treatment of anemia in cancer that is free of the risks associated with blood transfusion. The first approval in the United States for ESA treatment of cancer-related anemia came in 1993. This practice subsequently found favor in Europe and the rest of the world and is currently the standard of care.

Since 1989 three ESAs have been approved and marketed for use in cancer anemia: epoetin alfa, epoetin beta, and darbepoetin alfa. Epoetin alfa and epoetin beta are cloned versions of natural human erythropoietin and are marketed by different pharmaceutical companies.[36,37] Darbepoetin alfa is a version of human erythropoietin engineered to have five glycosylation side chains rather than the three that occur normally.[38] The therapeutic half-life of this product substantially exceeds that of natural human erythropoietin.[39]

ESAs are effective with either intravenous or subcutaneous administration (Table 5-4). However, the magnitude of the hematopoietic response differs dramatically for the two routes of delivery. Intravenous administration produces a sharp peak in the plasma drug level followed by a rapid decline. Erythroid precursors have relatively few erythropoietin receptors, generally as few as 1000 per cell.[40] This small number of receptors exists only during the BFU-E and CFU-E stages of development, a fairly narrow window in the progression of the erythroid lineage. Intravenously administered ESAs quickly saturate the erythropoietin receptors existing at the time of injection but dissipate before the next cohort of immature cells reach a receptive phase of development. Therefore, much of the intravenously administered ESA is effectively wasted.

In contrast, drug delivered subcutaneously forms a small depot. The ESA seeps from the depot site into the circulation, providing a more sustained presence of drug in the plasma. The drug does not attain the high peak plasma concentration seen with intravenous administration. However, with a miniscule number of erythropoietin receptors that are quickly saturated, peak plasma drug levels are less important than drug duration in the plasma.

TABLE 5-4	KEY MANAGEMENT POINTS WITH CANCER ANEMIA
Issue	*Comments*
ESA support	• Myeloid cancers such as acute leukemia are not eligible • Hemoglobin $\leq$ 11 g/dL • Best results with low serum erythropoietin • Replace iron if necessary • Twelve-week therapeutic trial • Validated only for anemia associated with chemotherapy • Transfusions as necessary • Higher hemoglobin values correlate with improved quality of life • Possible higher rate of thrombovascular events • Effect on survival is unsettled
Transfusion	• Indicated for severe anemia (Hb less than 8 g/dL) • Can be given along with ESA therapy • Transfusion products should be irradiated

ESA use differs in the settings of anemia due to CKD and cancer-related anemia both with respect to drug dose and interval between drug administrations. The anemia of CKD most closely approximates pure erythropoietin deficiency, meaning that ESA use in this setting produces the most robust erythropoietic response. The complicated nature of cancer-related anemia means that erythropoiesis in response to ESA treatment often is blunted and sometimes absent. Drug doses required for an acceptable response usually exceed by twofold or more than those needed to treat CKD.

Administration of ESAs for cancer-related anemia initially followed a thrice in a week (TIW) schedule. This routine grew out of the treatment approach for CKD where the first patients treated with ESAs underwent hemodialysis three times a week. TIW dosing in the hemodialysis setting matched a pre-existing requirement for medical encounters. Furthermore, this schedule appeared appropriate for the known short half-life of epoetin alfa and epoetin beta.

A TIW treatment schedule is extremely inconvenient for people with cancer-related anemia who, unlike their CKD counterparts, have no reason for such frequent medical attention. Experimentation with dosing schedules showed that effective hemoglobin rises occurred with once-weekly administration of these ESAs if the drug dose was sufficiently high.[41] Treatment of cancer-related anemia gradually shifted to the more convenient weekly schedule.

The engineering of darbepoetin alfa grew out of an effort to address the issue of dosing interval with the ESAs. Experiments with erythropoietin devoid of carbohydrate side chains showed the importance of glycosylation in erythropoietin biology. The bare erythropoietin protein disappears quickly from the circulation, apparently due to rapid degradation of the protein.[42] Nonglycosylated erythropoietin consequently has little activity in the whole animal despite an excellent in vitro activity profile.

Since erythropoietin without carbohydrate side chains has a short half-life in the circulation, the possibility existed that extra carbohydrate side chains might prolong the agent's survival in the circulation. The genetic modification of erythropoietin structure in darbepoetin alfa produces five rather than three carbohydrate side chains. The drug does indeed have a longer activity profile than the previously existing ESAs. The initial administration schedule for darbepoetin alfa was weekly. Higher dosing later allowed administration of darbepoetin once in 3 weeks for cancer-related anemia.[43] This is a far more palatable schedule for patients since obligate medical encounters for chemotherapy often are once every 3 weeks.

Experience with ESAs to treat cancer-related anemia has led to consensus definitions of drug efficacy. A positive response commonly is defined as an increase in hemoglobin level by 1–2 g/dL over the treatment course. The maximum hemoglobin level attained varies depending on the starting baseline hemoglobin value. Hemoglobin increments of less than 1 g/dL are unlikely to produce a clinically meaningful response (see below).

The hematopoietic response to ESAs in cancer-related anemia is irregular both in magnitude and rate of onset. Up to 40% of patients fail to respond significantly to these agents. The basis of this heterogeneity is unclear. The fact that cancer-related anemia often displays a chronic inflammatory state with substantial cytokine activation makes plausible the contention that a storm of circulating cytokines sometimes overwhelms erythropoiesis activation by ESAs. Therapeutic approaches that include efforts at cytokine suppression might prove beneficial to patients who are otherwise refractory to ESAs. Predictive markers to identify patients who a priori will not respond to ESAs would provide valuable direction in the targeting of ESA therapy. Such markers currently are nonexistent.

One possible approach to improving the therapeutic profile of ESAs is the administration of supplemental iron. Most patients with cancer-related anemia are not truly iron deficient. As noted earlier, however, hepcidin overexpression in response to cytokine activation often produces a relative degree of iron sequestration. Erythropoiesis is suboptimal due to the relative iron deficiency. Supplemental iron administration can partially overcome this trapping effect by providing transient surges in mineral availability in the circulation that can be used briefly for hematopoiesis before the iron is sequestered away.

Few published investigations directly address the question. In one study, patients given iron dextran either as total dose infusion or as smaller intermittent boluses had substantially better hemoglobin increments in response to ESA treatment than did control patients who received either no iron supplementation or iron as an oral preparation.[44] Assuming that corroborating data are forthcoming, the study suggests that iron bioavailability for erythropoiesis in cancer patients is a dynamic process. Boluses of parenteral iron create a brief crack in the wall of iron imprisonment created by high levels of hepcidin. During this wrinkle in time, the erythropoietic machinery has the opportunity to use some of this iron for new red cell production.

Iron supplementation in anemic cancer patients is not without risk. Since these patients usually are not deficient in total body iron, supplementation opens the possibility of iron overload as a complication. Careful monitoring along with the administration of the smallest quantity of parenteral iron that will temporarily perturb the block in hemoglobin synthesis should provide an adequate safety margin. A less well-defined risk is the possibility of tumor progression in response to supplemental iron. Although iron deficit can blunt tumor proliferation, little data support the contention that iron surfeit promotes tumor growth. Nonetheless, any study that assesses iron supplementation should address this issue. The conceptually related idea that excess iron could create an infection risk (a hypothesis with considerably more supporting data) also deserves exploration.

Malignancies that involve the primary blood-forming elements of the bone marrow are generally excluded from ESA treatment. Acute leukemia in particular is not eligible for this form of therapy. Lymphoma and multiple myeloma are malignancies that derive from the lymphoid branch of the hematopoietic system. Both commonly produce substantial anemia and both respond well to treatment with ESAs. Among the solid tumors, the incidence of anemia varies greatly, as noted above. The rate of response to ESA treatment does not appear to vary across the spectrum of cancer subtypes.[45]

Irrespective of tumor type or other obvious distinctions, ESA treatment produces poor responses in some patients and brisk responses in others. A rapid rise in the hemoglobin level, for instance an increase of more than 2 g/dL over 2 weeks, places patients at risk for complications, such as dangerous rises in blood pressure. Consequently, careful monitoring of the rate of hemoglobin rise and the blood pressure status is essential to the safe use of ESAs in the treatment of cancer-related anemia.

Similarly, the magnitude of the hemoglobin response can be a source of concern. Early studies of ESAs in the setting of cancer anemia often permitted the hemoglobin value to rise into the high normal range, namely 14–15 g/dL. However, patients with cancer are not normal. Reports of serious thrombovascular complications including strokes, myocardial infarctions, and deep venous thromboses prompted the imposition of a 13 g/dL ceiling on hemoglobin values deemed acceptable in this treatment setting (see below). For patients who exceed that value, ESA therapy is held until the hemoglobin value declines to an acceptable range. Treatment is restarted at a lower dose if continued therapy is necessary.

Although no existing test predicts patient response to ESAs, careful early monitoring provides guidance into the possible magnitude of the hemoglobin rise. About three-quarters of patients for whom hemoglobin values rise by 1 g/dL or more during the first 4 weeks of therapy eventually have a positive therapeutic response.[46] By contrast, only one-quarter of patients who fail to meet this milestone will have a positive response to continued ESA treatment. The 1-g/dL threshold augurs favorably for response to ESAs both in patients on chemotherapy and those who are treatment naïve.[47] An algorithm that combines a greater than 1 g/dL ESA response at 4 weeks, baseline transfusion independence and a favorable erythropoietin level predicts a favorable ESA response 85% of the time.

Baseline erythropoietin levels indicate the extent to which renal production of the hormone has risen in response to anemia. High erythropoietin levels at the start of treatment means that bone marrow erythroid precursor cells have substantial exposure to the hormone. Pharmacological intervention with an ESA consequently faces a serious challenge in the quest to further accelerate erythropoiesis. In contrast, the combination of a low baseline erythropoietin level (<100 mIU/mL) and a rise in hemoglobin of >0.5 g/dL at 2 weeks gives a 95% prediction of a positive erythropoietic response.[48]

ANEMIA SEVERITY AND ESA TREATMENT

The issue of effective ESA use in cancer-related anemia is a broadly important question in medicine. The problem has implications of both medical and economic importance. The former reflects the impact of ESAs on patient well-being. The latter reflects the impact of ESAs on health-care costs. The point of inflection between a net positive and a net negative scenario is an issue involving complex considerations. Additional careful consideration of the subject is warranted.

A plethora of studies address the issue of medical use of ESAs in cancer-related anemia. The quality of these studies varies greatly, along with the design and objectives of the work. At the behest of the Agency for Healthcare Research and Quality, the American Society of Clinical Oncology (ASCO) and the American Society of Hematology (ASH) convened an expert panel to review the data and make recommendations.

Over the course of several years, the panel evaluated the literature published between 1985 and 1999, and issued an evidence-based clinical practice guideline.[49] These voluntary guidelines recommended use of epoetin for cancer patients with anemia where the hemoglobin value was ≤10 g/dL. For cancer patients "with declining hemoglobin levels but less severe anemia (those with hemoglobin concentration below 12 g/dL but who never have fallen below 10 g/dL), the decision of whether to use epoetin immediately or to wait until hemoglobin levels fall closer to 10 g/dL should be determined by clinical circumstance." The latter recommendation reflected the fact that while existing data on the whole favored the use of epoetin in this setting, the studies were small and mainly unblinded. That along with inconsistent statistical treatments across the spectrum made impossible any definitive statement on the matter.

The initial large studies of ESAs in cancer anemia not surprisingly focused on patients with more severe degrees of anemia. Additional reports involving patients with milder anemia appeared after the ASCO/ASH panel disbanded. One review evaluated 69 publications from between 1999 and 2004, deeming 11 worthy of detailed analysis based on size, design, and completeness.[50] The composite data strongly supported the benefit of ESA therapy in patients with hemoglobin values exceeding 10 g/dL. The recommendation, which dovetailed with that of the National Comprehensive Cancer Network, was that clinicians consider ESA intervention for patients with hemoglobin values ≤11 g/dL. The European Organisation for Research and Treatment of Cancer Guidelines set a hemoglobin target range of 11–13 g/dL.

The key studies involving ESA use in cancer anemia have addressed patients undergoing chemotherapy. The role of ESAs in the management of the 30% of cancer patients who are anemic in the absence of myelosuppressive chemotherapy is unknown. The growing use of biological agents, such as monoclonal antibodies and hormones, along with directed therapies, such as drugs aimed at tyrosine kinase enzymes, means that the fraction of cancer patients who do not fit the vetted profile for ESA use will grow. Also outside the circle of defined use are the large number of people who receive myelosuppressive agents as part of adjuvant treatment regimens. Only additional investigation will provide the needed answers.

■ IMPACT OF ANEMIA IN CANCER

In the context of a pernicious and potentially fatal illness, anemia sometimes receives little attention from health-care providers. Recently, however, the increased weight given to issues of QoL in circumstances where cancer cure is not possible has brought greater attention to the impact of anemia.[51] Fatigue and dyspnea are the key manifestations in people with anemia of any cause, and this holds for anemia in the setting of cancer.[52] The impact of fatigue on the well-being of patients with cancer is often substantial.

No objective measure for fatigue exists, making its assessment difficult. The development of an objective scoring system for the problem has made possible the systematic investigation of the impact of fatigue on the well-being of patients in general and cancer patients in particular. A commonly used questionnaire is the Functional Assessment of Cancer Therapy (FACT).[53] The version of this instrument that assesses anemia (FACT-An) entails a series of questions that describe anemia along with related fatigue and assesses their effect on well-being relative to other problems commonly faced by cancer patients, including nausea, pain, and depression.[54,55] In addition, patients estimate the impact of fatigue on other aspects of their lives such as social functioning, ability to work, and dependence on the person(s) providing them with primary help and support. Open-ended questions allow patients to fill in other important aspects of their clinical experience.

Another tool used to determine the impact of fatigue is the Linear Analogue Scale Assessment (LASA).[56] Here, a 100-mm line represents the patient's sense of well-being, with one end indicating "worst" and the other "best." The line is segmented by nine small bars spaced 10 mm apart. At the start of the study, the patient marks the point along the line that best corresponds to his or her sense of well-being. Subsequent evaluations involve the patient placing indicators on new line with no previous assessment marking that the patient might use as a reference. Investigators can compare the scales at the end of the study, thereby gaining a feel for changes in the patient's sense of well-being over the interval. Pooled patient LASA data provides a window into the benefit of the treatment intervention. LASA data are easier to collect than that from FACT-An surveys. The penalty for the tool's simplicity is greater variability of outcome. Consequently, LASA instruments perform best when used in the setting of large study cohorts.[57]

ESA THERAPY AND PATIENT QUALITY OF LIFE

A key observation is that cancer patients with mild anemia, i.e., hemoglobin values in the 10–11 g/dL range, have significant symptoms and debility. Two studies of cancer patients in community treatment settings reviewed over 4000 patients and recorded responses to interventions designed to correct the anemia.[58,59] Substantial improvements in the QoL measures paralleled rises in hemoglobin values. Interestingly, the most marked improvement occurred with a hemoglobin rise from 11 to 12 g/dL, supporting the practice of intervening before severe anemia develops.[60] Hemoglobin values in this mild range commonly drew little notice in the past. A 1-g rise in hemoglobin values from 11 to 12 g/dL often would have been dismissed as an insignificant change. However, this degree of rise in hemoglobin level improved QoL measures even in patients whose underlying cancer progressed. This observation indicates that hemoglobin rise is not simply a surrogate for cancer treatment response with respect to enhanced patient well-being.

Over half of patients in one large study reported that fatigue had a significant negative impact on their lives.[61] Despite the clinical impact of fatigue, more than half of the patients never discussed the issue with their health-care providers. A sense of resignation existed among many of the patients in whom they assumed that chronic debilitating fatigue was a reality they simply had to live with. Interestingly, only 14% of patients who experienced fatigue reported that an intervention was prescribed or recommended for the problem. The most common recommendation was for the patient to "have a rest."

Fatigue produces significant difficulties for patients, including diminished energy levels, a need to slow down from a normal pace of living, and a general sense of sluggishness or tiredness. Ninety percent of patients in one study reported that fatigue prevented them from leading a normal life and forced an alteration in their normal daily routine.[62] Sixty percent of these patients reported that fatigue exceeded nausea, pain, and depression as a negative factor in their lives. Other problems associated with fatigue were decreased motivation or interest, difficulty concentrating, and difficulty remembering dates and "keeping things straight."

Ordinary activities such as walking or house cleaning become new challenges as a result of fatigue. Three-quarters of patients are forced to change their employment status and one-quarter discontinued work altogether due to fatigue. The caregivers for these individuals also suffer, with one in five taking more time off from work or accepting fewer responsibilities. Fatigue can reach such distressing proportions that 1 in 10 patients report an urge to die in the face of this problem.[63] Fatigue resulting from anemia clearly is a major problem in cancer.

Another trial failed to identify an optimal hemoglobin level for improvement of QoL.[64] Nonetheless, an increase in hemoglobin of at least 2 g/dL from baseline (without transfusion) correlated significantly with improvements in QoL. These results are in accord with another study in which increases in hemoglobin concentration (as opposed to reaching a predefined target hemoglobin level) produced the greatest improvement in QoL.[65] A study of over 300 patients in the Netherlands showed that ESA therapy for patients with hemoglobin values below 12 g/dL reduced the need for transfusion, increased aggregate hemoglobin levels, and improved QoL.[66] The lesson of these trials is that treatment intervention before severe anemia develops (Hb ≤10g/dL) averts side effects that greatly hamper patients with anemia.

ESA THERAPY AND TRANSFUSION REQUIREMENT

Elimination of the need for transfusion is a key goal in the use of ESAs in cancer-related anemia. Although complete abolition of transfusions often is not possible, trials with blood transfusion as a study end point generally show reductions that range between 10% and 50%.[67,68] Since as many as 40% of patients treated with ESAs fail to respond to the drugs, the benefit in transfusion avoidance is substantial for the group of people who do respond to these agents.

Chemotherapy regimes that use agents in the platinum family of drugs (e.g., cisplatinum) are mainstays in the treatment of many of the common solid tumors, including malignancies of lung, GI, and ovarian origin. These agents also have powerful myelosuppressive qualities, with severe anemia as a common sequel. In an investigation involving over 300 such patients, 36% of the ESA-treated group required transfusion, compared with 65% of controls.[69] Furthermore, the ESA group required only 1.5 units of blood on average, while the value was 3.1 for the controls. Finally, the ESA-treated patients had higher aggregate hemoglobin values during treatment and better QoL scores. The net result is strong support for the use of ESAs in these patients.

IMPACT OF ESA THERAPY ON SURVIVAL

The question of whether ESA therapy alters the survival of patients with cancer-related anemia has drawn great scrutiny and engendered intense debate. From a theoretical standpoint, arguments exist for ESAs prolonging or shortening survival. Correction of anemia might improve perfusion and oxygenation of tumors, making them more susceptible to anticancer treatments. Hypoxic tumors are more resistant to radiation therapy since the effect of this intervention depends in part on the generation of ROS.[70,71] ROS are important to the action of some chemotherapy agents, such as doxorubicin.[72] In addition, the improved sense of well-being associated with ESA therapy might allow some patients to adhere more closely to debilitating chemotherapy regimens.

On the other side of the equation lies the fact that erythropoietin is a growth promoting hormone.[73,74] Although erythropoietic precursors are the primary site of erythropoietin receptors, other tissues also express functional receptors.[75] Data suggesting possible erythropoietin receptor expression by tumor cells give pause for contemplation.[76] However, two studies in particular raised serious questions about the impact of ESAs on the survival of patients with cancer. One investigation with over 900 patients involved epoetin alfa treatment of women with metastatic breast cancer, most of whom were not anemic.[77] The investigation used a randomized, placebo-controlled, double-blind design. Higher mortality among the patients receiving epoetin alfa prompted early termination of the trial. No clear cause for the difference existed, although a larger number of deaths from thrombovascular events in the treated group contributed to some of the excess mortality.

The second study involving 350 patients with head and neck cancer treated with epoetin beta also used a randomized, placebo-controlled, double-blind design.[78] The hemoglobin response among the treated patients was excellent, paralleling that seen in previous similar investigations. What was not previously seen, however, was the effect on survival. The locoregional progression-free survival among the patients who received epoetin beta was substantially inferior to that of the controls. The overall patient cohort was similar to that used in other studies of head and neck cancer. No bias in subgroup assignment explained the survival differential.

The most comprehensive look at the issue of patient survival with ESA treatment comes from the Cochrane Collaborative Report, "Erythropoietin for Patients with Malignant Disease (Review)."[79] A subsequent update of the data in the report allowed coverage of 57 trials involving over 9000 patients published between 1985 and 2005.[80] The meta-analysis produced a result with no certainty as to whether therapy with epoetin or darbepoetin alters overall patient survival. A higher risk of thrombovascular events was apparent in patients treated with the ESAs. The report recommended careful monitoring for thrombovascular complications in patients treated with these compounds as well as continued investigation into the issue of ESAs and cancer patient survival.

References

1. Kyle RA. 1975. Multiple myeloma: Review of 869 cases. Mayo Clin Proc 50:29–40.
2. Gallagher CJ, Gregory WM, Jones AE, et al. 1986. Follicular lymphoma: Prognostic factors for response and survival. J Clin Oncol 4:1470–1480.
3. Moullet I, Salles G, Ketterer N, et al. 1998. Frequency and significance of anemia in non-Hodgkin's lymphoma patients. Ann Oncol 9:1109–1115.
4. Obemair A, Handisurya A, Kaider A, et al. 1998. The relationship of pretreatment serum hemoglobin level to the survival of epithelial ovarian carcinoma patients: A prospective review. Cancer 15:726–731.
5. Ludwig H, Van Belle S, Barrett-Lee P, et al. 2004. The European Cancer Anaemia Survey (ECAS): A large multinational, prospective survey defining the prevalence, incidence, and treatment of anaemia in cancer patients. Eur J Cancer 40:2293–2306.
6. Brugnara C. 2003. Iron deficiency and eropoiesis: New diagnostic approaches. Clin Chem 49:1573–1578.
7. Ebert BL, Bunn HF. 1999. Regulation of the erythropoietin gene. Blood 94:1864–1877.
8. Van Wyck DB, Stivelman JC, Ruiz J, et al. 1989. Iron status in patients receiving erythropoietin for dialysis-associated anemia. Kidney Int 35:712–716.
9. Cash JM, Sears DA. 1989. The anemia of chronic disease: Spectrum of associated diseases in a series of unselected hospitalized patients. Am J Med 87:638–644.
10. Finch C. 1994. Regulators of iron balance in humans. Blood 84:1697–1702.
11. Frazer DM, Wilkins SJ, Becker EM, et al. 2002. Hepcidin expression inversely correlates with the expression of duodenal iron transporters and iron absorption in rats. Gastroenterology 123:835–844.
12. Laftah AH, Ramesh B, Simpson RJ, et al. 2004. Effect of hepcidin on intestinal iron absorption in mice. Blood 103:3940–3944.

[13] Delaby C, Pilard N, Goncalves AS, et al. 2005. Presence of the iron exporter ferroportin at the plasma membrane of macrophages is enhanced by iron loading and down-regulated by hepcidin. Blood 106:3979–3984.

[14] Weinstein DA, Roy CN, Fleming MD, Loda MF, Wolfsdorf JI, Andrews NC. 2002. Inappropriate expression of hepcidin is associated with iron refractory anemia: Implications for the anemia of chronic disease. Blood 100:3776–3781.

[15] Nemeth E, Rivera S, Gabayan V, et al. 2004. Il-6 mediates hypoferremia in inflammation by inducing the synthesis of the iron regulatory hormone, hepcidin. J Clin Invest 113:1271–1276.

[16] Lee P, Peng H, Gelbart T, Beutler E. 2005. Regulation of hepcidin transcription by interleukin-1 and interleukin-6. Proc Natl Acad Sci U S A 1906–1910.

[17] McKeown DJ, Brown DJ, Kelly A, Wallace AM, McMillan DC. 2004. The relationship between circulating concentrations of C-reactive protein, inflammatory cytokines and cytokine receptors in patients with non-small-cell lung cancer. Br J Cancer 91:1993–1995.

[18] Scott HR, McMillan DC, Forrest LM, Brown DJ, McArdle CS, Milroy R. 2002. The systemic inflammatory response, weight loss, performance status and survival in patients with inoperable non-small cell lung cancer. Br J Cancer 87:264–267.

[19] Forrest LM, McMillan DC, McArdle CS, Angerson WJ, Dunlop DJ. 2003. Evaluation of cumulative prognostic scores based on the systemic inflammatory response in patients with inoperable non-small-cell lung cancer. Br J Cancer 89:1028–1030.

[20] Lauta VM. 2003. A review of the cytokine network in multiple myeloma: Diagnostic, prognostic and therapeutic implications. Cancer 97:2440–2052.

[21] Macciò A, Lai P, Santona MC, et al. 1998. High serum levels of soluble Il-2 receptor, cytokines and C-reactive protein correlate with impairment of T cell response in patients with advanced epithelial ovarian cancer. Gynecol Oncol 69:248–252.

[22] Thompson MA, Witzig TE, Kumar S, et al. 2003. Plasma levels of tumour necrosis factor alpha and interleukin-6 predict progression-free survival following thalidomide therapy in patients with previously untreated multiple myeloma. Br J Haematol 123:305–308.

[23] Scambia G, Testa U, Benedetti Panici P, et al. 1995. Prognostic significance of interleukin-6 serum levels in patients with ovarian cancer. Br J Cancer 71:354–356.

[24] Nieken J, Mulder NH, Buter J, et al. 1995. Recombinant human interleukin-6 induces a rapid and reversible anemia in cancer patients. Blood 86:900–905.

[25] Faquin WC, Schneider TJ, Goldberg MA. 1992. Effect of inflammatory cytokines on hypoxia-induced erythropoietin production. Blood 79:1987–1894.

[26] Means RT, Jr. 1999. Advances in the anemia of chronic disease. Int J Haematol 70:7–12.

[27] Rusten LS, Jacobsen SEW. 1995. Tumour necrosis factor (TNF)-(directly inhibits human erythropoiesis in vitro: Role of p55 and p75 TNF receptors. Blood 80:989–996.

[28] Toyokuni S, Okamoto K, Yodoi J, et al. 1995. Persistent oxedative stress in cancer. FEBS Lett 16:3581–3583.

[29] Guven M, Ozturk B, Sayal A, et al. 1999. Lipid peroxidation and antioxidant system in the blood of cancerous patients with metastasis. Cancer 17:155–162.

[30] Lusini L, Tripodi SA, Rossi R, et al. 2001. Altered glutathione anti-oxidant metabolism during tumor progression in human renal cell carcinoma. Int J Cancer 91:55–59.

[31] Estrin JT, Schocket L, Kregnow R, et al. 1999. A retrospective review of blood transfusions in cancer patients with anemia. Oncologist 4:318–324.

[32] Goodnough LT, Brecher ME, Kanter MH, AuBuchon JP. 1999. Transfusion medicine. First of two parts—blood transfusion. N Engl J Med 340:438–447.

[33] Skillings JR, Sridhar FG, Wong C, et al. 1993. The frequency of red cell transfusion for anemia in patients receiving chemotherapy: A retrospective cohort study. Am J Clin Oncol 16:22–25.

[34] Rizzo JD, Lichtin AE, Woolf SH, et al. 2002. Use of epoetin in patients with cancer: Evidence-based clinical practice guidelines of the American Society of Clinical Oncology and the American Society of Hematology. J Clin Oncol 20:4083–4107.

[35] Groopman JE, Itri LM. 1999. Chemotherapy-induced anemia in adults: Incidence and treatment. J Natl Cancer Inst 19:1616–1634.

[36] Bennett WM. 1991. A multicenter clinical trial of epoetin beta for anemia of end-stage renal disease. J Am Soc Nephrol 1:990–998.

[37] Delano BG. 1989. Improvements in quality of life following treatment with r-HuEPO in anemic hemodialysis patients. Am J Kidney Dis 14(2 Suppl 1):14–18.

[38] Egrie JC, Browne JK. 2001. Development and characterization of novel erythropoiesis stimulating protein (NESP). Br J Cancer 84(Suppl 1):3–10.

[39] Heatherington AC, Schuller J, Mercer AJ. 2001. Pharmacokinetics of novel erythropoiesis stimulating protein (NESP) in cancer patients: Preliminary report. Br J Cancer 84(Suppl 1):11–16.

[40] Broudy VC, Lin N, Brice M, Nakamoto B, Papayannopoulou T. 1991. Erythropoietin receptor characteristics on primary human erythroid cells. Blood 77:2583–2590.

[41] Shasha D, George MJ, Harrison LB. 2003. Once-weekly dosing of epoetin-alpha increases hemoglobin and improves quality of life in anemic cancer patients receiving radiation therapy either concomitantly or sequentially with chemotherapy. Cancer 98:1072–1079.

[42] Tsuda E, Kawanishi G, Ueda M, Masuda S, Sasaki R. 1990. The role of carbohydrate in recombinant human erythropoietin. Eur J Biochem 188:405–411.

[43] Boccia R, Malik IA, Raja V, et al. 2006. Darbepoetin alfa administered every three weeks is effective for the treatment of chemotherapy-induced anemia. Oncologist 11:409–417.

[44] Auerbach M, Ballard H, Trout RJ, et al. 2004. Intravenous iron optimizes the response to recombinant human erythropoietin in cancer patients with chemotherapy-related anemia: A multicenter, open-label, randomized trial. J Clin Oncol 22:301–301.

[45] Gabrilove JL, Cleeland CS, Livingston RB, et al. 2001. Clinical evaluation of once-weekly dosing of epoetin alfa in chemotherapy patients: Improvement in hemoglobin and quality of life are similar to three-times-weekly dosing. J Clin Oncol 19:2875–2882.

[46] Quirt I, Robeson C, Lau C, et al. and the Canadian Eprex Oncology Study Group. 2001. Epoetin alfa therapy increases hemoglobin levels and improves quality of life in patients with cancer-related anemia who are not receiving chemotherapy and patients with anemia who are receiving chemotherapy. J Clin Oncol 19:4126–4134.

[47] Henry D, Abels R, Larholt K. 1995. Prediction of response to recombinant human erythropoietin (r-HuEPO/epoetin-alpha) therapy in cancer patients. Blood 85(6):1676–1678.

[48] Ludwig H, Fritz E, Leitgeb C, Pecherstorfer M, Samonigg H, Schuster J. 1994. Prediction of response to erythropoietin treatment in chronic anemia of cancer. Blood 84(4):1056–1063.

[49] Rizzo JD, Lichtin AE, Woolf SH, et al. 2002. Use of epoetin in patients with cancer: Evidence-based practice guidelines of the American Society of Clinical Oncology and the American Society of Hematology. Blood 100:2303–2320.

[50] Lyman GH, Glaspy J. 2006. Are there clinical benefits with early erythropoietic intervention for chemotherapy-induced anemia? A systematic review. Cancer 106:223–233.

[51] Portenoy RK, Thaler HT, Korblith AB, et al. 1994. Symptom prevalence, characteristics, and distress in a cancer population. Qual Life Res 3:183–189.

[52] Blesch KS, Paice JA, Wickham R, et al. 1991. Correlates of fatigue in people with breast or lung cancer. Oncol Nurs Forum 18:81–87.

[53] Yellen SB, Cella DF, Webster K, et al. 1997. Measuring fatigue and other anemia symptoms with the functional assessment of cancer therapy (FACT) measurement system. J Pain Symptom Manage 13:63–74.

[54] Cella D. 1997. The Functional Assessment of Cancer Therapy-Anemia (FACT-An) scale: A new tool for the assessment of outcomes in cancer anemia and fatigue. Semin Hematol 34(Suppl 2):13–19.

[55] Cella D. 1998. Factors influencing quality of life in cancer patients: Anemia and fatigue. Semin Oncol 25(Suppl 7):43–46.

[56] Boyd NF, Selby PJ, Sutherland HJ, Hogg S. 1988. Measurement of the clinical status of patients with breast cancer: Evidence for the validity of self assessment with linear analogue scales. J Clin Epidemiol 41:243–250.

[57] Bernhard J, Sullivan M, Hurny C, Coates AS, Rudenstam CM. 2001. Clinical relevance of single item quality of life indicators in cancer clinical trials. Br J Cancer 84:1156–1165.

[58] Glaspy J, Bukowski R, Steinberg D, et al. 1997. Impact of therapy with epoetin alfa on clinical outcomes in patients with nonmyeloid malignancies during cancer chemotherapy in community oncology practice. J. Clin Oncol 15:1218–1234.

[59] Demetri GD, Kris M, Wade J, et al. 1998. Quality-of-life benefit in chemotherapy patients treated with epoetin alfa is independent of disease response and tumor type: Results from a prospective community oncology study. J Clin Oncol 16:3412–3425.

[60] Crawford J, Cella D, Cleeland CS, et al. 2002. Relationship between changes in hemoglobin level and quality of life during chemotherapy in anemic cancer patients receiving epoetin alfa therapy. Cancer 95:888–895.

[61] Stone P, Richardson A, Ream E, et al. 2000. Cancer-related fatigue: Inevitable, unimportant and untreatable? Results of a multi-centre patients survey. Ann Oncol 11:971–975.

[62] Curt GA, Breitbart W, Cella D, et al. 2000. Impact of cancer-related fatigue on the live of patients: New finding from the Fatigue Coalition. Oncologist 5:353–360.

[63] Harper P, Littlewood T. 2005. Anaemia of cancer: Impact on patient fatigue and long-term outcome. Oncology 69(Suppl 2):2–7.

[64] Österborg A, Brandberg Y, Molostova V, et al. 2002. Randomized, double-blinded, placebo-controlled trial of recombinant human erythropoietin (epoetin beta) in hematological malignancies. J Clin Oncol 20: 2486–2494.

[65] Glimelius B, Linne T, Hoffman K, et al. 1998. Epoetin beta in the treatment of anemia in patients with advanced gastrointestinal cancer. J Clin Oncol 16:434–440.

[66] Savonije JH, Van Groeningen CJ, Wormhoudt LW, et al. 2006. Early intervention with epoetin alfa during platinum-based chemotherapy: An analysis of quality-of-life results of a multicenter, randomized, controlled trial compared with population normative data. Oncologist 11:197–205.

[67] Cascinu S, Fedeli A, Del Ferro E, et al. 1994. Recombinant human erythropoietin treatment in cisplatin-associated anemia: A randomized, double-blind trial with placebo. J Clin Oncol 12:1058–1062.

[68] Oberhoff C, Neri B, Amadori D, et al. 1998. Recombinant human erythropoietin in the treatment of chemotherapy-induced anemia and prevention of transfusion requirement associated with solid tumors: A randomized, controlled study. Ann Oncol 9:255–260.

[69] Savonije JH, van Groegingen CJ, van Bochove A, et al. 2005. Effects of early intervention with epoetin alfa on transfusion requirement, hemoglobin level and survival during platinum-based chemotherapy: Results of a multicenter randomised controlled trial. Eur J Cancer 41:1560–1569.

[70] Renschler MF. 2004. The emerging role of reactive oxygen species in cancer therapy. Eur J Cancer 40:1934–1940.

[71] Cook JA, Gius D, Wink DA, et al. 2004. Oxidative stress, redox, and the tumor microenvironment. Semin Radiat Oncol 14:259–266.

[72] Porumb H, Petrescu I. 1986. Interaction with mitochondria of the anthracycline cytostatics adriamycin and daunomycin. Prog Biophys Mol Biol 48:103–125.

[73] Kaushansky K. 2006. Lineage-specific hematopoietic growth factors. N Engl J Med 354:2034–2045.

[74] Ogilvie M, Yu X, Nicolas-Metral V, et al. 2000. Erythropoietin stimulates proliferation and interferes with differentiation of myoblasts. J Biol Chem 275:39754–39761.

[75] Nagai A, Nakagawa E, Choi HB, et al. 2001. Erythropoietin and erythropoietin receptors in human CNS neurons, astrocytes, microglia, and oligodendrocytes grown in culture. J Neuropathol Exp Neurol 60:386–392.

[76] Acs G, Acs P, Beckwith SM, et al. 2001. Erythropoietin and erythropoietin receptor expression in human cancer. Cancer Res 61:3561–3565.

[77] Leyland-Jones B, Semiglazov V, Pawlicki M, et al. 2005. Maintaining normal hemoglobin levels with epoetin alfa in mainly nonanemic patients with metastatic breast cancer receiving first-line chemotherapy: A survival study. J Clin Oncol 23:5960–5972.

[78] Henke M, Lasig R, Rübe C, et al. 2003. Erythropoietin to treat head and neck cancer patients with anaemia undergoing radiotherapy: Randomized, double-blind, placebo-controlled trial. Lancet 362:1255–1260.

[79] Bohlius J, Langersiepen S, Schwarzer G, et al. 2005. Recombinant human erythropoietin and over survival in cancer patients: Results of a comprehensive meta-analysis. J Natl Cancer Inst 97:489–498.

[80] Bohlius J, Wilson J, Seidenfeld J, et al. 2006. Recombinant human erythropoietin and cancer patients: Updated meta-analysis of 57 studies including 9353 patients. J Natl Cancer Inst 98:708–714.

MALARIA AND THE RED CELL

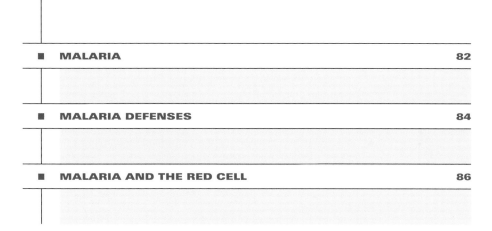

Malaria has had a greater impact on the human race than almost any other disease. The parasite continues to spread despair and death across wide swaths of the world to this very day. Malaria became a major problem for people about 10,000 years ago when the last ice age ended and humans began to move from a hunter–gatherer existence to one that involved agriculture. Stagnant pools of water, ideal breeding grounds for the mosquitoes that transmit malaria, were common byproducts of the slash and burn farming that marked the dawn of the agricultural age. The rice paddies still prevalent in Asia are excellent environments for mosquito propagation. By providing a controlled and dependable food source, agriculture gave humans important power over their fate. By providing an environment for mosquitoes to breed, agriculture simultaneously placed much of that power into the hands of a malevolent parasite.

Analysis of the genome map of *Plasmodium falciparum* provides insight into the origin and spread of the most deadly pathogen that confronts mankind.[1] The parasite appears to have arisen in Africa from a common ancestor sometime between 25,000 and 60,000 years ago.[2] The parasite population apparently increased dramatically approximately 10,000 years ago at the end of the Pleistocene era and the beginning of human horticulture.[3] The pathogen probably spread from Africa to other tropical and subtropical regions of the world in the last 6000 years. The human colonists in the New World, who arrived between 20,000 and 40,000 years ago, by then were isolated from their Old World origins and thus missed the expansion of *P. falciparum*.

Reports of severe febrile illness exist since the beginning of writing about 5000 years ago. Whether such reports concern malaria or other illnesses is a conjecture. However, Hippocrates wrote of severe febrile illness and divided the fever into different types: quotidian (daily), tertian (alternate days), and quartan (every fourth day). These fever patterns are characteristic of malaria. Malaria did not exist in the Americas prior to Columbus and European expansion. Interestingly, none of the surviving records from the Mayans or Aztecs describe febrile illness of a severity and pattern that is consistent with malaria.

Malaria came to the Americas through the blood of European colonists and the slaves they brought to the New World. The disease found fertile ground that included Anopheles mosquito species that could support the growth of malaria parasites and transmit the disease to human hosts in a fashion analogous to the mosquito vectors of the Old World. Malaria became firmly entrenched in the tropical regions of Central and South America and even spread into southern sections of North America.

Throughout human history, no effective countermeasure existed to the ravages of malaria. Amulets, incantations, and charms were all equally ineffective. The observation has been made, however, that "diseases desperate grown by desperate appliance are relieved, or not at all."* Only desperation could explain the attempt to treat malaria using an extract from the bark of the South American Cinchona tree that contained a toxic plant alkaloid. Fortunately, the gamble paid off. Jesuit missionaries in South America learned of the antimalarial properties of the extract and introduced it into Europe by the 1630s and into India by 1657. Not until 1820 was the active agent identified as quinine.

The cause of malaria remained a mystery, however. The breakthrough occurred on this front in Algeria when, in 1880, Alphonse Laveran through painstaking analysis and careful observation correlated fatal malaria with peculiar bodies that appeared to be parasites in the blood of the victims. His initial reports to the French Academy of Medicine met skepticism. Laveran later reviewed some of his material with Louis Pasteur who was instantly convinced of the matter. In 1907, Laveran received the Nobel Prize in Medicine for his discovery.

■ MALARIA

Four species of malaria, *P. falciparum*, *P. vivax*, *P. ovale,* and *P. malariae*, cause almost all human infections. The disorder occurs throughout tropical regions of the world. About 500 million cases of malaria occur each year with about 4 million of these classified as severe malaria. Approximately one million people die of the disease annually, with *P. falciparum* as the leading cause of death by far. Most deaths from malaria occur in Africa, with the vast majority of victims being children younger than 5 years. WHO estimates of the leading causes of death among children in developing countries in 2002 places malaria in fourth place, ahead even of HIV/AIDS (Figure 6-1).

The female Anopheles mosquito is the vector that transmits the malarial parasite to people as part of the complex life cycle of the organism (Figure 6-2). A bite by the mosquito releases sporozoites beneath the skin of the victim. The organisms make their way to the blood stream and from there into liver hepatocytes. Growth and division in the hepatocytes produces merozoites that eventually break out of these

---

* **Hamlet** Act IV, Scene III, 9–11

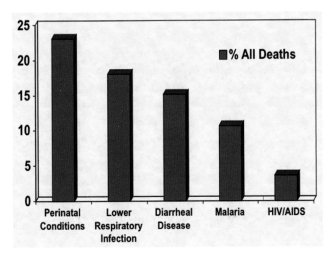

FIGURE 6–1 *Leading causes of death in children from developing countries (in 2002). (Data source: World Health Organization. The World Health Report 2003.)*

cells, enter the blood stream, and penetrate red cells. Here the parasites begin their second phase of growth and maturation.

Parasites in the trophozoite or ring stage are the usual form seen in the peripheral blood (Figure 6-3). The organisms grow and proliferate to the point that red cells burst and release a new wave of merozoites into the blood stream. Synchronous growth of the parasites in host red cells showers pyrogenic material into the blood stream when the cells lyse. The result is intermittent fever spikes that are a hallmark of malaria (tertian fever). A fraction of the red cell parasites form gametocytes (the sexual parasite stage). Mosquitoes feeding on the blood of humans infected with malaria ingest the gametocytes, thereby initiating a new cycle of disease.

Malaria most often produces an uncomplicated or mild illness characterized by fever, shaking chills, myalgia, and headache. Prominent splenic enlargement called "tropical splenomegaly" commonly develops after repeated bouts of malaria.[4] *P. vivax* and *P. ovale* typically produce mild malarial illness. Although *P. falciparum* most often produces a mild to moderately severe syndrome, this organism also produces a severe form of malaria in some of its victims, the likes of which occur with neither *P. vivax* nor *P. ovale*. The characteristics of severe malaria are high fever, lethargy, coma, seizures, respiratory distress, severe anemia, metabolic acidosis, and hypoglycemia. Infants and children often succumb to severe disease produced by *P. falciparum*, with a case fatality rate of 20%. Severe malaria in pregnant women can produce low birth weight infants who are more susceptible to death from other conditions and diseases.

Any natural defense against malaria would profoundly benefit victims of the disease. Such defenses would have a selective advantage that would raise their frequency in the population. A number of red cell mutations provide such an advantage by reducing the impact of malaria on its victims.

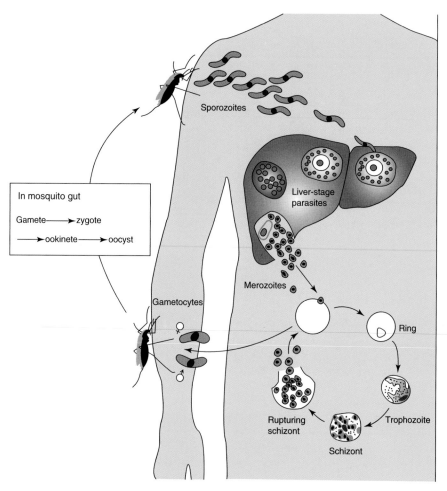

FIGURE 6–2 *Malaria life cycle. A bite from an Anopheles mosquito deposits malaria sporozoites beneath the skin. Some of the organisms reach the blood stream and home to hepatocytes where they multiply and mature into merozoites. Hepatocyte rupture releases merozoites into the blood stream where they invade erythrocytes becoming ring forms and trophozoites. Red cell rupture releases newly developed merozoites and a few gametocytes. The latter can be taken up by feeding mosquitoes, initiating a new cycle of parasite transmission. (From Greenwood et al. 2005. Lancet 365:1487–1498.)*

■ **MALARIA DEFENSES**

The complex nature of the malaria parasite life cycle in the human host presents several points at which the organism could be targeted for destruction. The sporozoites that enter the blood stream following the initial mosquito bite are attacked there by components of the immune system. These include antibodies, natural killer cells,

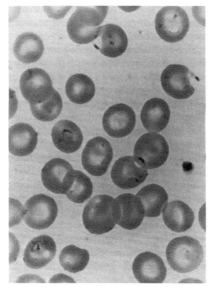
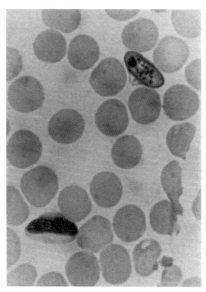

A   **B**

FIGURE 6–3 *The peripheral blood smear shows P. falciparum trophozoites visible as a delicate hoop-shaped rings near the margin of the erythrocytes. (From James H. Jandl. 1987. Blood: Textbook of Hematology. Boston: Little, Brown and Company, Figure 10-4A, p. 324. Used with permission of publisher.)*

as well as conditioned lymphocytes produced as a result of prior exposure to the organisms.

Host immunity is crucial to survival of people infected with the malaria parasite. This is particularly true in the case of the nocuous *P. falciparum* parasite. The immune system works best when it has been primed against the invader. Children who suffer their first or second bout of malaria have not developed the immune response needed to provide adequate defense against the parasite. This explains in part the high mortality seen in children infected with *P. falciparum*. In contrast, infants are more resistant to malaria up to the age of 6 or 7 months due to passive immunity transferred from the mother.

The intrahepatic phase of malarial parasite growth presents another potential point at which to attack the organism. No mutation in the structure or function of hepatic cells that kills the malarial parasite or retards its growth is known. An immune assault on malaria-infected hepatocytes is conceivable. Immune responses directed against hepatocytes can run awry, however, and produce more harm than good as witnessed by the chronic active hepatitis generated by hepatitis C infection.

The last point at which the life cycle of the malarial parasite can be frustrated in humans is in the phase of red cell invasion and multiplication. Red cells are constantly created and then destroyed as they age and senesce. A mutation that somehow destroys both the infected red cells and the parasite could eliminate the malaria parasite. Newly produced healthy cells would replace the infected cells destroyed by the defense response.

■ MALARIA AND THE RED CELL

The morbidity and mortality from malaria over the ages produced a great selective pressure in affected populations for mutations that reduce the impact of the disease. In noting the concordant distribution of malaria and thalassemia, J.B.S. Haldane first proposed that the high thalassemia gene frequency in certain populations reflected protection against infection afforded by heterozygous thalassemia.[5] Table 6-1 lists some of the red cell defenses against malaria that have arisen by natural selection. The mechanisms by which some of these alterations thwart the malaria parasite are well characterized while others are not. Studies by various investigators attribute specific antimalarial properties to individual red cell mutants. Most likely, however, multiple mechanisms contribute to malaria suppression with each of the red cell defense systems.

Perhaps the clearest mechanism of protection involves the Duffy red cell membrane antigen, which is a chemokine receptor. *P. vivax* merozoites attach to red cells using this molecule in the first phase of erythrocyte invasion. The high association of Duffy antigen null red cells in some groups of people with sickle cell trait suggested that the Duffy antigen might provide some protection against malaria.[6,7] Subsequent investigations showed that a point mutation in the *Duffy* gene promoter eliminates Duffy antigen expression.[8] People who lack the Duffy antigen (FY*O allele) are resistant to *P. vivax*.[9] The Duffy null phenotype is most common in people whose ancestors derive from regions in West Africa with endemic vivax malaria. A second Duffy null "hot spot" exists in Papua New Guinea where *P. vivax* is also a major problem.[10]

TABLE 6-1 | **RED CELL DEFENSES AGAINST MALARIA**

Cell Component	*Alteration*	*Global Distribution*
Membrane	Duffy antigen null	West Africa
	Melanesian elliptocytosis	Melanesia
	Hemoglobin S	Africa, Middle East, India
	Hemoglobin C	West Africa
	Hemoglobin E	S.E. Asia
Hemoglobin	β-thalassemia	Africa, Mediterranean, India, S.E. Asia, Melanesia
	α-thalassemia	Africa, India, S.E. Asia, Melanesia
Enzymes	G6PD deficiency	Africa, Mediterranean, India, S.E. Asia

Sickle hemoglobin provides an excellent example of a change in the hemoglobin molecule that impairs malaria growth and development. The initial hints of a relationship between the two came with the realization that the geographical distribution of the gene for hemoglobin S and the distribution of malaria in Africa virtually overlap. A further hint came with the observation that peoples indigenous to the highland regions of the continent did not display the high expression of the sickle hemoglobin gene seen in their lowland neighbors in the malaria belts. Malaria does not occur in the cooler, drier climates of the highlands in the tropical and subtropical regions of the world and neither does the gene for sickle hemoglobin.

Sickle trait provides a survival advantage over people with normal hemoglobin in regions where malaria is endemic. Sickle cell trait provides neither absolute protection nor invulnerability to the disease. Rather, people (and particularly children) infected with *P. falciparum* are more likely to survive the acute illness if they have sickle cell trait. When these people with sickle cell trait procreate, both the gene for normal hemoglobin and that for sickle hemoglobin are transmitted into the next generation.[11]

The genetic selection scenario in which a heterozygote for two alleles of a gene has an advantage over either of the homozygous states is called "balanced polymorphism." The key to the concept as applied to the Hb S gene is that selective advantage lies in sickle cell trait. A common misstatement is that malaria selects for sickle cell disease. People with sickle cell disease are at an extreme survival disadvantage because of the ravages both of sickle cell disease and malaria infection. Consequently, a negative selection exists for sickle cell disease. Sickle cell trait is the genetic condition selected for in regions of endemic malaria. Sickle cell disease is a necessary consequence of the existence of the trait condition due to the stochastic inheritance of two sickle cell genes in any population where sickle cell trait is common.

The precise mechanism by which sickle cell trait imparts resistance to malaria is unknown. A number of factors likely are involved and contribute in varying degrees to the defense against malaria. Sickle cell trait does not block or prevent infection by *P. falciparum*. Rather, the trait condition enhances the chance of surviving an acute malarial attack.

Red cells from people with sickle trait do not sickle to any significant degree at normal venous oxygen tension. Very low oxygen tensions will cause the cells to sickle. For example, extreme exercise at high altitude increases the number of sickled erythrocytes in venous blood samples from people with sickle cell trait.[12] Sickle trait red cells infected with the *P. falciparum* parasite deform, presumably because the parasite reduces the oxygen tension within the erythrocytes to very low levels as it carries out its metabolism. Deformation of sickle trait erythrocytes would mark these cells as abnormal and target them for destruction by phagocytes.[13]

In vitro experiments with sickle trait red cells show that under low oxygen tension, cells infected with *P. falciparum* parasites sickle much more readily than do uninfected cells.[14] Since sickle cells are removed from the circulation and destroyed in the reticuloendothelial system, selective sickling of infected sickle trait red cells would reduce the parasite burden in people with sickle trait. These people would be more likely to survive acute malarial infections.

Other investigations suggest that malaria parasites are damaged or killed directly in sickle trait red cells. *P. falciparum* parasites cultured in sickle trait red cells die when the cells are incubated at low oxygen tension.[15] In contrast, parasite health and growth were unimpeded in cells maintained at normal atmospheric oxygen tensions. The sickling process that occurs at low oxygen tensions is presumed to harm the parasite in some fashion. Ultrastructural studies show extensive vacuole formation in *P. falciparum* parasites inhabiting sickle trait red cells incubated at low oxygen tension, suggesting metabolic damage to the parasites.[16] Prolonged states of hypoxia are not physiological conditions, raising questions about degree to which such data can be extrapolated to human beings. However, they do suggest mechanisms by which sickle hemoglobin at the concentrations seen with sickle cell trait red cells could impair parasite proliferation.

Other studies suggest that oxygen radicals formed in sickle trait erythrocytes retard growth and even kill the *P. falciparum* parasite.[17] Sickle trait red cells produce higher levels of the superoxide anion (O_2^-) and hydrogen peroxide (H_2O_2) than do normal erythrocytes. Each compound is toxic to a number of pathogens, including malarial parasites. Homozygous hemoglobin S red cells produce hemin associated with the membrane due to repeated formation of sickle hemoglobin polymers. This membrane-associated hemin can oxidize membrane lipids and proteins.[18] Sickle trait red cells normally produce little in the way of such products. If the infected sickle trait red cells form sickle polymer due to low oxygen tension secondary to parasite metabolism, the cells might generate enough hemin to damage the parasites.[19]

The immune system is the key to weathering attacks by *P. falciparum*, illustrated by the protection afforded to infants by passive immunity from the mother. Elements of the complement system enhance phagocytosis of sickle trait red cells infected by ring-stage *P. falciparum*.[20] People with sickle trait also have augmented antibody responses to key *P. falciparum* antigens involved in malarial infection.[21,22] Analyses of individuals with sickle cell trait and people homozygous for hemoglobin A in the regions with endemic malaria in fact show a lower mean parasite burden in people with sickle cell trait relative to hemoglobin A homozygotes.[23] In contrast, children with sickle cell disease have a high fatality rate, with acute malarial infections being a chief cause of death.[24]

Hemoglobin C is also believed to protect against malaria, although data on this point were not conclusive until recently. Support for this hypothesis came with greater difficulty than in the case of Hb S. Hb C inhibits growth of *P. falciparum* with in vitro culture systems, but the effect is less dramatic than that seen with Hb S.[25] Some epidemiological studies found no evidence for protection against malaria in people with either homozygous or heterozygous hemoglobin C.[26] The relatively small number of patients with hemoglobin C in these studies left the conclusions open to question, however.

The issue was finally settled by an investigation that included more than 4000 subjects.[27] Hemoglobin C heterozygotes had significantly fewer episodes of *P. falciparum* malaria than did controls with only hemoglobin A. The risk of malaria was lower still in subjects who were homozygous for hemoglobin C. Homozygous hemoglobin C produces a mild hemolytic anemia and splenomegaly. The much milder phenotype of the condition relative to homozygous hemoglobin S led the investigators to speculate that without medical intervention for malaria, hemoglobin C would replace hemoglobin S over the next few thousand years as the dominant "antimalarial" hemoglobin in West Africa. Children with either heterozygous or homozygous Hb C suffer fewer episodes of severe malaria than do controls.[28] Moderation of the severity of *P. falciparum* infection appears to be a key antimalarial effect of Hb C.

The thalassemias likewise reached high levels of expression in human populations by providing protection against malaria. The imbalance in globin chain production characteristic of thalassemia produces membrane oxidation by hemichromes and the reactive oxygen species they generate.[29,30] These reactive oxygen species also injure and kill malaria parasites.[31]

Cells containing hemoglobin H (β-globin tetramers) provide the best in vitro evidence of malaria toxicity produced by thalassemic red cells.[32,33] Hemoglobin H occurs most often in people with three-gene-deletion α-thalassemia (see Chapter 14). The compound heterozygous condition of two-gene-deletion α-thalassemia and hemoglobin Constant Spring also produces erythrocytes that contain hemoglobin H.[34] Two-gene-deletion α-thalassemia alone also protects the host from malaria, apparently by retarding parasite growth in erythrocytes.[35] α-Thalassemia might provide additional protection against malaria in part by altering the immune response to parasitized red cells.[36] In any event, epidemiological studies show clear evidence of protection provided by two-gene deletion α-thalassemia.[37,38]

One of the key reasons for the high fatality rate in *P. falciparum* malaria is the occurrence of so-called cerebral malaria. Patients become confused, disoriented, and often lapse into a terminal coma. The *P. falciparum* parasite alters the characteristics of the red cell membrane, creating cells with a high propensity to adhere both to uninfected red cells as well as endothelial cells. Clusters of parasitized red cells can line the capillary circulation, blocking blood flow and exacerbating cerebral hypoxia. Thalassemic erythrocytes adhere to parasitized red cells much less readily than do their normal counterparts.[39,40] This alteration would lessen the risk of developing cerebral malaria.

Hemoglobin E produces a mild microcytic anemia in both heterozygotes (Hb AE) and homozygotes (Hb EE). Oxidant stress to the cells produces Heinz bodies to a greater degree than is seen with normal Hb AA cells, indicating that Hb E impairs red cell oxidant defense.[41] In vitro investigations show that both Hb AE and Hb EE cells are more resistant to invasion by *P. falciparum* parasites than are normal Hb AA red cells.[42] Linkage disequilibrium studies in the Thai population where Hb E is extremely prevalent suggest that the initial rise in gene frequency began between 1200 and 4400 years ago.[43] This explosive expansion is consistent with selective pressure from malaria beginning with the rise of agriculture.

Of all the red cell defenses against malaria, only Melanesian elliptocytosis produces erythrocyte resistance to invasion by *P. falciparum* (Duffy null red cells are resistant only to *P. vivax*.)[44] The membranes of these red cells are very rigid, creating an effective barrier to the parasites.[45] Melanesian elliptocytosis derives from a deletion of nine amino acids in band 3, the red cell membrane anion channel.[46,47] Defective anion transport by these red cells might also contribute to malarial resistance.[48,49]

People with Melanesian elliptocytosis are less prone to develop cerebral malaria, which would lessen the impact of *P. falciparum* infection.[50,51]

The rise to high frequency of alleles that produce red cells deficient in glucose-6-phosphate dehydrogenase (G6PD) activity is one of the most dramatic examples of the selective pressure of malaria on mankind.[52] Protection is afforded both to males who are hemizygous for the X-linked condition and to heterozygous females.[53] Two common G6PD mutants are the Mediterranean and A⁻ variants (see Chapter 15). Haplotype analysis and statistical modeling indicate that the A⁻ allele arose in the past 4,000 to 11,000 years.[54] Similar analysis brackets the origin of the Mediterranean allele at between 1500 and 6500 years ago. Random genetic drift cannot explain such rapid rises in gene frequency. Natural selective pressure by malaria is the most compelling explanation.

Reactive oxygen species are formed continually as erythrocytes take up oxygen from the lungs and release it to the peripheral tissues. As noted earlier, malaria parasites are easily damaged by these reactive oxygen species. G6PD prevents oxidation of the heme group. In its absence, hemichromes and other molecules that generate reactive oxygen species accumulate in erythrocytes.[55] These free radicals could directly injure the parasites. *P. falciparum* parasites in fact grow poorly in erythrocytes that are deficient in G6PD.[56] However, malaria continues to battle back in this struggle. The advent of *P. falciparum* parasites that produce their own G6PD provides ample evidence of the continuing moves and countermoves in the battle between man and malaria.[57]

References

[1] Hoffman SL, Subramanian GM, Collins FH, Venter JC. 2002. Plasmodium, human and Anopheles genomics and malaria. Nature 415:702–709.

[2] Rich SM, Licht MC, Hudson RR, Ayala FJ. 1998. Malaria's Eve: Evidence of a recent population bottleneck throughout the world populations of Plasmodium falciparum. Proc Natl Acad Sci U S A 95:4425–4430.

[3] Joy DA, Feng X, Mu J, et al. 2003. Early origin and recent expansion of Plasmodium falciparum. Science 300:318–321.

[4] Engwerda CR, Beattie L, Amante FH. 2005. The importance of the spleen in malaria. Trends Parasitol 21:75–80.

[5] Haldane JBS. 1949. The rate of mutation of human genes. Hereditas 35(Suppl 1):267–273.

[6] Gelpi AP, King MC. 1976. Association of Duffy blood groups with the sickle cell trait. Hum Genet 32:65–68.

[7] Miller LH, Manson SJ, Clyde DF, McGinniss MH. 1976. The resistance factor to Plasmodium falciparum in Blacks. N Engl J Med 295:302–304.

[8] Tournamille C, Colin Y, Cartron JP, Le Van Kim C. 1995. Disruption of a GATA motif in the Duffy gene promoter abolishes erythroid gene expression in Duffy-negative individuals. Nat Genet 10:302–304.

[9] Hamblin MT, Di Rienzo A. 2000. Detection of the signature of natural selection in humans: Evidence from the Duffy blood group locus. Am J Hum Genet 66:1669–1679.

[10] Zimmerman P, Woolley I, Masinde GL, et al. 1999. Emergence of FY*A(null) in a Plasmodium vivax-endemic region of Papua New Guinea. Proc Natl Acad Sci U S A 96(24):13973–13977.

[11] Ringelhann B, Hathorn MK, Jilly P, Grant F, Parniczky G. 1976. A new look at the protection of hemoglobin AS and AC genotypes against plasmodium falciparum infection: A census tract approach. Am J Hum Genet 28:270–279.

[12] Martin TW, Weisman IM, Zeballos RJ, Stephenson SR. 1989. Exercise and hypoxia increase sickling in venous blood from an exercising limb in individuals with sickle cell trait. Am J Med 87:48–56.

[13] Luzzatto L, Nwachuku-Jarrett ES, Reddy S. 1970. Increased sickling of parasitised erythrocytes as mechanism of resistance against malaria in the sickle-cell trait. Lancet 1(7642):319–321.

[14] Roth EF, Jr, Friedman M, Ueda Y, Tellez I, Trager W, Nagel RL. 1978. Sickling rates of human AS red cells infected in vitro with Plasmodium falciparum malaria. Science 202:650–652.

[15] Friedman MJ. 1978. Erythrocytic mechanism of sickle cell resistance to malaria. Proc Natl Acad Sci U S A 75:1994–1997.

[16] Friedman MJ. 1979. Ultrastructural damage to the malaria parasite in the sickled cell. J Protozool 26:195–199.

[17] Anastasi J. 1984. Hemoglobin S-mediated membrane oxidant injury: Protection from malaria and pathology in sickle cell disease. Med Hypotheses 14:311–320.

[18] Rank BH, Carlsson J, Hebbel RP. 1985. Abnormal redox status of membrane-protein thiols in sickle erythrocytes. J Clin Invest 75:1531–1537.

[19] Orjih AU, Chevli R, Fitch CD. 1985. Toxic heme in sickle cells: An explanation for death of malaria parasites. Am J Trop Med Hyg 34:223–227.

[20] Ayi K, Turrini F, Piga A, Arese P. 2004. Enhanced phagocytosis of ring-parasitized mutant erythrocytes: A common mechanism that may explain protection against falciparum malaria in sickle trait and beta-thalassemia trait. Blood 104:3364–3371.

[21] Cabrera G, Cot M, Migot-Nabias F, Kremsner PG, Deloron P, Luty AJ. 2005. The sickle cell trait is associated with enhanced immunoglobulin G antibody responses to plasmodium falciparum variant surface antigens. J Infect Dis 191:1631–1638.

[22] Tebo AE, Kremsner PG, Piper KP, Luty AJ. 2002. Low antibody responses to variant surface antigens of Plasmodium falciparum are associated with severe malaria and increased susceptibility to malaria attacks in Gabonese children. Am J Trop Med Hyg 67:597–603.

[23] Fleming AF, Storey J, Molineaux L, Iroko EA, Attai ED. 1979. Abnormal haemoglobins in the Sudan savanna of Nigeria. I. Prevalence of haemoglobins and relationships between sickle cell trait, malaria and survival. Ann Trop Med Parasitol 73:161–172.

[24] Fleming AF. 1989. The presentation, management and prevention of crisis in sickle cell disease in Africa. Blood Rev 3:18–28.

[25] Fairhurst RM, Fujioka H, Hayton K, Collins KF, Wellems TE. 2003. Aberrant development of Plasmodium falciparum in hemoglobin CC red cells: Implications for the malaria protective effect of the homozygous state. Blood. 101:3309–3315.

[26] Willcox M, Bjorkman A, Brohult J, Pehrson PO, Rombo L, Bengtsson E. 1983. A case-control study in northern Liberia of Plasmodium falciparum malaria in haemoglobin S and beta-thalassaemia traits. Ann Trop Med Parasitol 77:239–246.

[27] Modiano D, Luoni G, Sirima BS, et al. 2001. Haemoglobin C protects against clinical Plasmodium falciparum malaria. Nature 414:305–308.

[28] Mockenhaupt FP, Ehrhardt S, Cramer JP, et al. 2004. Hemoglobin C and resistance to severe malaria in Ghanaian children. J Infect Dis 190:1006–1009.

29 Grinberg LN, Rachmilewitz EA, Kitrossky N, Chevion M. 1995. Hydroxyl radical generation in beta-thalassemic red blood cells. Free Radic Biol Med 18:611–615.

30 Sorensen S, Rubin E, Polster H, Mohandas N, Schrier S. 1990. The role of membrane skeletal-associated alpha-globin in the pathophysiology of beta-thalassemia. Blood 75:1333–1336.

31 Clark IA, Chaudhri G, Cowden WB. 1989. Some roles of free radicals in malaria. Free Radic Biol Med 6:315–321.

32 Ifediba TC, Stern A, Ibrahim A, Rieder RF. 1985. Plasmodium falciparum in vitro: Diminished growth in hemoglobin H disease erythrocytes. Blood 65:452–455.

33 Yuthavong Y, Butthep P, Bunyaratvej A, Fucharoen S, Khusmith S. 1988. Impaired parasite growth and increased susceptibility to phagocytosis of Plasmodium falciparum infected alpha-thalassemia or hemoglobin Constant Spring red blood cells. Am J Clin Pathol 89:521–525.

34 Derry S, Wood WG, Pippard M, et al. 1988. Hematologic and biosynthetic studies in homozygous hemoglobin Constant Spring. J Clin Invest 173:1673–1682.

35 Pattanapanyasat K, Yongvanitchit K, Tongtawe P, et al. 1999. Impairment of Plasmodium falciparum growth in thalassemic red blood cells: Further evidence by using biotin labeling and flow cytometry. Blood 93:3116–3119.

36 Luzzi GA, Merry AH, Newbold CI, Marsh K, Pasvol G, Weatherall DJ. 1991. Surface antigen expression on Plasmodium falciparum-infected erythrocytes is modified in alpha- and beta-thalassemia. J Exp Med 173:785–791.

37 Flint J, Hill AV, Bowden DK, et al. 1986. High frequencies of alpha-thalassaemia are the result of natural selection by malaria. Nature 321:744–750.

38 Modiano G, Morpurgo G, Terrenato L, et al. 1991. Protection against malaria morbidity: Near-fixation of the alpha-thalassemia gene in a Nepalese population. Am J Hum Genet 48:390–397.

39 Carlson J, Nash GB, Gabutti V, al-Yaman F, Wahlgren M. 1994. Natural protection against severe Plasmodium falciparum malaria due to impaired rosette formation. Blood 84:3909–3814.

40 Udomsangpetch R, Sueblinvong T, Pattanapanyasat K, Dharmkrong-at A, Kittikalayawong A, Webster HK. 1993. Alteration in cytoadherence and rosetting of Plasmodium falciparum-infected thalassemic red blood cells. Blood 82:3752–3759.

41 Lachant NA, Tanaka KR. 1987. Impaired antioxidant defense in hemoglobin E-containing erythrocytes: A mechanism protective against malaria? Am J Hematol 26:211–219.

42 Chotivanich K, Udomsangpetch R, Pattanapanyasat K, et al. 2002. Hemoglobin E: A balanced polymorphism protective against high parasitemias and thus severe P falciparum malaria. Blood 100:1172–1176.

43 Ohashi J, Naka I, Patarapotikul J, et al. 2004. Extended linkage disequilibrium surrounding the hemoglobin E variant due to malarial selection. Am J Hum Genet 74:1198–1208.

44 Hadley T, Saul A, Lamont G, Hudson DE, Miller LH, Kidson C. 1983. Resistance of Melanesian elliptocytes (ovalocytes) to invasion by Plasmodium knowlesi and Plasmodium falciparum malaria parasites in vitro. J Clin Invest 71:780–782.

45 Mohandas N, Lie-Injo LE, Friedman M, Mak JW. 1984. Rigid membranes of Malayan ovalocytes: A likely genetic barrier against malaria. Blood 63:1385–1392.

46 Jarolim P, Palek J, Amato D, et al. 1991. Deletion in erythrocyte band 3 gene in malaria-resistant Southeast Asian ovalocytosis. Proc Natl Acad Sci U S A 88:11022–11026.

47 Schofield AE, Tanner MJ, Pinder JC, et al. 1992. Basis of unique red cell membrane properties in hereditary ovalocytosis. J Mol Biol 223:949–958.

48 Schofield AE, Reardon DM, Tanner MJ. 1992. Defective anion transport activity of the abnormal band 3 in hereditary ovalocytic red blood cells. Nature 355:836–838.

49 Sarabia VE, Casey JR, Reithmeier RA. 1993. Molecular characterization of the band 3 protein from Southeast Asian ovalocytes. J Biol Chem 268:10676–10680.

50 Genton B, al-Yaman F, Mgone CS, et al. 1995. Ovalocytosis and cerebral malaria. Nature 378:564–565.

51 Allen SJ, O'Donnell A, Alexander ND, et al. 1999. Prevention of cerebral malaria in children in Papua New Guinea by southeast Asian ovalocytosis band 3. Am J Trop Med Hyg 60:1056–1060.

52 Ruwende C, Khoo SC, Snow RW, et al. 1995. Natural selection of hemi- and heterozygotes for G6PD deficiency in Africa by resistance to severe malaria. Nature 376:246–249.

53 Ruwende C, Hill A. 1998. Glucose-6-phosphate dehydrogenase deficiency and malaria. J Mol Med 76:581–588.

54 Tishkoff SA, Varkonyi R, Cahinhinan N, et al. 2001. Haplotype diversity and linkage disequilibrium at human G6PD: Recent origin of alleles that confer malarial resistance. Science 293:455–462.

55 Janney SK, Joist JJ, Fitch CD. 1986. Excess release of ferriheme in G6PD-deficient erythrocytes: Possible cause of hemolysis and resistance to malaria. Blood 67:331–333.

56 Roth EF, Jr, Raventos-Suarez C, Rinaldi A, Nagel RL. 1983. Glucose-6-phosphate dehydrogenase deficiency inhibits in vitro growth of Plasmodium falciparum. Proc Natl Acad Sci U S A 80:298–299.

57 Usanga EA, Luzzatto L. 1985. Adaptation of Plasmodium falciparum to glucose 6-phosphate dehydrogenase-deficient host red cells by production of parasite-encoded enzyme. Nature 313:793–795.

Nutrition and Anemia

IRON DEFICIENCY

In contrast to many medical conditions whose discovery carries a specific date often associated with a particular investigator, iron deficiency is an ancient disorder that stretches to the dawn of human history. Iron deficiency is a reality despite the vast abundance of the mineral on the Earth. The characteristics of the element make it essential to many vital biological reactions. And yet some of those same characteristics make it elusive both to men and microbes. The most important of these is the formation of highly insoluble iron salts whose acquisition and use for biological purposes require complex uptake machinery.

At the other end of the spectrum, the lack of a physiological mechanism for iron excretion starkly underscores the central importance of iron in human biology. No excretory mechanism is needed, because acquiring and retaining sufficient iron for metabolic function is the daunting challenge that humans share with every organism on the planet. Lowly bacteria produce iron-binding molecules called siderophores that scavenge for the mineral when unleashed into the environment. The bacteria have intricate coupling mechanisms that capture the iron–siderophore complex at the completion of the mission. This intricate bacterial biology reflects billions of years of evolution. Iron deficiency is an ancient problem, indeed.

Iron is a central component of hemoglobin, making anemia a central manifestation of iron deficiency. However, anemia is neither the only nor necessarily the most important manifestation of iron deficiency. Heme, whose structure includes a (literally) central iron atom, is vital to a host of enzymes, many of which participate in energy generation through mitochondrial respiration. Other proteins, including enzymes vital to DNA synthesis, have nonheme iron prosthetic groups. These proteins are functional cripples in the absence of iron.

The ramifications of iron deficiency ripple through every aspect of metabolism. The manifestations depend both on the severity of the deficiency and stage of life of the victim. Iron deficiency during infancy produces neurocognitive injury that has no correlate in adults. Long-standing, severe iron deficiency in adults produces spooning of the nails, which is virtually diagnostic of the disorder. Women of childbearing age face additional pressure brought to bear by the physiological blood loss of menstruation. Iron deficiency is a disorder with many faces. The challenge to the clinician is to recognize and respond to each face.

■ IRON DEFICIENCY DURING CHILDHOOD

Iron deficiency anemia in neonates is fleetingly rare. The placenta provides the fetus with the material needed for growth and development, including iron. The organ's highly efficient iron extraction system will leach iron from the mother's stores in order to meet fetal demands. With the exception of neonates born to women who are iron deficient in the extreme, the placenta supplies sufficient mineral to maintain the hemoglobin value at the lower limit of normal. These newborns commonly have depleted or absent iron stores despite normal hemoglobin values, however. The challenge for these newborns derives from the lack for iron reserves needed to handle the buffeting that follows birth.

Low or absent iron stores manifest themselves during infancy as a failure appropriately to augment hemoglobin levels after birth. A physiological anemia develops during the initial 6–8 weeks after birth where the immediate postnatal hemoglobin value of 16–17 g/dL declines to the range of 11–12 g/dL. Thereafter the hemoglobin value rises to its early childhood mean of 12.5 g/dL. What appears to be a slight recovery to a new steady state is in fact a tremendous expansion in total body hemoglobin content. The rapid growth of the first months of life demands the rapid production of new hemoglobin, which requires iron.

The gut's immature iron absorption machinery places a high initial burden on iron stores of the infant.[1,2] The first sign of absent stores is a fall to lower than expected hemoglobin values in the first 6–8 weeks of life. In children whose iron stores are not so wanting, anemia often appears during the early childhood years.[3] Iron deficiency often becomes apparent during the growth spurts of childhood. The prevalence of iron deficiency rises sharply in adolescent girls. The combination of the growth spurt that occurs at this time with the onset of menstruation depletes the shallow iron stores that might exist.

Poverty exacerbates the issue of iron deficiency, since inadequate iron intake during childhood often mirrors low socioeconomic status.[4] Low energy levels and the easy onset of fatigue are common manifestations of iron deficiency anemia in these children. Severe manifestations of iron deficiency such as glossitis or koilonychias are uncommon, but can occur with severe, long-standing iron deficit. Iron deficiency anemia can also produce poor attention.

Iron deficiency can lower attention span for reasons that are much more sinister than anemia, however. Iron deficiency, with or without anemia, can impair growth and intellectual development in children. Studies of cognitive development in the setting of iron deficiency initially produced conflicting results. In some investigations, dietary iron supplementation in infants with iron deficiency anemia reversed cognitive dysfunction,[5] while other studies failed to show improvement.[6,7] Although some of the disparities could have resulted from differences in the analytical instruments used or differences in the populations examined, these unsettling questions remained open.[8]

Information on the long-term effects of iron deficiency during infancy added new urgency to the issue of childhood iron deficiency. A key investigation in this regard involved a group of children with iron deficiency anemia (hemoglobin less than 10 g/dL) treated during infancy and whose Mental Development Index test scores then improved. The investigators reexamined these children at 5 years of age to assess their cognitive development.[9] The children who were initially iron deficient during infancy scored lower on tests of mental and motor functioning than did normal counterparts. This discrepancy existed despite correction of the iron deficiency in the pediatric subjects during infancy. Adjustments for differences in socioeconomic background failed to eliminate the disparate test scores.

The chilling conclusion of this work is that iron deficiency during infancy places children at risk of persistent developmental disadvantage relative to peers with better iron status.[10] Other studies of iron deficiency during infancy have produced similar results.[11,12] Correction of iron deficiency during infancy clearly improves scores in short-term tests, such as the Bayles Scales of Infant Development, without preventing longer-term, and possibly more serious, impairment of cognitive function. Prevention of iron deficiency during infancy must therefore be a major goal of health-care providers.[13,14]

Severe iron deficiency can affect growth during childhood, although the effect is often difficult to separate from overall nutritional deficiency. The high prevalence of childhood iron deficiency among less affluent people has yoked deficiencies of iron and general nutrients. When the two factors are separated, correction of iron deficiency improves growth and development independently of nutritional status.

■ IRON DEFICIENCY IN ADULTS

Complaints related to anemia most often prompt adults with iron deficiency anemia to seek medical advice. These include dyspnea, fatigue, and lethargy. These problems are not specific to iron deficiency; rather they occur with any anemia whose onset is slow and whose progression is persistent. People with severe, long-standing folate deficiency, for instance, give a story similar to those with iron deficiency. Other manifestations of iron deficiency can provide more direction regarding the underlying problem, however.

Iron deficiency in adults almost invariably reflects chronic bleeding. A history of dark or tarry stools (melena) suggests bleeding from the upper gastrointestinal tract. Blood is digested like any other protein, particularly when released into the stomach. The duodenum and jejunum absorb the resulting peptides and heme byproducts. Brisk bleeding produces these components at rates exceeding the gut's absorption capacity.

The patient history can provide clues to the specific source of the bleeding. Postprandial fullness, pain, or nausea, for instance, raises the possibility that a peptic ulcer is the culprit. Chest discomfort or indigestion that worsens after meals and with recumbency suggests gastric reflux with associated erosive injury to the esophagus. Generalized abdominal pain and diarrhea are common complaints from people with an inflammatory bowel disorder such as Crohn's disease. Crohn's disease in particular has systemic manifestations, reflecting its inflammatory nature. Fever, sweating, and weakness are common associated problems.

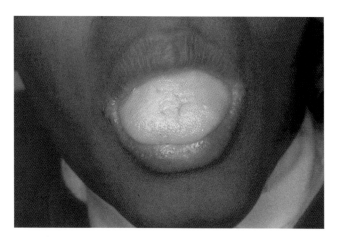

FIGURE 7-1 *Atrophic glossitis and angular stomatitis due to iron deficiency. The shiny, smooth appearance of the tongue represents the loss of papillae caused by the iron deficit. The white cracks at the angle of the mouth are due to angular stomatitis. The patient complained of a burning tongue and great sensitivity to spicy foods. Symptoms such as weakness and fatigue came to light only in retrospect.*

Bright red blood in the stool, in contrast, points to bleeding from the lower gastrointestinal tract. Bleeding rectal hemorrhoids with alarmingly scarlet blood coating the stool and tingeing the toilet bowl water is a vivid example of the problem. The blood is clearly distinct from stool since excreta forms in the upper gastrointestinal tract and coalesces in the colon with the removal of water. Blood released at the level of the rectum or below coats the outside of stool solid. Free blood in the toilet bowl also points to the terminus of the gastrointestinal tract as the source of bleeding.

Pain involving the tongue and mouth occasionally prompts people with iron deficiency to seek medical attention. These symptoms are due to the glossitis and angular stomatitis that can develop with severe, long-standing iron deficiency (Figure 7-1). The smooth shiny tongue reflects loss of papillae on the upper lingual surface. Occasionally, patients present complaining of sensitivity to spicy foods and even of frank lingual pain.[15] Angular stomatitis represents a breakdown of the buccal mucosa at the corners of the mouth. This alteration reflects thinning of the epithelial covering in this area. Patients complain most frequently of painful cracking at the angles of the mouth.

Koilonychia is a striking change in the character of the fingernails that points to iron deficiency. The basal cells in the nail bed require iron to generate keratin. With severe iron deficiency the nail substance is thin and soft, allowing molding as the nail grows. The concave deformations of the surface of the fingernail characteristic of koilonychia most likely result from pressure on the fingertips during ordinary daily activities. The changes of koilonychia often are particularly pronounced in the thumb of the dominant hand. This probably reflects the pressure applied to the digit by activities such as writing and holding eating utensils.

Iron deficiency also blunts keratin formation by hair follicle cells.[16] The result is brittle hair that breaks easily. Hair production by some follicles markedly declines causing an overall thinning that is most pronounced over the scalp.[17] Women notice these changes more often than do men since for them hair thinning and loss occur less commonly than in males. Pointed questioning about hair often is needed to elicit information on these changes. Permanents for instance greatly stress hair integrity thereby accentuating its loss. Detailed questioning reveals that some women with severe iron deficiency have foresworn permanents because of hair damage.

Blue sclerae occur in some patients with severe iron deficiency anemia.[18] The thinning of the epithelial lining over the eye highlights the bluish coloration of the subepithelial surface of the sclerae. The low level of venous blood oxygenation with severe anemia possibly magnifies the effect. Oxygenated blood is bright red while deoxygenated blood in tissue capillaries and veins has a bluish color. The effect often is striking in the forearm veins of relatively pale people. The soubriquet "blue blood" as applied to royalty relates to this phenomenon. Medieval European nobility avoided the sun in part to distinguish themselves from the tanned peasants who toiled in the fields. Their pale skin highlighted the bluish color of the venous blood.

Very rarely, a patient who presents to a physician for difficulty with swallowing has the Plummer-Vinson syndrome. Severe iron deficiency can produce a postcricoid web that creates an esophageal stricture.[19] The condition can cause dysphasia. Although the Plummer-Vinson abnormality is usually described in adults, the syndrome occasionally occurs in children.[20] This unusual complication of iron deficiency also predisposes victims to esophageal cancer.[21]

Pica occurs variably in people with iron deficiency. Patients consume unusual items, such as laundry starch, ice, and soil clay.[22] Both clay and starch can bind iron in the gastrointestinal tract, exacerbating the deficiency.[23,24] Pica is an often unrecognized problem during pregnancy.[25] The associated maternal iron deficiency places the neonate at great risk of accumulating insufficient iron stores.

PERIPHERAL BLOOD SMEAR

Iron deficiency produces microcytic, hypochromic red cells (Figure 7-2). Central pallor can comprise 90% of the cell diameter, leaving only a small rim of hemoglobin around the edges. Severe iron deficiency also produces a cohort of extremely small erythrocytes that appear almost to be cell fragments. Many of these cells have irregular shapes with contours resembling schistocytes.

The respective diameters of erythrocytes and lymphocyte nuclei provide the best visual estimate of red cell size. The diameter of normal red cells roughly equals that of lymphocyte nuclei. Red cells generated in an iron-deficient environment often are smaller than lymphocyte nuclei and sometimes substantially so. Target cells can also develop with iron deficiency. While the finding is less common than in thalassemia, the number of target cells cannot be used to distinguish iron deficiency from thalassemia.

Iron deficiency frequently produces thrombocytosis. The high number of platelets can be visually striking and supports iron deficiency as a diagnosis. The platelets are

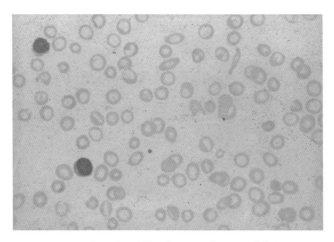

FIGURE 7–2   *Peripheral blood smear of an iron deficiency anemia. The red cells are small and pale with large areas of central pallor. The lymphocyte in the field provides a size reference. Some cells are very small, nearly to the point of being red cell fragments.*

normal in size and shape, lacking abnormalities such as giant size seen in some hematological disorders.

LABORATORY TESTS

Iron deficiency substantially depresses the mean corpuscular volume (MCV). The MCV usually is lower than 80 fL and values sometimes reach the mid-60s. Red cell size varies markedly with iron deficiency making an elevated RDW virtually universal. Iron deficiency depresses both the mean corpuscular hemoglobin (MCH) and the mean corpuscular hemoglobin concentration (MCHC). The cell size and the mean cell hemoglobin define the MCHC. The MCHC is low because iron deficiency suppresses cellular hemoglobin content more profoundly than it reduces cell size. A proportional reduction in cell size and hemoglobin content would produce small erythrocytes with a normal MCHC.

Thrombocytosis with platelet counts in the range of 600,000–700,000 cells/μL is common. Careful laboratory investigations disproved the hypothesis that thrombocytosis with iron deficiency results from megakaryocyte activation by erythropoietin due to cross-reactivity with the structurally similar thrombopoietin.[26,27] Values rarely exceed 1,000,000 cells/μL due solely to iron deficiency. A concomitant disorder should be considered in cases with extraordinarily high platelet counts.

Absence of the iron stores on bone marrow examination is the gold standard for iron deficiency. This invasive procedure rarely merits a place in the diagnosis of iron deficiency, however. New noninvasive tests in concert with older tests almost always establish the diagnosis of iron deficiency. The three stalwarts in the assessment of iron status are the serum iron, total iron-binding capacity (TIBC), and serum ferritin level (Table 7-1).

TABLE 7-1 | **TESTS THAT ASSESS IRON STATUS**

Test	Measurement	Comment
Serum iron	Chemical determination of serum iron content.	The spread of normal values is high. The level typically is low with iron deficiency, but can fall into the normal range with modest deficiency.
TIBC	Total capacity of the serum to bind iron.	Transferrin specifically binds serum iron, meaning that the TIBC reflects transferrin in the serum.
Transferrin saturation	The fraction of the iron binding sites in the serum occupied by iron.	The ratio of serum iron to TIBC gives the transferrin saturation. This ratio is more useful than serum iron or TIBC in isolation.
Serum ferritin	Quantity of ferritin protein in the circulation.	Serum ferritin level is proportional to body iron stores. Inflammation independently increases serum ferritin values. Serum ferritin transports *no* iron.
Soluble transferrin receptors	Quantity of transferrin receptors circulating in the serum.	Both iron deficiency and chronic hemolytic anemias increase the test readout.
Red cell ZPP	ZPP content of red cells	Iron-deficient erythropoiesis increases red cell ZPP values. Conditions that interfere with iron insertion into heme also raise ZPP, including lead intoxication and myelodysplasia.

TIBC, total iron-binding capacity; ZPP, zinc protoporphyrin.

The serum iron level normally ranges between 50 and 150 mg/dL, all of it bound to transferrin. The TIBC reflects the maximum quantity of iron that serum transferrin can bind. The normal value ranges between 250 and 375 mg/dL. The broad range of normal values for both the serum iron and the TIBC diminishes the utility of isolated values for either parameter. These tests instead are best used to determine the transferrin saturation, which is the ratio of the serum iron to the TIBC. The transferrin saturation usually ranges between 20% and 50%. Adult males have higher normal values than do females. Severe iron deficiency often drives the transferrin saturation to below 10%.

Some laboratories measure the quantity of transferrin protein in the serum and report results in milligrams of protein per deciliter of serum. Health-care providers sometimes assume incorrectly that the serum transferrin value is the same as the TIBC. The two are related but not synonymous. Transferrin is the sole plasma protein that binds iron. The TIBC therefore depends on the quantity of transferrin in the plasma. A mathematical conversion is needed to directly connect the two, however.

The serum ferritin value expressed in nanograms of protein per milliliter is proportional to body iron stores. Normal values range between 10 and 200 ng/mL for reproductive-age women and between 15 and 400 ng/mL for men.[28] Ethnic and racial variations in serum ferritin levels likely represent population trends in body iron stores.[29] Serum ferritin levels in postmenopausal women approximate those of their male counterparts. The serum ferritin value alone often can be used to estimate the iron status of a patient.

A common point of confusion regarding the relationship of serum ferritin and serum iron arises from the fact that ferritin is the storehouse for intracellular iron.[30] Ferritin molecules within cells are multi-subunit spherical shells that can sequester more than 4000 iron atoms. A widespread misconception is that serum ferritin is the same as intracellular ferritin and consequently transports iron in the serum. Serum ferritin is a secreted protein that contains essentially *no* iron.[31] Cellular iron stores modulate the secretion of this virtually iron-free form of ferritin. Consequently, serum ferritin is merely a surrogate marker of body iron stores.[32]

A particularly important adventitious response of serum ferritin is its natural rise during pregnancy.[33] Pregnant women are particularly susceptible to iron deficiency and the condition must be corrected when it occurs to prevent the previously noted complications of neonatal iron deficiency. Chapter 4 reviews the approach to possible iron deficiency in pregnant women.

Comorbid conditions sometimes conspire to obscure the diagnosis of iron deficiency as determined either by transferrin saturation or serum ferritin values. The most important of these is chronic inflammation. Ferritin is an acute phase protein whose levels rise as a part of the inflammatory response.[34] Baseline ferritin values are high in patients with inflammatory disorders irrespective of body iron stores, meaning that ferritin cannot be used to assay for iron deficiency. Serum transferrin levels also rise with inflammation while the serum iron value tends to fall. Consequently, the condition produces a lower than expected transferrin saturation. Chronic inflammation therefore severely compromises information gained from the two tests most commonly used in the noninvasive assessment of iron stores.

The soluble transferrin receptor assay provides information on iron status independently of serum ferritin or transferrin saturation values.[35] Transferrin binds to specific receptors on the cell surface and delivers iron in a process termed *receptor-mediated endocytosis*.[36,37] The transferrin receptor is an intrinsic membrane protein, meaning that it is anchored securely in the plasma membrane bilayer.[38] Proteases can clip the receptor protein just above its membrane insertion point, releasing a soluble form of the receptor into the circulation.[39,40] Iron deficiency increases the number of transferrin receptors on cells, which secondarily increases the number of soluble transferrin receptors in the circulation. Most transferrin receptors in the body reside on erythroid precursors, meaning that iron-deficient erythropoiesis greatly raises the soluble transferrin receptor value.

Important caveats exist with respect to the soluble transferrin receptor assay and body iron stores. First, the soluble transferrin receptor level increases markedly with hemolytic anemias and with ineffective erythropoiesis. The soluble transferrin receptor level is high in patients with sickle cell disease as well as those with thalassemia.[41,42] The rise in the number of erythroid precursors with hemolytic anemias boosts the quantity of soluble transferrin receptor.[43] The increase in erythroid precursors associated with ineffective erythropoiesis also increases the quantity of soluble transferrin receptors.[44]

A second issue with the assay is the lack of standard parameters that define normal values with respect to soluble transferrin receptor levels. A number of commercial kits exist for this ELISA-based technique. Kits from different manufacturers can give different results when used to assay a single blood sample. The variability likely reflects factors such as differences in antibody affinity for the transferrin receptor and the technical approaches recommended for different kits. Rigorous in-house testing and standardization is essential in order to derive useful information from the soluble transferrin receptor assay.

Another test that sometimes provides insight into iron status in murky situations is the zinc protoporphyrin (ZPP) level.[45] Heme synthesis is a complex biochemical process that begins in mitochondria, moves to the cytoplasm, and finally returns to mitochondria for the final reactions (Figure 12-2, Chapter 12). The enzyme ferrochelatase inserts iron into the protoporphyrin IX ring as the last step in the process. Iron deficiency deprives ferrochelatase of its substrate, inhibiting heme formation from protoporphyrin IX.

Zinc is the second most abundant cation in the red cell. In the absence of sufficient iron, zinc couples noncatalytically to the protoporphyrin ring to produce ZPP in normoblasts. ZPP is fluorescent, making it easy to detect in erythrocytes derived from iron-deficient normoblasts.[46] Accumulation of ZPP in erythrocytes is not exclusive to iron deficiency, however. Drugs that interfere with ferrochelatase function, such as isoniazid, also produce ZPP-laden red cells. Lead or aluminum intoxication likewise markedly raises erythrocyte ZPP levels.[47] The assay is in fact a common screening tool for lead poisoning.[48] The ZPP value can be very useful in the assessment of iron deficiency in some clinical circumstances.

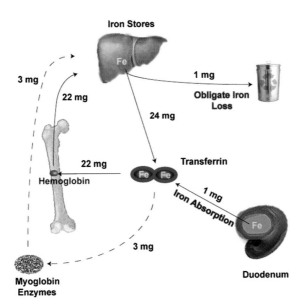

Iron Stores

3 mg

22 mg

1 mg

Obligate Iron Loss

24 mg

22 mg

Transferrin

Hemoglobin

Iron Absorption 1 mg

3 mg

Duodenum

Myoglobin Enzymes

FIGURE 7-3   *Iron homeostasis. Approximately 1 mg of iron is absorbed daily from the gastrointestinal tract, which precisely balances obligate iron losses. The absorbed iron joins a large pool of iron flowing from storage sites to the bone marrow for the production of new red cells. This quantity of iron balances that entering storage sites from senescent red cells. A small amount of iron is directed to myoglobin and enzymes.*

■ ETIOLOGY OF IRON DEFICIENCY

With the exception of fetal development when the placenta mediates iron transfer from the mother to the fetus, the gastrointestinal tract is the vehicle for all iron entry in the body (Figure 7-3). The daily absorption of 1 mg of iron precisely balances the obligate daily loss of the mineral. Eighty percent of body iron resides in red cells. A tremendous flux of iron occurs each day as senescent red cells break down with the iron mainly deposited in liver storage sites. At the same time, the mobilization of storage iron allows production of new red cells that replace the retiring erythrocytes. The balance between iron uptake and loss rests on a fine edge. Factors that disturb this balance produce iron deficiency. Impaired iron uptake reflects problems in the upper gastrointestinal tract. Bleeding, which is the primary cause of iron loss, can occur anywhere along the gastrointestinal tract (Table 7-2).

■ IMPAIRED IRON UPTAKE FROM THE GASTROINTESTINAL TRACT

POOR BIOAVAILABILITY

Most environmental iron exists as insoluble salts such as ferric hydroxide, $Fe(OH)_3$ (also called rust). Ionic iron (iron salts) is absorbed almost exclusively in the

TABLE 7-2 | **CAUSES OF IRON DEFICIENCY**

Basis	Cause	Example
Impaired iron intake	Poor iron availability	Diets low in animal protein
	Impaired iron absorption	• Iron chelators in diet, e.g., tannins
		• Histamine H_2 blockers
	Disrupted GI mucosa	• Celiac disease
		• Crohn's disease
	Loss of functional bowel	• Surgical resection
		• Peptic ulcer
Blood loss	GI tract bleeding	• Aspirin ingestion
		• Colonic diverticali
		• Colonic arteriovenous malformations
	GU tract bleeding	• Stag horn renal calculi
		• Menstruation
	Reproductive system	• Childbirth
		• Endometriosis

duodenum and upper jejunum. As shown in Figure 7-4, the mineral translocates into enterocytes for processing and eventual coupling to plasma transferrin in a process that involves several proteins. Gastric acidity assists conversion of iron salts to absorbable forms, but the process is inefficient.[49] Many plants produce powerful chelators, such as the phytates (organic polyphosphates) found in wheat products, that further impair iron absorption.[50–52] The iron deficiency seen commonly in people for whom cereals are the dietary staple derives in part from the effects of these chelators.[53] Animal proteins are a rich source of heme that is well-absorbed by mechanisms different from those involving iron salts.[54,55]

Conditions that raise the gastric pH also impede iron absorption. Surgical interventions, such as vagotomy or hemigastrectomy for peptic ulcer disease, formerly were the major causes of impaired gastric acidification with secondary iron deficiency.[56,57] Today, the histamine H_2 blockers used to treat peptic ulcer disease and acid reflux are more common causes of defective iron absorption.[58–60] Consequently, the chance of physicians encountering this particular problem is good.

Iron deficiency often accompanies and exacerbates pernicious anemia.[61] The impaired function of the gastric parietal cells in pernicious anemia both reduces the production of intrinsic factor and lowers the degree of gastric acidity. Impaired iron absorption can result from the lack of gastric acid. Iron balance is further complicated by the fact that megaloblastic enterocytes resulting from cobalamin deficiency of the gastrointestinal lining cells absorb iron poorly. The net result is a complicated multifactorial nutritional anemia.[62]

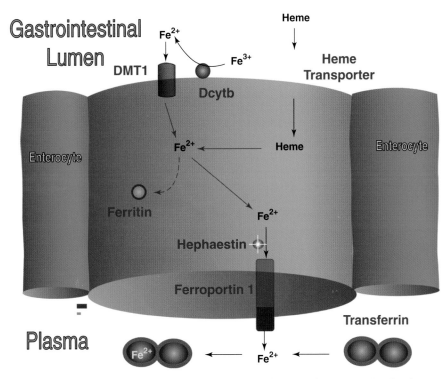

FIGURE 7–4 *Gastrointestinal iron absorption. Dcytb (a membrane-associated reductase enzyme structurally related to mitochondrial cytochrome B) reduces ferric iron in the gastrointestinal tract (Fe^{3+}) to the ferrous form (Fe^{2+}), allowing the divalent metal ion transport channel DMT1 to move the mineral into the enterocyte. Most of the iron exits at the basolateral surface through the action of hephaestin and ferroportin 1 with immediate complexing to plasma transferrin. A yet-to-be characterized heme transport molecule takes up heme independently of the ionic iron absorption mechanism. Heme oxygenase degrades the molecule and releases its iron into the general metabolic pool of the enterocyte. Ferritin sequesters a small quantity of iron that is lost with senescence and sloughing of the enterocyte into the gut lumen.*

INHIBITION OF IRON ABSORPTION

Both coffee and tea contain compounds that inhibit iron absorption. Tannins found in teas are powerful iron chelators.[63,64] These chelators form tight complexes with ionic iron that elude the iron absorption apparatus. The complex of iron and chelator passes through the gastrointestinal tract without being taken into the body.[65] Black tea contains iron-binding compounds called tannins that can produce iron deficiency with heavy consumption of the beverage.[66] Tea consumed with meals disrupts iron absorption more profoundly than when use is confined to periods between meals.[67]

The iron chelation compounds in coffee enter body fluids, including milk produced by lactating mothers. Chelation of iron in the milk reduces the availability of the mineral to the infant and can exacerbate neonatal iron deficiency.[68] Coffee consumption by young children is common practice in some cultures. The result can be aggravation of the iron deficit with the most malefic consequences in poor children who have additional reasons for iron deficiency.[69,70]

A number of other environmental factors, including metals that share the iron absorption machinery, such as lead, cobalt, zinc, and strontium contribute to dietary iron deficiency by retarding iron absorption.[71–74] Of these, only lead is a significant problem. The threat is particularly marked for children. Iron deficiency increases uptake both of iron and lead from the gastrointestinal tract. Iron deficiency and lead intoxication, consequently, are common companions.[75]

DISRUPTION OF THE ENTERIC MUCOSA

Sprue, of both the tropical and nontropical variety (celiac disease), can also disrupt iron absorption.[76,77] Celiac disease is common and often is surprisingly subtle in character. Degeneration of the intestinal lining cells along with chronic inflammation causes profound malabsorption with severe celiac disease. The anemia in these patients is often complicated by a superimposed nutritional deficiency. Some patients with deranged iron absorption, however, lack gross or even histologic changes in bowel mucosal structure.[78] The disease can be mild to the point that few or no symptoms exist.[79,80] In some patients, iron deficiency sufficiently severe to produce secondary manifestations such as pica or Plummer-Vinson syndrome exists for years before celiac disease is revealed as the cause of the mineral deficit.[81,82] A gluten-free diet improves bowel function in such patients, with secondary correction of the anemia. A trial period with a gluten-free diet is a reasonable intervention for suspected celiac disease.

Whole cow's milk contains proteins that can irritate the lining of the gastrointestinal tract in infants. The result commonly is impaired iron absorption with associated low-grade hemorrhage that can produce iron deficiency.[83,84] The lower bioavailability of iron from cow's milk despite an iron content that roughly equals that of milk from humans can aggravate the problem.[85] The intersection of blood loss, decreased iron uptake, and high iron demand makes iron deficiency a significant problem for children nourished with whole cow's milk.[86] Although supplemental dietary iron can reduce the degree of iron deficiency associated with consumption of cow's milk, refraining from this source of nutrition is the wisest course.[87]

Some disorders hamper iron absorption by disrupting the integrity of the enteric mucosa. Inflammatory bowel disease, particularly Crohn's disease, can injure extensive segments of the small intestine.[88] The disorder primarily affects the distal small intestine and colon, but occasionally extends to the jejunum and duodenum. Invasion of the submucosa by inflammatory cells and disruption of tissue architecture impair absorption both of iron and dietary nutrients. Occult gastrointestinal bleeding exacerbates the disturbed iron balance. The result is iron deficiency anemia often superimposed on anemia due to cobalamin deficiency and chronic inflammation.

LOSS OF FUNCTIONAL BOWEL

Substantial segments of bowel are sometimes removed surgically, with consequent disruption of iron absorption. Intractable inflammatory bowel disease occasionally is treated by surgical excision. Traumatic abdominal injury, such as one that occurs with motor vehicle accidents, at times also requires extensive bowel resection. Structural complications, such as intestinal volvulus or intussusception, can necessitate removal of significant stretches of bowel in children. Hemigastrectomy to alleviate the problem of ulcers virtually obliterates gastrointestinal iron absorption. Postsurgical iron deficiency usually develops slowly and often is unrecognized for several years after the surgical procedure.

■ BLOOD LOSS

PHYSIOLOGICAL BLOOD LOSS

Menstrual blood loss is the most common cause of iron deficiency in reproductive-age women. In contrast to gastrointestinal bleeding that always is pathologic, menstrual bleeding is physiologic. The cardinal question is whether the blood loss is *excessive*. Unfortunately, precise quantification of menstrual blood loss is impossible. Clinicians often apply qualitative terms with murky meanings such as "light," "normal," or "heavy" to describe menstrual blood flow. Subjective interpretations of these categories by individual women further complicate the use of these imprecise terms. Estimating blood loss by the number of days of menstrual flow per month, the number of changes of sanitary pads in an average day, and the occurrence of bleeding between menstrual cycles provides a better appraisal of blood loss.

Menstrual bleeding is not an automatic explanation of iron deficiency in women. *Woman and men are equally susceptible to colonic adenocarcinoma.* The fact that reproductive-age women have a physiological explanation for blood loss does not obviate the need to consider minatory etiologies such as colonic adenocarcinoma. The physician who omits an in-depth search for other bleeding sources must clearly justify that position. Postmenopausal woman with iron deficiency anemia always merit a full bleeding evaluation.

STRUCTURAL DEFECTS

Blood loss due to gastrointestinal structural faults is a common cause of iron deficiency.[89,90] The most frequent congenital defect in the gastrointestinal tract is Meckel's diverticulum, a persistent omphalomesenteric duct. The flaw can produce abdominal pain and, occasionally, intestinal obstruction in young children. Occult blood loss with secondary iron deficiency is a concern in adolescents and even adults with Meckel's diverticulum.[91,92] Otherwise, unexplained iron deficiency anemia in adults occasionally reflects a persistent and previously undetected Meckel's diverticulum.

Peptic ulcer disease in adults is a common cause of gastrointestinal blood loss. The stomach and duodenum are affected most often.[93,94] Inflammation and erosion are prominent at affected sites. The discovery that many cases of peptic ulcer disease are associated with *Helicobacter pylori* infection prompted the use of antibiotics as part of the treatment regimen.[95,96] The result is enhanced healing of the ulcer and reduced blood loss. Bleeding hemorrhoids are another common cause of gastrointestinal blood loss in adults. The lesions can cause perianal pain and itching, but often are asymptomatic. Bright red blood in the toilet bowl quickly brings hemorrhoidal hemorrhage to the attention of most affected people. Colonic diverticali that bleed and produce iron deficiency occur most commonly in older adults.

Other structural defects of the gastrointestinal tract that produce bleeding are much less common. Arteriovenous malformations involving the superficial blood vessels along the gastrointestinal tract occur with hereditary hemorrhagic telangiectasia (the Osler-Weber-Rendu syndrome.) These defective vessels frequently bleed to a degree that engenders iron deficiency. Although the disorder displays an autosomal dominant mode of transmission, the pathognomonic lesions rarely attain clinical significance prior to young adulthood. The condition is not a diagnostic enigma, since the mucosal lining of the oropharynx and nasal cavity exhibit characteristic telangiectasia.

DYSFUNCTIONAL UTERINE BLEEDING

Dysfunctional uterine bleeding is the most common cause of iron deficiency in postmenopausal women. The problem often reflects endometriosis. Some women suffer intermittent heavy episodes of bleeding. Others experience spotty bleeding that at times becomes an almost daily phenomenon. Dysfunctional uterine bleeding can produce very severe iron deficiency anemia with hemoglobin values that descend to 3 g/dL in the most severe cases. The physiological adjustments to the slow decline in hemoglobin permit survival in the face of such extraordinary anemia.

Low body iron stores due to menstruation exacerbate the effect of dysfunctional uterine bleeding. Pica involving substances such as starch that bind gut iron and block its uptake can magnify the problem. A variety of medical interventions can dampen the severity of dysfunctional uterine bleeding. Sometimes, however, hysterectomy is the only option that controls the problem.

PARASITES

The world's leading cause of gastrointestinal blood loss is parasitic infestation. Hookworm infection, produced primarily by *Necator americanus* or *Ancylostoma duodenale,* is endemic to much of the world and often is asymptomatic.[97,98] Microscopic blood loss leads to significant iron deficiency, most commonly in children.[99-101] Severe persistent anemia in some children produces bony changes reminiscent of thalassemia major, including frontal bossing and maxillary prominence. Over one billion people, most in tropical or subtropical areas, are infested with parasites.[102] Daily blood losses exceed 11 million liters. The larvae spawn in moist soil and penetrate the skin of unprotected feet. Hookworm infection, once prevalent in the southeastern United States, declined precipitously with better sanitation and the routine use of footwear out-of-doors. Treatment programs to reduce worm infestation in children substantially lower the incidence and severity of iron deficiency.[103,104]

Trichuris trichiura, the culprit in trichuriasis or whipworm infection, is believed to infest the colon of 600–700 million people. Only about 10–15% of these people have worm burdens sufficiently great to produce clinically apparent disease. *Trichuris trichiura* infestation produces less pronounced gastrointestinal bleeding than does hookworm. Iron deficiency tends to be a part of generalized problems with malnutrition and dysentery.[105] Most victims are children between the ages of 2 and 10 years. Heavy infestations retard overall growth and development in these children in addition to producing iron deficiency.[106] Trichuriasis is the most common helminthic infection encountered in Americans returning from visits to tropical or subtropical regions of the world.

■ EFFECTS OF IRON DEFICIENCYY

ERYTHROPOIESIS AND IRON DEFICIENC

Eighty percent of absorbed iron flows to the bone marrow for hemoglobin synthesis (Figure 7-3). Erythrocyte production is therefore an early casualty of iron deficiency. Iron-deficient erythropoiesis develops in several steps as indicated in Table 7-3. Prelatent iron deficiency occurs when stores are depleted without a change in hematocrit or serum iron levels. This stage of iron deficiency is rarely detected. Latent iron deficiency occurs when the serum iron drops and the TIBC increases without a change in hematocrit. This stage is occasionally detected by a routine check of transferrin saturation. Overt iron deficiency anemia shows erythrocyte microcytosis and hypochromia.

The microcytic, hypochromic anemia impairs tissue oxygen delivery, producing weakness, fatigue, palpitations, and light-headedness. The microcytosis seen with thalassemia trait can be confused with iron deficiency. Iron deficiency produces small cells with a broad range of sizes.[107] Some cells are almost normal in size while others are miniscule (Figure 7-2). The result is a higher than normal RDW. In contrast, thalassemia trait affects all cells equally, producing microcytic cells whose size

TABLE 7-3	STATES OF IRON DEFICIENCY
Stage	*Manifestation*
Prelatent	• Depleted iron stores • Normal serum iron • Normal hemoglobin
Latent	• Depleted iron stores • Low serum iron • Normal hemoglobin
Overt	• Depleted iron stores • Low serum iron • Low hemoglobin

distribution and RDW are normal (see Chapter 14). The RDW value therefore provides valuable information that helps the clinician distinguish iron deficiency from thalassemia.[108] Importantly, an RDW comes with every electronic red cell readout.[109] Other common features of thalassemia trait are basophilic stippling and target cells. These characteristics are not sufficiently unique to distinguish thalassemia trait from iron deficiency, however.

The plasma membranes of iron-deficient red cells are abnormally rigid.[110] This inflexibility could contribute to poikilocytic changes, seen particularly with severe iron deficiency. These small, stiff, misshapen cells are cleared by the reticuloendothelial system, contributing to the low-grade hemolysis that often accompanies iron deficiency. The basis of this alteration in erythrocyte membrane fluidity is unknown.

■ FUNCTIONAL IRON DEFICIENCY

Recombinant human erythropoietin (rHepo) was one of the first clinically useful agents produced by commercial DNA technology. Used to correct the anemia of end-stage renal disease (ESRD), this hormone provided new insight into the kinetic relationship between iron and erythropoietin in red cell production. Erythropoietin treatment of anemia in patients with ESRD also underscored the variable nature of storage iron. The shifting states of storage iron contribute to the inconsistency with which erythropoietin corrects the anemia of renal failure.

With steady-state erythropoiesis, iron and erythropoietin flow to the bone marrow at constant, low rates. Patients with ESRD receive rHepo in intermittent surges, as either as intravenous or subcutaneous boluses. The procedure produces markedly aberrant kinetics of erythropoiesis that strains the production machinery. Erythropoietin, the accelerator of erythroid proliferation, is not coordinated with the supply of iron, the fuel for hemoglobin production (Figure 7-5). This imbalance almost never occurs naturally. The rHepo jars previously quiescent cells to proliferate and produce hemoglobin. The requirement for iron jumps dramatically, and outstrips iron delivery by transferrin.[111]

Erythropoietin prompts proliferation and differentiation of erythroid precursors, with an upsurge in heme synthesis.[112] Cells take up iron from transferrin by cell surface transferrin receptors, transport the mineral to the mitochondria, and insert it into the protoporphyrin IX ring in a reaction catalyzed by ferrochelatase. The number of transferrin receptor increases with differentiation, peaking at over 10^6 per cell in the late pronormoblasts. The number subsequently declines, to the point that mature erythroid cells lack transferrin receptors altogether. This variable expression of transferrin receptors means that iron delivery must be synchronized both with proliferation and stage of erythroid development. Late normoblasts, for instance, cannot compensate for iron that was not delivered to basophilic normoblasts earlier in the maturation sequence. These cells have fewer transferrin receptors, and those receptors are busy supplying iron for heme molecules currently under production.

Transferrin-bound iron is the only important source of the element for erythroid precursors.[113,114] Even with normal body iron stores and normal transferrin

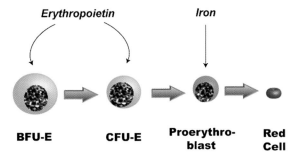

Erythropoietin   **Iron**

BFU-E   **CFU-E**   **Proerythro-blast**   **Red Cell**

FIGURE 7–5 *The interplay of iron and erythropoietin in erythropoiesis. The schematic shows the late stages in red cell development, going from the CFU-E (colony forming unit-erythroid) to the mature erythrocyte. Erythropoietin promotes growth and maturation both of the CFU-E and BFU-E (burst forming unit-erythroid). Iron is needed for hemoglobin production, which begins in earnest with the proerythroblast. Erythropoietin stimulation and iron delivery must be coordinated for optimal hemoglobin production. Iron without erythropoietin manifests as markedly dampened red cell production. Erythropoietin without the timely and concomitant delivery of adequate iron produces erythroid cells that are deficient in hemoglobin. This is "functional iron deficiency." Iron might be present in liver iron stores, for instance, but is functionally useless to the developing erythroid cells.*

saturation, robust proliferation of erythroid precursors can create a demand that outstrips the capacity of the iron delivery system.[115,116] Transferrin iron saturation falls as voracious erythroid precursors strip the element from plasma transferrin.[117] Plasma iron turnover rises, as does erythron iron turnover and erythron transferrin uptake. The late arrival of newly mobilized storage iron fails to prevent production of hypochromic cells. This is "iron-erythropoietin kinetic imbalance" or "functional iron deficiency."[118,119]

New erythroid cells in the form of reticulocytes emerge from the bone marrow in 3 days following exogenous rHepo activation of BFU-E and CFU-E precursors. A number of advanced blood cell analyzers can estimate the hemoglobin content of reticulocytes (CHr). Hypochromic reticulocytes following treatment with rHepo are the sine qua non of functional iron deficiency. These cells arise from bone marrow normoblasts that experience a mismatch between rHepo and iron-loaded transferrin during development.[120,121] Injection of rHepo into a person with normal iron stores produces a window of functional iron deficiency. The hypochromic reticulocytes (low CHr) generated by the maneuver are a red flag that cannot be hidden.[122]

■ TREATMENT OF IRON DEFICIENCY ANEMIA

ORAL IRON SUPPLEMENTATION

Oral iron administration is optimal for correction of iron deficiency. The iron absorption capacity of the duodenum and upper jejunum is limited, however. The 1 mg of iron normally absorbed each day by the gastrointestinal tract precisely balances

TABLE 7-4	EXAMPLES OF ORAL IRON PREPARATIONS			
Supplement Category	**Formulation**	**Elemental Iron Content (mg)**	**Advantages**	**Disadvantages**
Iron salts	Ferrous sulfate	65	Low cost	Poor tolerance
	Ferrous gluconate	50	Lost cost; good tolerance	-
	Ferrous fumarate	50	Good tolerance	High cost
Iron saccharates	Ferric polymaltose	150	Good tolerance	High cost
Elemental iron	Carbonyl iron	50	Good tolerance; high iron absorption	High cost
Heme iron	Meats; health food extracts	-	Excellent bioavailability of iron	-

iron loss from the sloughing of epithelial cells from the skin and gastrointestinal and genitourinal tracts. Each month menstruating women lose on average an additional 20–40 mg of iron. Higher daily iron absorption averaging 2 mg compensates in large part for the higher rate of iron loss.

Iron deficiency anemia boosts daily iron absorption to the range of 4–6 mg. The net positive iron uptake of 3–5 mg is nonetheless small relative to the 2–4 g iron deficit seen with severe iron deficiency. Correction of a 2-g iron deficit at the rate of 4 mg per day, for instance, would require 500 days of oral supplemental iron. A typical tablet used for iron repletion, such as ferrous gluconate, contains 50 mg of elemental iron. The iron content of a single tablet exceeds the absorption capacity of the gastrointestinal tract, meaning that administration of more than a single tablet at a time only increases possible side effects without increasing absorption. Iron absorption does increase with multiple tablets administered over the course of the day, but the price is a possible increase in the incidence of side effects. Since poor patient compliance is the major problem with oral iron supplementation, the commonly recommended thrice daily administration of iron tablets often is counter productive. Patients commonly find the oral iron to be disagreeable and cease its use.

Oral iron supplements fall into three categories. The first group consists of iron salts in which cationic iron bonds with any of a variety of anionic moieties (Table 7-4). The most commonly used formulation is ferrous sulfate, which provides about 65 mg of elemental iron per tablet. The drug is inexpensive but is tolerated poorly by many people due to abdominal cramping, bloating, or constipation. The sulfate anion likely is the major offender with respect to these side effects. Ferrous gluconate is a good alternative and its cost is similar to that of ferrous sulfate. Although each tablet contains only 50 mg of elemental iron, the difference is inconsequential since most of the iron from either formulation passes through the gastrointestinal tract without being absorbed. (The dark stool seen with oral iron replacement reflects unabsorbed iron in the excrement.) Most people likewise tolerate ferrous fumarate well. However, this agent generally costs more than ferrous gluconate.

A second iron replacement formulation, polysaccharide–iron complex, has ionic iron in a coordinated complex with polar oxygen groups in the polysaccharide. The well-hydrated microspheres of polysaccharide iron remain in solution over a wide pH range. Most patients tolerate this form of iron better than ferrous sulfate, even though the 150 mg of elemental iron per tablet is substantially greater than that provided by iron salts. The higher cost of polysaccharide–iron complex is its primary disadvantage. No information exists on the efficacy of iron absorption with this formulation. However, anecdotal information suggests efficient iron replacement.

Carbonyl iron, a third available formulation, provides the mineral in a nonionic form as part of a macromolecular complex. Carbonyl iron, a form of iron that is nontoxic and well tolerated even in large doses, is highly purified elemental iron produced by the decomposition of iron pentacarbonyl as a dark gray powder. Carbonyl iron has a minimum 98% iron content. What distinguishes the formulation is its fine spherical size of 2-μm which is an order of magnitude smaller than other commercial iron forms. Pinocytosis by cells lining the gastrointestinal tract brings carbonyl iron into the body from the gut. Patients tolerate the formulation extremely well. Some people who are unable to use any of the iron salts can use carbonyl iron without problem.

The gastrointestinal uptake apparatus has a much higher avidity for ferric iron, Fe(III), than it does for ferrous iron, Fe(II). Oxidizing compounds that convert ferrous iron to the ferric form augment gastrointestinal iron absorption. Ascorbic acid is an excellent agent in this regard.[123] Ascorbic acid has the additional advantage of being a weak iron chelator.[124] As a weak chelator, the vitamin prevents the formation of insoluble iron salts in the gastrointestinal tract thereby maintaining iron in a soluble form that is easily absorbed.[125,126]

Combined supplementation of oral iron salts with ascorbic acid substantially boosts gastrointestinal iron absorption. A useful approach is to take one iron tablet at bedtime along with an ascorbic acid tablet in orange juice. Reduced nocturnal gastrointestinal motility increases the residence time of the iron in the upper portion of the gut, further aiding absorption. The net result is iron uptake superior to that with thrice daily ingestion of tablets and superior tolerance by patients. Although combination tablets with iron and ascorbic acid are available, the best approach is to purchase separate stocks. The cost of individual drugs is significantly lower than that of the combination tablets.

Physicians faced with the dilemma of a patient who fails to respond to oral iron must be certain that the patient takes the medication properly (Table 7-5). Iron salts work best when taken on an empty stomach. Patients commonly forget to take their medication. Gastrointestinal side effects discourage many people who require iron supplements. Detailed questioning often is the only way to bring these difficulties to light. Changing to a different iron formulation or moving to bedtime administration often solves problems related to poor patient tolerance. Every alternate avenue should be exhausted before oral iron supplements are deemed to be failures.

TABLE 7-5 | **CAUSES OF A POOR RESPONSE TO ORAL IRON**

Noncompliance

Ongoing blood loss
    Peptic ulcer disease
    Meckel's diverticulum
    Parasites
    Gastrointestinal cancer
Insufficient duration of therapy
    Mixing iron and milk in infant bottle

High gastric pH
    Vagotomy
    Antacids
    Histamine H_2 blockers (e.g., Tagamet®)

Inhibitors of iron absorption/utilization
    Lead
    Iron-binding substances in food (such as phytates)
    Chronic inflammation
    Neoplasia
Incorrect diagnosis

    Thalassemia
    Sideroblastic anemia

Heme is the most readily absorbed form of iron. Meat products are the most abundant source of dietary heme. Heme absorption does not depend on the machinery used for the uptake of ionic iron and therefore is not shackled by the daily limits of iron absorption seen with iron salts (Figure 7-4). Unfortunately, meat often is not an option due sometimes to dietary preferences and at other times to limited finance means.

PARENTERAL IRON SUPPLEMENTATION

Parenteral iron replacement circumvents the limited iron absorption capacity of the gastrointestinal tract. Parenteral formulations can rapidly correct extremely severe iron deficits. Parenteral iron is the only option available to correct iron deficits in people who lack small bowel function due to disease or surgical resection. Both intravenous and intramuscular formulations provide vehicles for parenteral iron administration. The two common drug classes used for parenteral iron replacement

TABLE 7-6 | **PARENTERAL IRON REPLACEMENT FORMULATIONS**

	Iron Dextran	*Iron Saccharates*
Maximum dose	6 g	about 250 mg
Total dose infusion	yes	no
Reported anaphylaxis	yes	no
Side effects (other than anaphylaxis)	frequent	rare

are iron dextran and a variety of formulations where polar interactions with oxygen groups in saccharate compounds stabilize ionic iron. Each class has advantages and shortcomings (Table 7-6).

Iron dextran was the first formulation widely available for parenteral iron repletion. The drug can be administered intravenously in doses of up to 6 g at a single sitting, allowing complete repletion of body iron stores in even the most severe case of iron deficiency.[127] The obligatory test dose screens for possible anaphylactic response to the therapeutic infusion. The risk of anaphylaxis with iron dextran is low, contrary to popular belief.[128]

In contrast to the intravenous route, intramuscular iron dextran administration cannot exceed 1 g in a single sitting. The drug is administered bilaterally as depot injections of 500 mg into the gluteus maximus muscles. A "Z-tract" must be used for the intramuscular injection to prevent seepage of drug into the dermis. The areas of black skin discoloration produced by iron dextran are unsightly and persist for years. Pain at the site of the injection is another common source of often-bitter patient complaints.[129]

The most frequent systemic problems with iron dextran therapy are fevers, myalgias, and arthralgias 12–24 hours after administration. These difficulties occur in about 20% of the patients. They were once believed to be an immune response and were likened to serum sickness. The reactions probably instead reflect release of cytokines such as interleukin-1 and tumor necrosis factor by macrophages activated in the process of engulfing and processing the iron dextran particles in the blood stream. Parenteral steroids almost completely abrogate these reactions. An accepted approach is intravenous bolus administration of 125 mg of methylprednisolone prior to the iron dextran.[130] The steroid must be given *after* the test dose of iron dextran so as not to mask an adverse reaction to the test.

Iron dextran is a farraginous amalgam of iron and dextran that reticuloendothelial cells clear from the circulation with a half-time of about 2 days.[131] The macrophage cellular machinery strips the iron from the dextran polymer and places it on circulating transferrin. The transferrin iron can then be used for erythropoiesis. Iron dextran is otherwise inert with respect to providing iron for erythropoiesis. Routine laboratory testing for serum iron will detect iron dextran in the circulation. The result is a specious transferrin saturation far in excess of 100%, making serum iron values useless for a couple of weeks following parenteral iron replacement.[132]

When introduced into clinical practice 40 years ago, iron dextran routinely was given as an intramuscular depot injection. In addition to pain, this approach has several disadvantages relative to intravenous administration. The most important is that ongoing exposure to iron dextran cannot be stopped should an adverse reaction develop. Removing the material from the intramuscular depot is impossible. The nightmare scenario is an anaphylactic reaction to the intramuscular test dose of iron dextran. Anaphylaxis can occur with exposure to a few micrograms of drug. The intramuscular test dose of iron dextran is 10 mg. A patient with an anaphylactic reaction will continue to react to the drug even after the physician recognizes the adverse event and initiates appropriate supportive therapy. A rocky stay in the intensive care unit can result. Death can occur even with optimal support.

In contrast, an intravenous iron dextran infusion can be terminated with the first indication of anaphylaxis or other adverse response. Prevenient events usually appear after only a few milligrams of the intravenous test drug. These include flushing, faintness, and hypertension. Immediate cessation of the test dose in concert with intravenous administration of diphenhydramine can terminate the adverse reaction prior to serious events such as hypotension or shock. Patients who receive intravenous test doses of iron dextran rarely require hospitalization after an adverse reaction. For this reason, an intravenous test dose of iron dextran should be administered even when intramuscular therapy is planned.

One of the several iron saccharate compounds can be used as an alternative to iron dextran for parenteral iron administration. While these compounds are relatively new to the American market, the European medical community has used the drugs for more than 30 years with remarkably few adverse reactions. Most striking is the absence of reports of anaphylaxis with these agents.[133] The one shortcoming relative to iron dextran is the limited quantity of iron saccharate that can be administered intravenously during a single session (Table 7-6). The standard dose for these agents is about 125 mg as an intravenous infusion. Reports exist of uncomplicated bolus administration of up to 250 mg of some formulations. No report exists of administration of gram quantities of these drugs, however. Correction of a severe iron deficit therefore is not possible in a single sitting with the iron saccharate formulations.

■ ANEMIA OF CHRONIC DISEASE

As a cause of anemia, the anemia of chronic disease (ACD) is both common and complex. Sometimes called the "anemia of chronic inflammation," the condition reflects deranged iron metabolism produced by a host of conditions that include infections such as tuberculosis, autoimmune disorders such as rheumatoid arthritis, and cancers. The mind-boggling complexity of ACD falls into better focus with a step back from the particular conditions, which allows a wide-angle snapshot of iron metabolism.

| TABLE 7-7 | IRON DYSREGULATION STATES |

Condition	Body Iron Stores	Support Network Disturbance	Diagnosis	Complexity of Treatment
Iron deficiency	Low	None	Simple	Simple
Erythropoietin deficiency	Normal	None/Mild	Simple	Moderate
Anemia of chronic disease	Normal/High	Extensive	Complex	Complex

The gastrointestinal tract, kidney, bone marrow, and liver all have key roles in maintaining a steady-state hemoglobin value based on balanced iron metabolism. The key molecular components of this system are iron and erythropoietin. Undergirding this relatively simple superstructure is a complex support network of hormones, cytokines, and ancillary cells that facilitate the smooth operation of the iron metabolic pathways shown in Figure 7-3. The members of this network are numerous, their functions are variegated, and their interactions are promiscuous. Detailed diagrammatic representations often resemble a complex circuit diagram. A reductionist approach to the issue, however, allows construction of the simple summary shown in Table 7-7.

In the upper stratum of iron dysregulation outlined in Table 7-7 is iron deficit. A solitary defect perturbs the iron metabolism edifice without altering structural integrity. The effects of iron deficiency are relatively simple and the approaches to correction are straightforward.

Erythropoietin deficiency occupies the next rung in the ladder and is also conceptually simple. Rare conditions that selectively eliminate renal erythropoietin production while preserving kidney function provide the purest representation of this scenario. Most often a decline in erythropoietin production reflects a general compromise of kidney function due to a disorder such as diabetic nephropathy that destroys the renal parenchyma. The metabolic disturbances of kidney dysfunction can spill out to compromise the iron metabolism support network beyond the effect on erythropoietin production. Such disturbances usually are mild. Treating the condition is a moderately complex endeavor due to the timing issues of erythropoietin replacement involved in the previously discussed functional iron deficiency.

ACD stands in sharp contrast to either of these two states. A disturbance in the iron metabolism support network is the primary problem, which produces complex issues both with respect to diagnosis and treatment. Most importantly, ACD is not a single entity but a collection of syndromes that fracture the iron metabolism support network. The primary location of the rent in the net, its extent, and ultimate impact on iron metabolism vary depending on the nature of the primary process. ACD due to non small cell lung cancer differs significantly from ACD due to leprosy. Therapeutic approaches and responses likewise will vary sharply. The single statement that applies

TABLE 7-8 | **EFFECTS OF CYTOKINES IN THE ANEMIA OF CHRONIC DISEASE**

Cytokine	Iron Absorption	Erythropoiesis	RE Iron Stores	Erythropoietin Production
Hepcidin	↓	↓	↑	-
Interleukin 6	-	-	↑	-
Interleukin 1	-	-	↑	↓
TNF-α	-	↓	↑	↓
Interferon-γ	-	↓	↑	↓

The cytokines listed are the best characterized to date. Others will undoubtedly be uncovered.

TABLE 7-9 | **KEY DIAGNOSTIC POINTS WITH IRON DEFICIENCY**

Issue	Manifestation	Approach
Iron deficiency in the newborn	Exaggerated physiological anemia at 8 weeks	Assess serum transferrin saturation. Use iron-supplemented formula. Avoid cow's milk.
Etiology of iron deficiency in adults	Hypochromic, microcytic anemia	Look for an occult bleeding source. Rule out drugs that interfere with iron uptake such as histamine H_2 blockers. Rule out mild celiac disease.
Iron deficiency with coexisting inflammation	• Spuriously high ferritin • Spuriously low transferrin saturation	Assess iron status using the soluble transferrin receptor assay. Assess red cell ZPP levels, looking for high values.
Iron deficiency in menstruating females	Hypochromic, microcytic anemia	Check stool guaiacs for evidence of GI bleeding. Daily oral iron replacement. Full bleeding evaluation for persistent or intractable iron deficiency.
Iron deficiency versus thalassemia trait	Hypochromic, microcytic anemia	Check the RDW value; high with iron deficiency, normal with thalassemia. Hemoglobin electrophoresis.

| TABLE 7-10 | **KEY MANAGEMENT POINTS WITH IRON DEFICIENCY** |

Issue	*Comments*
Iron replacement in children	Use iron supplemented formula in infants. Use oral iron supplements in older children.
Oral iron replacement in adults	Use ferrous gluconate rather than ferrous sulfate for initial therapy. One tablet at bedtime with orange juice or an ascorbic acid tablet works best. Continue oral iron after correction of the anemia in order to replete iron stores.
Parenteral iron replacement in adults	Iron saccharates allow safe, well-tolerated replacement of 125–250 mg of iron per treatment. Iron dextran allows administration of up to 4 g of iron per treatment. The iron dextran test dose should always be given as an IV infusion.
Iron deficiency producing severe anemia	Use parenteral iron saccharates initially followed by oral ferrous gluconate. Transfusion is rarely needed. With transfusions, slowly infuse one-half unit aliquots of blood with close monitoring of fluid status to avoid fluid overload.
Anemia of chronic disease	Eliminate the underlying cause of the iron disturbance if possible. Eliminate iron deficiency. Replacement of erythropoietin might be useful, but will vary by cause. Transfusion support might be necessary in severe cases refractory to other intervention.
Iron deficiency with hepatocellular disease	Necrotic hepatocytes release ferririn into the circulation, thereby raising measures of serum ferritin. Hepatocellular disease can raise serum ferritin values astronomically.

to all ACD is that correction of the primary defect is the most effective way to correct the problem. Unfortunately, control of the primary disorder often is not possible. This leaves patchwork attempts to support the network using drugs, hormones, and iron as the only alternative.

The most important global disturbance of ACD is sequestration of iron in macrophages of the reticuloendothelial system.[134] Trapped in storage, the mineral cannot participate in hemoglobin synthesis. Transferrin saturation is low despite a normal or high total body iron content. Some of the cytokines in the malfunctioning network raise the level of plasma ferritin without reference to body iron content. Assessment of true iron status is difficult using standard assessment tools.

Table 7-8 lists some of the key hormones and cytokines involved in ACD. Hepcidin is the central operator in the process (see Chapter 5, Figure 5-4).[135] The liver produces the polypeptide hormone most avidly in response to bacterial lipopolysaccharide.[136,137] The hormone has a role in host cell's defense against infection that includes physiological changes that starve bacteria of the iron essential to their proliferation. Limits on iron of course limit erythropoiesis secondarily.[138] The other cytokines listed modify iron metabolism and erythropoiesis both directly and indirectly. Crosstalk and feedback between these cytokines creates truly complex disturbances in iron metabolism. Other yet unknown cytokines and metabolic perturbations will further complicate this picture. Recommendations on diagnosis and treatment of ACD (beyond correction of the underlying problem) will evolve as more experimental and clinical data become available[139] (Tables 7-9 and 7-10).

References

1   Rao R, Georgieff M. 2001. Neonatal iron nutrition. Semin Neonatol 6:425–435.

2   Saarinen U. 1978. Need for iron supplementation in infants on prolonged breast feeding. J Pediatr 93:177.

3   Katzman R, Novack A, Pearson H. 1972. Nutritional anemia in an inner-city community. Relationship to age and ethnic group. JAMA 222:670–673.

4   Zee P, Walters T, Mitchell C. 1970. Nutrition and poverty in preschool children. A nutritional survey of preschool children from impoverished black families, Memphis. JAMA 213:739–742.

5   Oski FA, Honig AS. 1978. The effects of therapy on the developmental scores of iron-deficient infants. Pediatrics 92:21–25.

6   Delinard A, Gilbert A, Dodds M, Egeland B. 1981. Iron deficiency and behavioral deficits. Pediatrics 68:828–833.

7   Yalcin SS, Yurdakok K, Acikgoz D, Ozmert E. 2000. Short-term developmental outcome of iron prophylaxis in infants. Pediatr Int 42:625–630.

8   Pollitt E. 2001. The developmental and probabilistic nature of the functional consequences of iron-deficiency anemia in children. J Nutr 131(2S-2):669S–675S.

9   Lozoff B, Jimenez E, Wolf A. 1991. Long-term developmental outcome of infants with iron deficiency. N Engl J Med 325:687–694.

10 Lozoff B, De Andraca I, Castillo M, Smith JB, Walter T, Pino P. 2003. Behavioral and developmental effects of preventing iron-deficiency anemia in healthy full-term infants. Pediatrics 112(4):846–854.

11 Friel JK, Aziz K, Andrews WL, Harding SV, Courage ML, Adams RJ. 2003. A double-masked, randomized control trial of iron supplementation in early infancy in healthy term breast-fed infants. Pediatrics 143:582–586.

12 Pollitt E, Saco-Pollitt C, Leibel R, Viteri F. 1986. Iron deficiency and behavioral development in infants and preschool children. Am J Clin Nutr 43:555–565.

13 Oski F, Honig A, Helu B, Howanitz P. 1983. Effect of iron therapy on behavior performance in nonanemic, iron-deficient infants. Pediatrics 71:877–880.

14 Dallman PR. 1989. Iron deficiency: Does it matter? J Intern Med 226(5):367–372.

15 Osaki T, Ueta E, Arisawa K, Kitamura Y, Matsugi N. 1999. The pathophysiology of glossal pain in patients with iron deficiency and anemia. Am J Med Sci 318:324–329.

16 Bisse E, Renner F, Sussmann S, Scholmerich J, Wieland H. 1996. Hair iron content: Possible marker to complement monitoring therapy of iron deficiency in patients with chronic inflammatory bowel diseases? Clin Chem 42:1270–1274.

17 Kantor J, Kessler LJ, Brooks DG, Cotsarelis G. 2003. Decreased serum ferritin is associated with alopecia in women. J Invest Dermatol 121:985–988.

18 Kalra L, Hamlyn A, Jones B. 1986. Blue sclerae: A common sign of iron deficiency? Lancet 2:1267–1269.

19 Uygur-Bayramicli O, Tuncer K, Dolapcioglu C. 1999. Plummer-Vinson syndrome presenting with an esophageal stricture. J Clin Gastroenterol 29:291–292.

20 Anthony R, Sood S, Strachan D, Fenwick J. 1999. A case of Plummer-Vinson syndrome in childhood. J Pediatr Surg 34:1570–1572.

21 Jessner W, Vogelsang H, Puspok A, et al. 2003. Plummer-Vinson syndrome associated with celiac disease and complicated by postcricoid carcinoma and carcinoma of the tongue. Am J Gastroenterol 98:1208–1209.

22 Talkington K, Gant N, Jr, Scott D, Pritchard J. 1970) Effect of ingestion of starch and some clays on iron absorption. Am J Obstet Gynecol 108:262–267.

23 Smulian J, Motiwala S, Sigman R. 1995. Pica in a rural obstetric population. South Med J 88:1236–1240.

24 Roselle H. 1970. Association of laundry starch and clay ingestion with anemia in New York City. Arch Intern Med 125:57.

25 Keith L, Rosenberg C, Brown E. 1969. Pica, pagophagia, and anemia. JAMA 208:535.

26 Racke F. 2003. EPO and TPO sequences do not explain thrombocytosis in iron deficiency anemia. J Pediatr Hematol Oncol 25:919.

27 Geddis A, Kaushansky K. 2003. Cross-reactivity between erythropoietin and thrombopoietin at the level of Mpl does not account for the thrombocytosis seen in iron deficiency. J Pediatr Hematol Oncol 25:919–920.

28 Liu JM, Hankinson SE, Stampfer MJ, Rifai N, Willett WC, Ma J. 2003. Body iron stores and their determinants in healthy postmenopausal US women. Am J Clin Nutr 78:1160–1167.

29 McLaren CE, Li KT, Gordeuk VR, Hasselblad V, McLaren GD. 2001. Relationship between transferrin saturation and iron stores in the African American and US Caucasian populations: Analysis of data from the third National Health and Nutrition Examination Survey. Blood 98:2345–2351.

30 Bonkovsky H. 1991. Iron and the liver. Am J Med 301:32–43.

31 Dorner MH, Salfeld J, Will H, Leibold EA, Vass JK, Munro HN. 1985. Structure of human ferritin light subunit messenger RNA: Comparison with heavy subunit message and functional implications. Proc Natl Acad Sci 82:3139–3143.

32 Halliday J, Cowlishaw J, Russo A, Powell L. 1977. Serum-ferritin in diagnosis of haemachromatosis: A study of 43 families. Lancet 2:621–624.

33 Guldholt I, Trolle B, Hvidman L. 1991. Iron supplementation during pregnancy. Acta Obstet Gynecol Scand 70:9–12.

34　Rogers J, Bridges K, Durmowicz G, Glass J, Auron P, Munro H. 1990. Translational control during the acute phase response. Ferritin synthesis in response to interleukin-1. J Biol Chem 265:14572–14578.

35　Kohgo Y, Torimoto Y, Kato J. 2002. Transferrin receptor in tissue and serum: Updated clinical significance of soluble receptor. Int J Hematol 76:213–218.

36　Karin M, Mintz B. 1981. Receptor-mediated endocytosis of transferrin in developmentally totipotent mouse teratocarcinoma stem cells. J Biol Chem 256:3245–3252.

37　Klausner RD, van Renswoude J, Ashwell G, et al. 1983. Receptor-mediated endocytosis of transferrin in K562 cells. J Biol Chem 258:4715–4724.

38　Iacopetta B, Rothenberger S, Kuhn L. 1988. A role for the cytoplasmic domain in transferrin receptor sorting and coated pit formation during endocytosis. Cell 54:485–489.

39　Shih Y, Baynes R, Hudson B, Cook J. 1993. Characterization and quantitation of the circulating forms of serum transferrin receptor using domain-specific antibodies. Blood 81:234–238.

40　Rutledge EA, Enns CA. 1996. Cleavage of the transferrin receptor is influenced by the composition of the O-linked carbohydrate at position 104. J Cell Physiol 168:284–293.

41　Beguin Y. 1992. The soluble transferrin receptor- biological aspects and clinical usefulness as quantitative measure of erythropoiesis. Haematologie 77:1–10.

42　Mast AE, Blinder MA, Gronowski AM, Chumley C, Scott MG. 1998. Clinical utility of the soluble transferrin receptor and comparison with serum ferritin in several populations. Clin Chem 44:45–51.

43　Rees DC, Williams TN, Maitland K, Clegg JB, Weatherall DJ. 1998. Alpha thalassaemia is associated with increased soluble transferrin receptor levels. Br J Haematol 103:365–369.

44　Kuiper-Kramer EP, Coenen JL, Huisman CM, Abbes A, van Raan J, van Eijk HG. 1998. Relationship between soluble transferrin receptors in serum and membrane-bound transferrin receptors. Acta Haematol 99:8–11.

45　Braun J. 1999. Erythrocyte zinc protoporphyrin. Kidney Int Suppl 69:S57–S60.

46　Paton T, Lembroski G. 1982. Fluorometric assay of erythrocyte protoporphyrins: Simple screening test for lead poisoning and iron deficiency. Can Med Assoc J 127:860–862.

47　Donnelly SM, Smith EK. 1990. The role of aluminum in the functional iron deficiency of patients treated with erythropoietin: Case report of clinical characteristics and response to treatment. Am J Kidney Dis 16(5):487–490.

48　Yip R, Dallman P. 1984. Developmental changes in erythrocyte protoporphyrins: Roles of iron deficiency and lead toxicity. J Pediatr 104:710–713.

49　Skikne B, Lynch S, Cook J. 1981. Role of gastric acid in food iron absorption. Gastroenterology 81:1068–1071.

50　Gillooly M, Bothwell T, Charlton R, et al. 1984. Factors affecting the absorption of iron from cereals. Br J Nutr 51:37–46.

51　Davidsson L, Galan P, Kastenmayer P, et al. 1994. Iron bioavailability studied in infants: The influence of phytic acid and ascorbic acid in infant formulas based on soy isolate. Pediatr Res 36:816–822.

52　Hallberg L, Rossander L, Skanberg AB. 1987. Phytates and the inhibitory effect of bran on iron absorption in man. Am J Clin Nutr 45:988–996.

53　Fuchs G, Farris R, DeWier M, et al. 1993. Iron status and intake of older infants fed formula vs cow milk with cereal. Am J Clin Nutr 58:343–348.

54　Uzel C, Conrad M. 1998. Absorption of heme iron. Semin Hematol 35:27–34.

55　Bwibo N, Neumann C. 2003. The need for animal source foods by Kenyan children. J Nutr 133:3936S–3940S.

56 Magnusson B, Faxen A, Cederblad A, Rosander L, Kewenter J, Hallberg L. 1979. The effect of parietal cell vagotomy and selective vagotomy with pyloroplasty on iron absorption. A prospective randomized study. Scand J Gastroenterol 14:177–182.

57 Rieu P, Jansen J, Joosten H, Lamers C. 1990. Effect of gastrectomy with either Roux-en-Y or Billroth II anastomosis on small-intestinal function. Scand J Gastroenterol 25:185–192.

58 Aymard J, Aymard B, Netter P, Bannwarth B, Trechot P, Streiff F. 1988. Haematological adverse effects of histamine H2-receptor antagonists. Med Toxicol Adverse Drug Exp 3:430–448.

59 Koop H, Bachem M. 1992. Serum iron, ferritin, and vitamin B12 during prolonged omeprazole therapy. J Clin Gastroenterol 14:288–292.

60 Koop H. 1992. Review article: Metabolic consequences of long-term inhibition of acid secretion by omeprazole. Aliment Pharmacol Ther 6:399–406.

61 Carmel R, Weiner J, Johnson C. 1987. Iron deficiency occurs frequently in patients with pernicious anemia. JAMA 257:1081–1083.

62 Demiroglu H, Dundar S. 1997. Pernicious anaemia patients should be screened for iron deficiency during follow up. N Z Med J 110:147–148.

63 Disler P, Lynch S, Charlton R, et al. 1975. The effect of tea on iron absorption. Gut 16:193–200.

64 Davis S, Murray J. 1996. One for tea, not two. Clin Lab Haematol 18:289–290.

65 Layrisse M, Garcia-Casal MN, Solano L, et al. 2000. Iron bioavailability in humans from breakfasts enriched with iron bis-glycine chelate, phytates and polyphenols. J Nutr 130:2195–2199.

66 Mahlknecht U, Weidmann E, Seipelt G. 2001. The irreplaceable image: Black tea delays recovery from iron-deficiency anemia. Haematologica 86, 559.

67 Nelson M, Poulter J. 2004. Impact of tea drinking on iron status in the UK: A review. J Hum Nutr Diet 17:43–54.

68 Munoz L, Lonnerdal B, Keen C, Dewey K. 1988. Coffee consumption as a factor in iron deficiency anemia among pregnant women and their infants in Costa Rico. Am J Clin Nutr 48:645–651.

69 Dewey K, Romero-Abal M, Quan de Serrano J, et al. 1997. A randomized intervention study of the effects of discontinuing coffee intake on growth and morbidity of iron-deficient Guatemalan toddlers. J Nutr 127:306–313.

70 Engle P, VasDias T, Howard I, et al. 1999. Effects of discontinuing coffee intake on iron deficient Guatemalan toddlers' cognitive development and sleep. Early Hum Dev 53:251–269.

71 Barton J, Conrad M, Holland R. 1981. Iron, lead, and cobalt absorption: Similarities an dissimilarities. Proc Soc Exp Biol Med 166:64–69.

72 Schade S, Felsher B, Bernier G, Conrad ME. 1970. Interrelationship of cobalt and iron absorption. Journal of Laboratory and Clinical Medicine 75:435–441.

73 Goddard W, Coupland K, Smith J, Long R. 1997. Iron uptake by isolated human enterocyte suspensions in vitro is dependent on body iron stores and inhibited by other metal cations. J Nutr 127:177–183.

74 Lutter C, Rivera J. 2003. Nutritional status of infants and young children and characteristics of their diets. J Nutr 133:2941S–2949S.

75 Yip R, Dallman P. 1984. Developmental changes in erythrocyte protoporphyrins: Roles of iron deficiency and lead toxicity. J Pediatr 104:710–713.

76 Anand B, Callender S, Warner G. 1977. Absorption of inorganic and haemoglobin iron in coeliac disease. Br J Haematol 37:409–414.

77 Annibale B, Capurso G, Chistolini A, et al. 2001. Gastrointestinal causes of refractory iron deficiency anemia in patients without gastrointestinal symptoms. Am J Med 111:439–445.

78 Egan-Mitchell B, Fottrell P, McNicholl B. 1981. Early or pre-coeliac mucosa: Development of gluten enteropathy. Gut 22:65–69.

79 Corazza G, Valentini R, Andreani M, et al. 1995. Subclinical coeliac disease is a frequent cause of iron-deficiency anaemia. Scand J Gastroenterol 30:153–156.

80 Cordum N, McGuire B, Nelson D. 1995. Celiac sprue in an asymptomatic elderly man. Minn Med 78:29–30.

81 Dickey W, McConnell B. 1999. Celiac disease presenting as the Paterson-Brown Kelly (Plummer-Vinson. syndrome. Am J Gastroenterol 94:527–529.

82 Korman S. 1990. Pica as a presenting symptom in childhood celiac disease. Am J Clin Nutr 51:139–141.

83 Tunnessen W, Jr, Oski F. 1987. Consequences of starting whole cow milk at 6 months of age. J Pediatr 111:813–816.

84 Bramhagen A, Virtanen M, Siimes M, Axelsson I. 2003. Transferrin receptor in children and its correlation with iron status and types of milk consumption. Acta Paediatr 92:671–675.

85 Picciano M, Deering R. 1980. The influence of feeding regiments on iron status during infancy. Am J Clin Nutr 33:746–753.

86 Nutrition Committee, American Academy of Pediatrics. 1992. The use of whole cow's milk in infancy. Pediatrics 89:1105–1109.

87 Virtanen M, Svahn C, Viinikka L, Raiha N, Siimes M, Axelsson I. 2001. Iron-fortified and unfortified cow's milk: Effects on iron intakes and iron status in young children. Acta Paediatr 90:724–731.

88 Beeken W. 1973. Absorptive defects in young people with regional enteritis. Pediatrics 52:69–74.

89 Annibale B, Capurso G, Delle Fave G. 2003. The stomach and iron deficiency anaemia: A forgotten link. Dig Liver Dis 35:288–295.

90 Pennazio M, Santucci R, Rondonotti E, et al. 2004. Outcome of patients with obscure gastrointestinal bleeding after capsule endoscopy: Report of 100 consecutive cases. Gastroenterology 126:643–653.

91 Baumgartner F, White G, Colman P, Marcus C, Salahi W. 1990. Bleeding Meckel's diverticulum in an adult. J Natl Med Assoc 82:585–588.

92 Lin S, Suhocki P, Ludwig K, Shetzline M. 2002. Gastrointestinal bleeding in adult patients with Meckel's diverticulum: The role of technetium 99 m pertechnetate scan. South Med J 95:1338–1341.

93 Gordon S, Smith R, Power G. 1994. The role of endoscopy in the evaluation of iron deficiency anemia in patients over the age of 50. Am J Gastroenterol 89:1963–1967.

94 Maleki D, Cameron A. 2002. Plummer-Vinson syndrome associated with chronic blood loss anemia and large diaphragmatic hernia. Am J Gastroenterol 97:190–193.

95 Hentschel E, Brandstatter G, Dragosics B, et al. 1993. Effect of ranitidine and amoxicillin plus metronidazole on the eradication of Helicobacter pylori and the recurrence of duodenal ulcer. N Engl J Med 328:308–312.

96 Marignani M, Angeletti S, Bordi C, et al. 1997. Reversal of long-standing iron deficiency anaemia after eradication of Helicobacter pylori infection. Scand J Gastroenterol 32:617–622.

97 Stephenson L, Latham M, Kurz K, Kinoti S, Oduori M, Crompton D. 1985. Relationships of Schistosoma hematobium, hookworm and malarial infections and metrifonate treatment to hemoglobin level in Kenyan school children. Am J Trop Med Hyg 34:519–528.

98 Hopkins R, Gracey M, Hobbs R, Spargo R, Yates M, Thompson R. 1997. The prevalence of hookworm infection, iron deficiency and anaemia in an aboriginal community in northwest Australia. Med J Aust 166:241–244.

99 Crompton D, Whitehead R. 1993. Hookworm infections and human iron metabolism. Parasitology 107:S137–S145.

100 Pritchard D, Quinnell R, Moustafa M, et al. 1991. Hookworm (Necator americanus) infection and storage iron depletion. Trans R Soc Trop Med Hyg 85:235–238.

101 Stoltzfus RJ, Chwaya HM, Tielsch JM, Schulze KJ, Albonico M, Savioli L. 1997. Epidemiology of iron deficiency anemia in Zanzibari schoolchildren: The importance of hookworms. Am J Clin Nutr 65:153–159.

102 Albonico M, Stoltzfus R, Savioli L, et al. 1998. Epidemiological evidence for a differential effect of hookworm species, Ancylostoma duodenale or Necator americanus, on iron status of children. Int J Epidemiol 27:530–537.

103 Olds G, King C, Hewlett J, et al. 1999. Double-blind placebo-controlled study of concurrent administration of albendazole and praziquantel in schoolchildren with schistosomiasis and geohelminths. J Infect Dis 179:996–1003.

104 Stoltzfus R, Dreyfuss M, Chwaya H, Albonico M. 1997. Hookworm control as a strategy to prevent iron deficiency. Nutr Rev 55:223–232.

105 Raj SM. 1999. Fecal occult blood testing on Trichuris-infected primary school children in northeastern peninsular Malaysia. Am J Trop Med Hyg 60(1):165–166.

106 Ramdath DD, Simeon DT, Wong MS, Grantham-McGregor SM. 1995. The relationship between varying intensities of Trichuris trichiura infection and iron status was examined in Jamaican schoolchildren, aged 7 to 11 years. Parasitology 110:347–351.

107 Bessman J, Gilmer P, Jr, Gardner F. 1983. Improved classification of anemias by MCV and RDW. Am J Clin Pathol 80:322–326.

108 Lin C, Lin J, Chen S, Jiang M, Chiu C. 1992. Comparison of hemoglobin and red blood cell distribution width in the differential diagnosis of microcytic anemia. Arch Pathol Lab Med 116:1030–1032.

109 Uchida T. 1989. Change in red blood cell distribution width with iron deficiency. Clin Lab Haematol 11:117–121.

110 Tillmann W, Schroter W. 1980. Deformability of erythrocytes in iron deficiency anemia. Blut 40:179–186.

111 Adamson J, Eschbach J. 1990. Treatment of anemia of chronic renal failure with recombinant human erythropoietin. Annu Rev Med 41:349–360.

112 Weiss G, Houston T, Kastner S, Johrer K, Grunewald K, Brock J. 1997. Regulation of cellular iron metabolism by erythropoietin: Activation of iron-regulatory protein and upregulation of transferrin receptor expression in erythroid cells. Blood 89:680–687.

113 Iacopetta B, Morgan E. 1983. The kinetics of transferrin endocytosis and iron uptake from transferrin in rabbit reticulocytes. J Biol Chem 258:9108–9115.

114 Hodgson L, Quail E, Morgan E. 1995. Iron transport mechanisms in reticulocytes and mature erythrocytes. J Cell Physiol 162:181–190.

115 Brugnara C, Colella G, Cremins J, et al. 1994. Effects of subcutaneous recombinant human erythropoietin in normal subjects: Development of decreased reticulocyte hemoglobin content and iron-deficient erythropoiesis. J Lab Clin Med 123:660–667.

116 Brugnara C, Chambers LA, Malynn E, Goldberg MA, Kruskall MS. 1993. Red blood cell regeneration induced by subcutaneous recombinant erythropoietin: Iron-deficient erythropoiesis in iron-replete subjects. Blood 81:956–964.

[117] Biesma D, Van de Wiel A, Beguin Y, Kraaijenhagen R, Marx J. 1994. Erythropoietic activity and iron metabolism in autologous blood donors during recombinant human erythropoietin therapy. Eur J Clin Invest 24:426–432.

[118] Thomas C, Thomas L. 2002. Biochemical markers and hematologic indices in the diagnosis of functional iron deficiency. Clin Chem 48:1066–1076.

[119] Mittman N, Sreedhara R, Mushnick R, et al. 1997. Reticulocyte hemoglobin content predicts functional iron deficiency in hemodialysis patients receiving rHuEPO. Am J Kidney Dis 30(6):912–922.

[120] Mast AE, Blinder MA, Lu Q, Flax S, Dietzen DJ. 2002. Clinical utility of the reticulocyte hemoglobin content in the diagnosis of iron deficiency. Blood 99(4):1489–1491.

[121] Patteril MV, Davey-Quinn AP, Gedney JA, Murdoch SD, Bellamy MC. 2001. Functional iron deficiency, infection and systemic inflammatory response syndrome in critical illness. Anaesth Intensive Care 29:473–478.

[122] Parisotto R, Gore CJ, Emslie KR, et al. 2000. A novel method utilising markers of altered erythropoiesis for the detection of recombinant human erythropoietin abuse in athletes. Haematologica 85:564–572.

[123] Hungerford D, Jr, Linder M. 1983. Interactions of pH and ascorbate in intestinal iron absorption. J Nutr 113:2615–2622.

[124] Plug C, Dekker D, Bult A. 1984. Complex stability of ferrous ascorbate in aqueous solution and its significance for iron absorption. Pharm Weekbl Sci 6:245–258.

[125] Siegenberg D, Baynes R, Bothwell T, et al. 1991. Ascorbic acid prevents the dose-dependent inhibitory effects of polyphenols and phytates on nonheme-iron absorption. Am J Clin Nutr 53:537–541.

[126] Lynch S, Stoltzfus R. 2003. Iron and ascorbic Acid: Proposed fortification levels and recommended iron compounds. J Nutr 133, 2978S–2984S.

[127] Auerbach M, Witt D, Toler W, Fierstein M, Lerner R, Ballard H. 1988. Clinical use of the total dose intravenous infusion of iron dextran. J Lab Clin Med 111:566–570.

[128] Prakash S, Walele A, Dimkovic N, Bargman J, Vas S, Oreopoulos D. 2001. Experience with a large dose (500 mg) of intravenous iron dextran and iron saccharate in peritoneal dialysis patients. Perit Dial Int 21:290–295.

[129] Fuller J, Williams H, McRorie T. 1988. Necrotic bilateral buttocks ulcerations occurring after multiple intramuscular iron dextran injections. Arch Dermatol 124:1722–1723.

[130] Auerbach M, Chaudhry M, Goldman H, Ballard H. 1998. Value of methylprednisolone in prevention of the arthralgia-myalgia syndrome associated with the total dose infusion of iron dextran: A double blind randomized trial. J Lab Clin Med 131:257–260.

[131] Kanakakorn K, Cavill I, Jacobs A. 1973. The metabolism of intravenously administered iron-dextran. Br J Haematol 25:637–643.

[132] Duke A, Kelleher J. 1974. Serum iron and iron binding capacity after total dose infusion of iron-dextran for iron deficiency anaemia in pregnancy. J Obstet Gynaecol Br Commonw 81:895–900.

[133] Van Wyck D, Cavallo G, Spinowitz B, et al. 2000. Safety and efficacy of iron sucrose in patients sensitive to iron dextran: North American clinical trial. Am J Kidney Dis 36:88–97.

[134] Finch C. 1994. Regulators of iron balance in humans. Blood 84:1697–1702.

[135] Ganz T. 2003. Hepcidin, a key regulator of iron metabolism and mediator of anemia of inflammation. Blood 102:783–788.

[136] Park CH, Valore EV, Waring AJ, Ganz T. 2001. Hepcidin, a urinary antimicrobial peptide synthesized in the liver. J Biol Chem 276:7806–7810.

[137] Krause A, Neitz S, Magert HJ, et al. 2000. LEAP-1, a novel highly disulfide-bonded human peptide, exhibits antimicrobial activity. FEBS Lett 480:147–150.

[138] Nemeth E, Valore EV, Territo M, Schiller G, Lichtenstein A, Ganz T. 2003. Hepcidin, a putative mediator of anemia of inflammation, is a type II acute-phase protein. Blood 101:2461–2463.

[139] Weiss G, Goodnough LT. 2005. Anemia of chronic disease. NEJM 352:1011–1023.

NUTRITIONAL ANEMIAS

■ **COBALAMIN AND FOLATE DEFICIENCY**

Deficiencies of cobalamin (vitamin B_{12}) or folate produce some of the most insidious yet dramatic cases of anemia seen in medicine. Complaints of modest fatigue and shortness of breath can belie a hemoglobin value of 3 g/dL. The decline from normal hemoglobin values to levels barely compatible with life reflects the slow evolution of anemia, particularly with cobalamin deficiency. The extended time over which the anemia develops allows compensatory adjustments that sustain the patients, the most important of which is plasma volume expansion. The vitamins are vital to a host of metabolic activities, meaning that anemia never exists in isolation. Low hemoglobin values are often a smoky pall, concealing an inferno that threatens to consume the patient from within. Early extinction of the flame prevents morbidity and irreversible injury.

Since they are vitamins, both cobalamin and folate are dietary essentials. Each produces anemia with similar characteristics, reflecting metabolic pathways common to both. Impaired DNA synthesis is the nexus of deficiency of either vitamin with a consequent imbalance between nuclear and cytoplasmic maturation in developing hematopoietic cells. The morphological aberrations in developing cells, termed "megaloblastic" maturation, are hallmarks of cobalamin or folate deficiency. Despite hematological similarities that can sometimes cause diagnostic confusion, deficiencies of cobalamin or folate differ vastly with respect to mode of onset and associated nonhematological manifestations. Correct diagnosis and treatment can be the difference between life and death.

Many if not most clinical disorders are initially discovered in their most extreme form. Milder variations surface as physicians expand their ken with respect to the disease process. Cobalamin and folate deficiency fits this pattern. The severe deficiency that first brought attention to cobalamin was called pernicious anemia, reflecting the invariably fatal nature of the condition. Today the medical community has broadened its concern to include possible problems produced by modest deficits of cobalamin or folate. In fact, uncertainty now exists as to the values that should encompass the "normal" serum ranges for these vitamins. Decisions concerning these questions will be vital to the health not only of the individuals but also whole populations.

COBALAMIN

Clinical Presentation of Cobalamin Deficiency

Although cobalamin deficiency can produce a host of problems, symptoms associated with anemia most often bring patients to medical attention. Fatigue, shortness of breath, light-headedness, and complaints of palpitations are common but nonspecific indications of depressed hemoglobin values. Furthermore, patients sometimes feel depressed or "all in." A sibilant sound in the ears particularly at night often is a bothersome feature that reflects blood whizzing through the great arteries of the cranium due to the severe anemia. Ankle swelling or edema occurs in some patients, particularly those with a history of cardiac insufficiency. The severe anemia can produce angina in patients with atherosclerotic coronary artery disease as the low hemoglobin value teams with the fixed obstruction to blood flow to produce cardiac ischemia.

Neurological disturbances in conjunction with anemia are a singular aspect of cobalamin deficiency that distinguishes this condition from folate deficiency. Anemia and neurological abnormalities are not directly linked, meaning that some patients with severe anemia due to cobalamin deficiency have no neurological problems. Conversely, neurological damage due to insufficient cobalamin can arise in the absence of anemia. Patient complaints often center on numbness and paresthesias in the feet and sometimes the fingers. Touching coarse surfaces such as an emery board can elicit exquisitely unpleasant sensations. Some patients develop an unsteady gait that can degenerate into spastic ataxia, particularly with severe and advanced cases of cobalamin deficiency.

Forgetfulness and inability to concentrate are problems that sometimes surface only with careful questioning. Family members often notice that the patient has

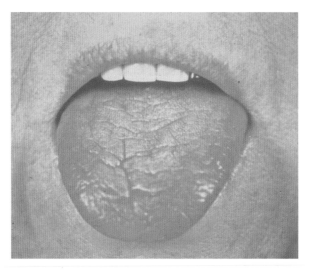

FIGURE 8–1 *Glossitis with cobalamin deficiency. The smooth shiny tongue results from loss of papillae over the lingual surface. Thinning of the epithelium sometimes gives the tongue a red "beefy" appearance.*

become more irritable and emotionally labile. These problems reflect the diffuse neurocognitive disturbances that can arise with cobalamin deficiency. Such disturbances along with the paranoia that sometimes arises create a picture that resembles Alzheimer's disease, adding another source of possible diagnostic confusion.

Physical examination produces findings often useful to diagnosis. Occasional patients develop an enlarged, smooth, and shiny tongue (Figure 8-1). The peculiar appearance of the organ reflects the loss of papillae over the surface of the tongue as part of the general injury to gastrointestinal epithelial cells. The changes often are most apparent at the tip of the tongue and along the sides. In contrast to the situation with folate deficiency, glossitis or soreness usually does not arise in association with these changes in patients with cobalamin deficiency.

Extreme pallor reflects the very low hemoglobin level. The manifestation is most apparent in patients with light complexion. In patients with dark skin, pallor is most readily visible in the mucous membranes, conjunctivae, and nail beds. Close examination often reveals mild or modest jaundice along with scleral icterus due to low-grade hemolysis. A rapid and bounding pulse reflects the severity of the anemia, as does the flow murmur common to the cardiac examination. Cobalamin deficiency does not produce palpable splenomegaly, although noninvasive examinations such as liver–spleen scan usually show enlargement of the organ. Dependent edema is another manifestation of severe anemia which underlying congestive heart failure can magnify substantially.

A less common abnormality associated with cobalamin deficiency is retinal hemorrhage. This injury can occur with any extreme anemia. The lesions often develop in the retinal periphery and elude detection in the absence of indirect ophthalmoscopy.

Optic atrophy is a rare complication limited to the most extreme cases of cobalamin deficiency.

Neurological examination at times uncovers reduced pain sense and dysesthesia in the feet and toes. Diminished proprioception commonly accompanies these disturbances. Loss of vibration sense often occurs in only a few toes, but can encompass the entire foot with more severe neurological injury. Patients are unable to perform heel-to-toe walking and the Romberg test is positive. Spasticity and hyperactive reflexes can develop in advanced cases of cobalamin-induced neurological injury.

Cognitive defects most commonly manifest as short-term memory deficits. Simple maneuvers, such as having the patient repeat a series of words in reverse order, can highlight the problems. Some people with neurocognitive deficits have difficulty recalling at the end of the examination three words they were asked to memorize at the start. During the history taking, patients can show loose associations in their train of thought or forget the topic of a question after they begin the answer.

Peripheral Blood Smear

Cobalamin deficiency produces a strikingly abnormal peripheral blood smear with changes in all three cell lines (Table 8-1). The characteristically large red cells vary tremendously in size with some nearly double the size of normal erythrocytes (Figure 8-2). Typically the cells are also oval shaped. These "macroovalocytes" are classical manifestations of cobalamin deficiency. Macroovalocytes also occur with folate deficiency and do not distinguish deficits of the two vitamins.

Sometimes the anemia is erroneously labeled as "megaloblastic" on the basis of erythrocyte size. The condition is properly termed "macrocytic" anemia. "Megaloblastic" is the description applied to the aberrant pattern of hematopoietic cell maturation seen on bone marrow examination. In the absence of bone marrow examination, the peripheral smear associated with cobalamin deficiency can only be called macrocytic. An exception occasionally occurs with nucleated red cells in the peripheral blood. Some of theses cells can be identified as megaloblastic normoblasts, allowing proper use of the designation "megaloblastic" anemia.

TABLE 8-1	PROMINENT PERIPHERAL BLOOD CHANGES WITH DEFICIENCY OF COBALAMIN OR FOLATE
Red Cells	• Macroovalocytes • Howell-Jolly bodies • Coarse basophilic stippling • Megaloblastic nucleated red cells
Neutrophils	• Hypersegmented neutrophils (6 or more lobes) • Giant neutrophils
Platelets	• Giant platelets

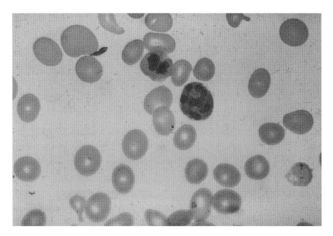

FIGURE 8–2   *Peripheral blood in megaloblastic anemia. The red cells are large and have an oval shape. The most striking feature is the neutrophil with seven nuclear lobes. The nucleated red cell has two irregular nuclei while other cells have Howell-Jolly bodies.*

The potpourri of peripheral blood erythrocytes includes teardrop forms, cell fragments, and even microspherocytes on occasion. Howell-Jolly bodies are common as is coarse basophilic stippling. Polychromatic erythrocytes, the characteristic appearance of reticulocytes on Wright Geimsa staining, are infrequent. Staining with new methylene blue, a procedure that directly highlights reticulocytes, confirms the dearth of these cells. A plethora of peripheral blood nucleated red cells with megaloblastic features sometimes occurs with cobalamin deficiency. The large number of immature nucleated cells in the peripheral blood has led at times to an incorrect preliminary diagnosis of leukemia. Further testing quickly corrects this misimpression.

Peripheral blood neutrophils are as striking in appearance as are the erythrocytes. Although the cells are large, the most prominent feature is a nucleus with numerous lobes (Figure 8-2). Rather than the usual three or four segments, cells with five or six lobes occur commonly with cobalamin deficiency. Rare cells have as many as twelve lobes. Normally, four or more segments occur in fewer than 5% of neutrophils. The color and pattern of cytoplasmic granulation within the neutrophils is normal despite the nuclear aberrations. In the sequence of events that characterize evolving cobalamin deficiency, hypersegmented neutrophils usually appear in the peripheral blood before the red cell macroovalocytes.

Cobalamin deficiency commonly depresses the number of peripheral blood platelets. Except in extreme cases, however, the low number of platelets is apparent only with close examination of the peripheral smear. Some of the platelets are large with bizarre morphology.

Laboratory Values

Cobalamin deficiency profoundly alters the CBC. Impaired erythrocyte production dramatically lowers the total red cell count, hemoglobin, and hematocrit. The large size of the red cells translates into MCV values that routinely exceed 110 fL and sometimes reach levels as high as 140 fL. Extremely high RDW values reflect the variable size and shape of the erythrocytes produced in the face of cobalamin deficiency. Depressed reticulocyte values, sometimes lower than 30,000 cells per cubic millimeter in the face of extremely low hemoglobin levels, are an invariant feature of cobalamin deficiency. Nucleated red cells appear in the peripheral blood with more severe cases of cobalamin deficit.

Although the neutrophil counts are less severely affected than are those of the erythrocytes, values are often depressed particularly with severe cobalamin deficiency. Peripheral blood nucleated red cells can raise the total nucleated blood cell count determined by automated cell analysis, but a correction will show the low number of neutrophils. Mild to modest thrombocytopenia is another feature common to the condition.

A low-serum haptoglobin level reflects both the ineffective erythropoiesis and mild hemolysis that exist with cobalamin deficiency. These abnormalities also substantially raise the serum LDH level. The serum iron value is high along with the transferrin saturation. These changes reflect the poor incorporation of iron into hemoglobin due to laggardly erythropoiesis. Also, much of the iron that accumulates in the marrow reticuloendothelial (RE) cells due to ineffective erythropoiesis recycles quickly back onto transferrin, helping to keep the saturation value high.

Diagnosis of Cobalamin Deficiency

Measurement of the quantity of cobalamin in the plasma was the first test used to assess cobalamin status and remains to this day the favored approach to the issue (Table 8-2). Although direct determination of serum vitamin levels has clear intellectual appeal, the methodology for the assay has changed drastically over the years, which has unfortunately clouded the meaning of the results. Prior to the 1970s, biological assays were the basis for assessing serum cobalamin levels. The most commonly used technique involved the growth characteristics of the cobalamin-dependent bacterium, *Lactobacillus leichmannii*, in culture medium supplemented with aliquots of patient serum. By current standards the technique was time consuming and labor intensive, with a consequent high cost. On the other hand, the growth assay was well standardized, sensitive, and reproducible.

The advent of the radioimmunoassay (RIA) opened the window to a faster and more cost effective means of assessing serum cobalamin levels. In the best research laboratories, the RIA compared favorably with the biological assay with respect to sensitivity for cobalamin. Problems sometimes arose with specificity because antibody preparations vary between lots, and some bind both cobalamin and metabolically inert cobalamin analogues. The resulting test results overestimated serum cobalamin levels relative to the touchstone biological assay.

An effective alternative to antibodies used intrinsic factor to recognize cobalamin in the radioisotope tag test. This eliminated the issue of antibody variability as well as cobalamin analogues since intrinsic factor is the natural cobalamin binding protein produced by gastric parietal cells (see below). The difficulty in producing

TABLE 8-2 | **DETECTION OF COBALAMIN DEFICIENCY**

Test	Specificity	Sensitivity	Comments
Serum Cobalamin	4+	3+	Multiple immunoassay techniques exist without standardization. Inexpensive.
Plasma methylmalonic acid	3+	4+	Test results changed by renal insufficiency, intravascular volume depletion. Expensive.
Plasma total homocysteine	1+	4+	Test results changed by renal insufficiency, intravascular volume depletion. Exacting sample collection and processing are required.

sufficient intrinsic factor for the procedure limits the degree to which the test is used.

RIA is the more simple approach to radioisotope tag testing for cobalamin and is the almost exclusive method used in commercial laboratories. Standardization does not exist for issues known to alter the effects of RIA such as reaction temperatures, time of incubation, etc. The tests are reproducible for a specific technique, but must be viewed carefully, particularly when comparing results from different times or from different laboratories.

Cobalamin is essential to a number of metabolic pathways as detailed below. Vitamin deficiency impedes these processes, causing an accumulation of intermediary metabolites, some of which spill over into the plasma and urine. These metabolites arise only with functionally important cobalamin deficiency. Clinical situations exist in which the serum cobalamin level is low but the availability of the vitamin for metabolic functions is normal. An example is the rare disorder in which the plasma transport protein for cobalamin, transcobalamin II, is low due to a genetic variation. The serum cobalamin level is low but the functional measures of cobalamin sufficiency are normal and patients experience no problems.

The two metabolites assessed most commonly in this context are plasma methylmalonic acid (MMA) and plasma total homocysteine (tHcy). As indicated in Table 8-2, both are very sensitive to cobalamin deficiency.[1] However, MMA is the more specific of the two. A number of conditions unrelated to cobalamin status perturb tHcy levels, including alcohol abuse, folate deficiency, and a number of drugs. The kidneys are the primary means of clearing both metabolites, meaning that levels are unreliable in the face of renal insufficiency.[2,3] The levels of both MMA and tHcy vary significantly during childhood, meaning that the appropriate age standard must be used for data interpretation.[4]

A reasonable approach to assessing clinical cobalamin status in a patient is to first determine the serum cobalamin level. Patients with the appropriate clinical picture in whom the values are well below the normal range (200 ng/L to 600 ng/L) have cobalamin deficiency and can move on to treatment. Since the standards for serum cobalamin levels are not absolute values and substantial biological variability exists between individuals, the finding of *functional* cobalamin deficiency with serum vitamin levels that are in the "low normal" range is not surprising.[5] Assessment of the plasma MMA in such cases supports or undermines the biological importance of a marginal serum cobalamin level.[6]

In the final analysis, however, the key to the patient assessment is an integrated analysis that includes the overall clinical picture, patient history, and manifestations. One tactic sometimes involves a trial of parenteral cobalamin replacement. The anemia corrects quickly and dramatically in people with clinically significant cobalamin deficiency. Vitamin replacement in such cases is both diagnostic and therapeutic.

Bone Marrow in Cobalamin Deficiency

Cobalamin deficiency strikingly impairs the balance between the maturation of the nucleus and the cytoplasm in rapidly growing cells. The bone marrow hematopoietic cells provide the most vivid examples of aberrations that exist in many tissues. For instance, gastric or duodenal biopsies performed in the past as part of the evaluation of pernicious anemia revealed megaloblastic changes in the rapidly growing enterocytes of the gastrointestinal epithelium. The striking megaloblastic maturation of hematopoietic cells is typical of cobalamin deficiency but not diagnostic. Folate deficit produces identical bone marrow changes. Other conditions, such as myeloproliferative disorders, produce some megaloblastic alterations in maturing hematopoietic cells, but never to the extent seen with cobalamin or folate deficiency.

Not surprisingly, megaloblastic changes are particularly dramatic in cells further along the developmental pathway since more time has elapsed to permit divergence in the degree of nuclear and cytoplasmic maturation. The earliest cells in the erythroid pathway, proerythroblasts, are slightly larger than normal but are otherwise relatively unremarkable. Dramatic deviations from normal maturation occur in the middle and late normoblasts. The cells are large and often oblong with sometimes gargantuan nuclei. The nuclear chromatin has a speckled pattern with an appearance resembling ground glass, which is called an "open chromatin" pattern (Figure 8-3). The changes reflect delayed DNA production due to a dearth of deoxyribonucleotides. Irregular regions of chromatin condensation coexist within the overall flecked pattern of the nuclei. Small, condensed segments often fragment from the nucleus, producing Howell-Jolly bodies.

Impaired nuclear maturation reduces the viability of these late erythroid cells, leading to their destruction within the bone marrow. The early death of erythroid cells is the basis of the marked ineffective erythropoiesis characteristic of cobalamin deficiency. The large number of normoblasts in the marrow with stalled maturation produces a myeloid-to-erythroid ratio (M:E ratio) close to 1:1 rather than the typical 5:1 ratio. The overall cellularity of the marrow is high for the same reason. The small

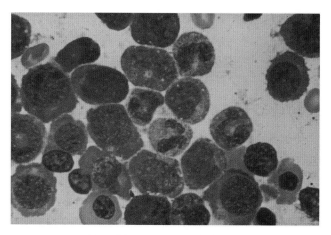

FIGURE 8–3   *Bone Marrow in megaloblastic anemia. The dissociation between nuclear and cytoplasmic development is most striking in the erythroid precursors. Some of the late normoblasts have open nuclear chromatin along with abundant hemoglobin in the cytoplasm. Many of the cells have irregular, ragged-appearing edges.*

trickle of late normoblasts that complete maturation accounts for the extremely low peripheral blood reticulocyte count.

As these sickly cells approach their demise, bare nuclei break free into the marrow stroma. Marrow RE cells consume cell remnants and in the process accumulate large quantities of iron through digestion of hemoglobin from the senescent cells. Perl's Prussian blue staining of the marrow shows substantial iron accumulation in these fixed tissue macrophages. Small quantities of hemoglobin escape into the plasma during phagocytosis of the moribund normoblasts. Plasma haptoglobin clears this hemoglobin, producing the low serum haptoglobin levels characteristic of cobalamin deficiency.

Myeloid cells also acquire striking megaloblastic characteristics during maturation. Giant metamyelocytes and bands are the centerpieces of megaloblastic myeloid maturation. The nuclei of these commonly colossal cells have a mottled pattern similar to that seen in the erythroid series. Vacuoles are frequent features, along with bizarre misshapen cellular morphology. Nucleoli often exist even at relatively late developmental stages. When assessed, granulopoiesis also proves to be ineffective in the setting of cobalamin deficiency. The low peripheral blood neutrophil count typical of cobalamin deficiency results directly from these problems with maturation.

The megaloblastic features of megakaryocytes are often more difficult to appreciate than those of the two other cell lines, perhaps due to the intrinsic irregularity of these cells. However, some cells demonstrate peculiar patterns of nuclear hypersegmentation. Large segments of megakaryocytes can separate from the main cell body producing the giant platelets or megakaryocytic fragments often seen in the peripheral blood.

Cobalamin Biology

Cobalamin is a dietary essential with an obligate daily requirement of about 3μg. The primary sources of the vitamin are meats, milk, and other foods of animal origin. Cobalamin absorption from the gastrointestinal tract involves a series of complex steps beginning in the stomach. Gastric acidity promotes separation of cobalamin from the constituents of ingested food. A polypeptide called an R protein initially binds the vitamin. Pepsin in the stomach and upper duodenum subsequently releases cobalamin from the R protein.

Gastric parietal cells produce intrinsic factor, a protein with both a high binding affinity and specificity for the vitamin. Intrinsic factor couples cobalamin following its release from the R protein and shepherds the vitamin in its journey through the small intestine. Receptors for intrinsic factor in the epithelial cells of the terminal ileum mediate uptake of the vitamin and delivery to the plasma transport protein, transcobalamin II (TCII).[7] A second binding protein in the plasma, transcobalamin I (TCI), has a greater capacity for cobalamin but does not mediate cellular vitamin uptake, as does TCII.

Free cobalamin can cross the gastrointestinal tract by passive diffusion. Not surprisingly, the process is far less efficient than that mediated by intrinsic factor, encompassing about 1% of the total quantity of ingested vitamin. Consumption of pharmacological quantities of cobalamin can provide minimal amounts of vitamin by passive uptake, but in general is not a recommended means of cobalamin replacement.

Following its transit through the circulation, the TCII/cobalamin complex binds to a specific cell surface receptor and is taken up by receptor-mediated endocytosis (Figure 8-4). Following fusion of the endosome with a lysosome, cobalamin separates from TCII and traverses the lysosomal membrane to enter the cytoplasm proper. Two important and independent metabolic pathways exist for cobalamin, one in the cytoplasm and the other in mitochondria. Mitochondrial cobalamin is converted to adenosylcobalamin (Adocbl), which is a cofactor in the conversion of methylmalonyl-CoA to succinyl-CoA. The conversion does not occur with cobalamin deficiency, producing a build up of methylmalonyl-CoA in the cell. This metabolite is the source of the elevated plasma MMA levels seen with cobalamin deficiency.

Cytoplasmic cobalamin enters a complex series of reactions as outlined in Figure 8-4. As seen on the right hand side of the figure, conversion of homocysteine to methionine depends on the smooth operation of these metabolic pathways. Cobalamin deficiency disrupts the cycle, leading to the accumulation of homocysteine in the cell. This metabolite is the source of the elevated plasma homocysteine levels seen with cobalamin deficiency. Neither methylmalonyl-CoA nor homocysteine accumulates if the cell has sufficient cobalamin, irrespective of the plasma level of the vitamin. Plasma MMA and tHcy are thus markers of cellular cobalamin sufficiency for essential metabolic pathways.

For the sake of clarity, Figure 8-4 does not include the many important metabolic steps that branch out from those shown. For instance, the synthesis of dTMP for DNA production critically depends on cobalamin metabolism. The delay in nuclear

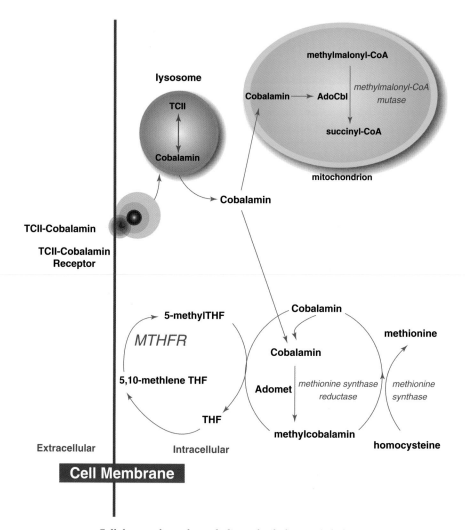

FIGURE 8–4 *Cellular uptake and metabolism of cobalamin. Cobalamin travels in the circulation as a complex with transcobalamin II (TCII). Cell surface receptors for the complex mediate its internalization and fusion with lysosomes. Cobalamin separates from TCII within the lysosome and translocates to the cytosol proper. A fraction of the vitamin cohort enters mitochondria. Following conversion to adenosylcobalamin (AdoCbl), the vitamin participates in metabolic reactions that include the conversion of methylmalonyl-CoA to succinyl-CoA. Cobalamin deficiency delays this conversion with the consequent accumulation of methylmalonyl-CoA. Its derivative, methylmalonic acid (MMA), spills into the blood and reflects functional cobalamin deficiency. Cytosolic cobalamin participates in a number of reactions that are key to the production of substrate for DNA synthesis. As shown in the lower right figure, methionine synthase converts homocysteine to methionine in one of the coupled reactions in the process. Cobalamin deficiency causes an accumulation of homocysteine that also spills into the blood. Adocbl, adenosylcobalamin; Adomet, S-adenosylmethionine; THF, tetrahydrofolate; 5-methyl-THF, methyltetrahydrofolate; TCII, transcobalamin II.*

maturation that characterizes megaloblastic cell maturation reflects impaired DNA synthesis due to the shortage of deoxyribonucleotides.

Healthy people have substantial body stores of cobalamin usually in the range of 3,000–4,000 μg. Since the daily requirement for the vitamin approximates 3 μg, the storage depot would suffice for several years even with absolutely no cobalamin intake. More than half of the vitamin reserves exist in the liver. The rich liver content of cobalamin was the basis of the Nobel Prize winning observation by Minot and Murphy that meals heavy in liver content averted the otherwise invariably fatal course of pernicious anemia.[8] The mass action absorption of a fraction of the immense quantity of cobalamin in these diets rescued the heretofore doomed patients.

Etiology of Cobalamin Deficiency

Cobalamin deficiency derives from a failure to get the vitamin into the body from dietary components. The Institute of Medicine's Food and Nutrition Board recommends a daily cobalamin allowance of 2.4 μg. Cobalamin deficiency due to low vitamin content in food occurs only with strict vegetarians who also abstain from eggs and milk (vegans), but is uncommon even in this selected group of people. On rare occasion, deficiency arises in vegetarians who are less strict but who cook their eggs and milk. Heating can destroy up to half the cobalamin in these foods, placing people with precarious intakes at risk of vitamin deficiency.

In nonvegetarians, cobalamin deficiency results almost invariably from defective operation of the complex processes required for vitamin absorption. Of these cases, the vast bulk relate to problems surrounding the stomach and its role in cobalamin absorption. Pernicious anemia, the clinical condition that prompted the work leading to the discovery of cobalamin, arises from an autoimmune process that destroys the cells in the stomach that normally produce gastric acid and intrinsic factor. The gastritis associated with the injury is designated "type A." The more common form of gastritis that impairs cobalamin uptake is designated "type B" and is associated with a degenerative and erosive process that commonly includes *Helicobacter pylori* infection. The specific factors that produce cobalamin deficiency differ in the two conditions, as does the severity of the vitamin deficit.

Pernicious Anemia.   Pernicious anemia is an autoimmune process in which antibodies directed against the gastric parietal cells trigger an inflammatory response that produces chronic atrophic gastritis. A hereditary predisposition to the disorder exists with some studies showing pernicious anemia in one-fifth of the siblings of probands with the condition. The frequent occurrence of serum antibodies to gastric parietal cells in relatives without pernicious anemia also supports the hereditary nature of the condition.

Pernicious anemia sometimes appears in association with other autoimmune conditions. Autoantibodies to thyroid tissue are common. Clinically apparent autoimmune disease, such as Hashimoto's thyroiditis, hypothyroidism, and Addison's disease coexist in some patients.[9,10] Vitiligo due to autoantibodies directed against melanin-producing cells in the skin occasionally also coexists with pernicious anemia.[11] The basis of these associations is unknown. Pernicious anemia also arises in a significant fraction of patients with polyglandular Glandular Syndrome Type I, an autoimmune condition with failure of multiple endocrine glands.

The fundus and body of the stomach are the primary regions of disease involvement with pernicious anemia. The loss of the parietal cells lowers acid secretion into the stomach in addition to reducing the production of intrinsic factor. These disturbances have multiple effects on cobalamin uptake.

Gastric acidity promotes cobalamin separation from the structural components of food, which is necessary to the ultimate formation of the complex between cobalamin and intrinsic factor. Gastric achlorhydria in pernicious anemia impairs this activity. Some of the cobalamin in food therefore passes through the gastrointestinal tract with no chance of uptake.

The deficit of intrinsic factor is, of course, the major problem that impairs cobalamin absorption in people with pernicious anemia. Without this protein the receptors in the terminal ileum neither recognize cobalamin nor promote its uptake. The autoimmune process can also generate antibodies to intrinsic factor that directly block cobalamin binding to the protein. Secretion of these antibodies into the gastric juices further impairs vitamin uptake. These blocking antibodies against intrinsic factor also appear in the blood and are diagnostic of pernicious anemia.

Hyperplasia of gastrin-producing cells also develops with pernicious anemia. High serum gastrin levels along with low serum levels of pepsinogen I and gastric achlorhydria are a frequent triad in pernicious anemia. Biopsy shows inflammation and gastric atrophy particularly in the fundus and body of the stomach.

The portions of the cobalamin absorption mechanism beyond the stomach are normal in patients with pernicious anemia. The receptors in the terminal ileum that recognize the complex between intrinsic factor and cobalamin are fully functional. The impaired uptake of the vitamin reflects solely the lack of intrinsic factor.

Concepts concerning the epidemiology of pernicious anemia have evolved significantly in recent years. Many of the early reports and much of the early work on the condition was done in Scandinavia and the United Kingdom. This research gave the impression that pernicious anemia was most common in people of northern European background. The early hints of a familial predisposition for the disease reinforced this impression. More recent studies show that pernicious anemia occurs in people of all ethnic backgrounds.[12] Studies of larger cohorts are needed to assign more precise risk values to various groups of people. The important fact, however, is that the possibility of pernicious anemia should never be dismissed or downplayed due to ethnic considerations.

Type A chronic atrophic gastritis associated with pernicious anemia often evolves into gastric carcinoma. The relative risk of gastric cancer in patients with pernicious anemia exceeds normal by as much as threefold. Successful replacement of cobalamin does not alter the cancer risk since the atrophic gastritis continues despite this intervention. People with pernicious anemia should be monitored in order to detect any cancer at the earliest stages.

The Schilling test provides unequivocal evidence of pernicious anemia in patients with cobalamin deficiency. A patient with pernicious anemia will not absorb orally administered cobalamin due to the lack of intrinsic factor. On the other hand, the patient will take up cobalamin from an orally administered complex of cobalamin and intrinsic factor since the receptors in the terminal ileum are intact. The Schilling test exploits this difference in the patterns of cobalamin absorption. An abnormal Schilling test in a patient with cobalamin deficiency makes the diagnosis of pernicious anemia.

A large quantity of cobalamin administered parenterally prior to the Schilling test saturates the TCI and TCII carrier proteins. Radiolabeled cobalamin given orally without intrinsic factor passes through the gastrointestinal tract. No label appears in the urine. In contrast, uptake of radiolabeled cobalamin administered as a complex with intrinsic factor is brisk. Since the binding sites on the carrier proteins are already filled with unlabeled cobalamin, a fraction of the labeled vitamin will appear in the urine. Thus, the addition of intrinsic factor to the radiolabeled cobalamin corrects an otherwise abnormal pattern of cobalamin absorption in the Schilling test.

Despite its unparalleled ability to pinpoint pernicious anemia as the basis of cobalamin deficit, the Schilling test has fallen into disuse because it is both cumbersome and expensive. The basic test consumes several days of patient, technician, and physician time with administration of labeled intrinsic factor, collection of urine, and injection of unlabeled intrinsic factor. The logistics of testing requires a skilled technician, a dedicated facility, and expertise in the interpretation of such data. The use of radioactive compounds in the patient setting is an issue of increasing concern and regulation.

Table 8-3 outlines more readily available approaches to the diagnosis of pernicious anemia. Detection of serum antibody to intrinsic factor provides the strongest evidence in favor of pernicious anemia. Elevated serum gastrin levels are common in pernicious anemia as are depressed levels of serum pepsinogen I. Neither finding is unique to pernicious anemia. Coexistence of the two in a suggestive clinical setting supports pernicious anemia as a diagnosis, however. Gastric achlorhydria in the face of histamine stimulation is powerful evidence for pernicious anemia. This approach to diagnosis has also fallen into disuse.

Chronic Atrophic Gastritis.   The most common cause of cobalamin deficit by far is type B chronic atrophic gastritis.[13] The frequency of the condition rises with age and often is associated with *H. pylori* infection.[14] The clinical significance of cobalamin deficit associated with chronic atrophic gastritis is an ongoing topic of debate with a key question being the extent to which the process produces clinically significant cobalamin deficiency.[15,16]

Type B chronic atrophic gastritis is a patchy process that often begins in the antrum of the stomach, but spreads to involve much of the gastric structure. The primary impact is low production of acid and pepsinogen due to invasion of the epithelial lining by inflammatory cells. Type B chronic atrophic gastritis has relatively little impact on the production of intrinsic factor. However, achlorhydria causes suboptimal release of cobalamin from food constituents. Furthermore, cobalamin that is released and initially bound by R proteins is not then properly transferred to intrinsic factor due to the depressed pepsin levels in the gastric juices.

TABLE 8-3	DIAGNOSIS OF PERNICIOUS ANEMIA
Test	*Comment*
Schilling test	Once the gold standard in the diagnosis of pernicious anemia, the test in now rarely performed. Extensive time requirements and the use of radioactive intrinsic factor make the test very expensive. Radiation in the urine and feces creates extreme logistical difficulties.
Antibody to intrinsic factor	Commonly elevated and diagnostic of pernicious anemia when present.
Serum gastrin	Elevated in most cases of pernicious anemia. Not specific to pernicious anemia.
Serum pepsinogen I	Depressed in most cases of pernicious anemia. Not specific to pernicious anemia.
Gastric achlorhydria with histamine stimulation	Strongly supportive of pernicious anemia. Rarely performed.

Type B chronic atrophic gastritis therefore manifests most strikingly as impaired uptake of food-bound cobalamin. Administration of crystalline cobalamin alone produces a normal pattern of vitamin uptake. This result indicates that the patients have relatively normal baseline production of intrinsic factor. With oral administration of preformed cobalamin and intrinsic factor also, patients show a normal pattern of vitamin uptake. This reaffirms the normal operation of the cobalamin uptake machinery in the terminal ileum. Interestingly, some patients with severe malabsorption of food cobalamin have relatively little in the way of atrophic gastritis.[17]

Uptake of labeled cobalamin from food sources typically is low, however, due to the impaired separation of cobalamin from the food components. Assessment of the absorption of food-bound cobalamin usually involves mixing radiolabeled vitamin with an egg yolk extract that the patient then consumes. Unfortunately, this technique by and large is a research tool. The diagnosis of food cobalamin malabsorption in a patient with cobalamin deficit usually involves eliminating pernicious anemia by the tests outlined in Table 8-3.

Gastric acid that enters the small intestine is one of the factors that keep the structure relatively free of bacteria. The gastric achlorhydria secondary to type B chronic atrophic gastritis can foster bacterial overgrowth of the small bowel. Many bacteria require cobalamin for proliferation. With overgrowth of the small bowel, these organisms can capture dietary cobalamin before it reaches the terminal ileum, further exacerbating the patient's cobalamin deficit.

The clinical murkiness that surrounds chronic atrophic gastritis and cobalamin deficiency relates to the common occurrence of this gastric abnormality in older adults along with the fact that most affected people do not have a cobalamin deficit. The important question is which subgroup in a large population that could number millions is at risk of clinically important cobalamin deficiency.[18] Serum cobalamin levels decline with age while MMA levels increase. Studies that combine assays of serum cobalamin with measurements either of MMA or tHcy often show evidence of functional cobalamin deficiency in 10–15% of subjects 65 years of age or older.[19] The subjects lack hematological or neurological manifestation that would have attracted clinical attention. The answer to the critical question of whether subclinical cobalamin deficiency of this type will evolve to produce significant morbidity awaits further investigation.

Structural Defects in the Gastrointestinal Tract.   A variety of defects involving the gastrointestinal tract can impair cobalamin uptake. Surgical interventions that can produce cobalamin deficiency include partial (or total) gastrectomy, vagotomy, and resection of the terminal ileum.[20] The latter intervention removes the absorption site for the intrinsic factor/cobalamin complex. The first two interventions markedly diminish or eliminate acid production and intrinsic factor by the stomach, producing the problems with cobalamin absorption reviewed earlier.[21] Both surgical procedures are now rare, as the severe peptic ulcer disease for which they were once used fortunately has more palatable alternatives. A key point with these patients is to remember that they are at risk of cobalamin deficiency since the onset can occur years after the surgical procedure.

Blind loops of small bowel sometimes harbor regions with bacterial overgrowth that produce cobalamin deficiency. These structures sometimes remain following emergency surgery for blunt abdominal trauma, such as might occur with a motor vehicle accident. A blind loop of bowel is a minor issue during the emergency surgery where the patient's life might be at issue. The cobalamin deficit then appears years later after the surgery and the blind loop is forgotten. Most often the patient presents to an internist whose ability to piece the puzzle together depends greatly on a detailed history.

Inflammatory disease of the small bowel produces cobalamin deficiency on occasion. Crohn's disease particularly affects the upper colon and terminal ileum, placing patients at risk of cobalamin deficiency. Gluten-sensitive enteropathy (Celiac disease) is an often more subtle condition that produces small bowel inflammation. Cobalamin deficiency is uncommon in patients with the disorder, fortunately. With either Crohn's disease or gluten-sensitive enteropathy, the associated cobalamin deficiency is one of the many metabolic disturbances.

Other Causes of Cobalamin Deficiency.   Dietary deficiency is a rare cause of cobalamin deficiency in adults, occurring in strict vegetarians (vegans) if at all. In contrast, dietary deficit is the most common cause of cobalamin deficiency among infants and neonates.[22] The affected child usually is breastfed after being born to a mother who is a vegan or who has pernicious anemia. Often the mother has borderline vitamin deficiency without clinical manifestations of cobalamin deficit. Breast milk does not replete the low body cobalamin stores in the newborn. Rapid growth during infancy consumes cobalamin at a prodigious rate that cannot be sustained in the face of marginal stores and meager intake. Clinical manifestations arise within a few months of birth. Low birth weight infants are also at risk of cobalamin deficiency.[23]

Delay in developmental progression or developmental regression most commonly brings the child to clinical attention, usually some months after birth.[24] Some infants develop movement disorders as well. Others are labeled as "failure to thrive," with the correct diagnosis remaining elusive for months. A variable degree of pancytopenia usually points to a hematological disturbance in the child. Subsequent work-up that includes a serum cobalamin level leads to the correct diagnosis. Assay for MMA or tHcy can help with the diagnosis but usually is not required.[25]

The Imerslund-Gräsbeck syndrome is an autosomal recessive disorder in which patients fail to absorb the complex of intrinsic factor and cobalamin. The problem reflects diminished or absent expression of the receptor for this complex in the terminal ileum. Although initial descriptions of the disorder involved children between the ages of 1 and 5 years, some reports describe an initial onset and diagnosis in older children. Reports of the condition exist for people of various racial and ethnic backgrounds. In addition to megaloblastic anemia, proteinuria of varying severity is virtually universal in patients with the Imerslund-Gräsbeck syndrome.

Imerslund-Gräsbeck syndrome arises from defects involving either of the proteins cubilin or amnionless (AMN).[26] Cubilin is the ileal receptor for the intrinsic factor/cobalamin complex.[27] However, cubilin alone does not foster receptor-mediated endocytosis of the complex. AMN associates with cubilin to form the functionally competent receptor that ushers the intrinsic factor/cobalamin complex into the enterocyte for subsequent delivery to TCII.[28]

A less well-characterized form of cobalamin deficiency that occurs in children has been termed "juvenile/congenital pernicious anemia."[29] The central defect is failure to secrete intrinsic factor into the gastric juices. The disorder differs from true pernicious anemia in its lack of an autoimmune component and its autosomal recessive mode of inheritance.[30] Interestingly, following the initial reports involving young children, the disorder is now discovered occasionally in older children and even adults.[31] The clinical syndrome might, in fact, be a cluster of disorders with different causes for failed secretion of intrinsic factor.[32]

Treatment of Cobalamin Deficiency.   With rare exceptions, such as deficiency of TCII, parenteral replacement corrects cobalamin deficiency. One effective approach to cobalamin replacement is administration of 1000 μg of the vitamin weekly for 4 weeks followed by monthly injections of 1000 μg. The initial retention of the replacement dose is only about 15% with the excess spilling into the urine. However, the vitamin is inexpensive and the surplus produces no problems. Failure to adequately replace cobalamin, in contrast, is a serious issue.

Cobalamin replacement in a patient with a deficit of the vitamin produces one of the most exuberant examples of erythropoiesis in medicine. The reticulocyte count rises within 3 days and peaks by 5 or 6 days with values that can approach 40%. The hemoglobin value can double in 10 days. The achlorhydria associated with cobalamin deficiency also dampens iron absorption and creates a cryptic iron deficit (see Chapter 7). The serum iron level and transferrin saturation can drop precipitously as the luxuriant erythropoiesis commandeers iron from the circulation. The accelerated erythropoiesis unmasks previously unrecognized iron deficiency that was obscured by the artifactually high transferrin saturation. Iron replacement is essential when a combined nutritional deficit exists.[33]

Rapid correction of the anemia in patients with cobalamin deficiency obviates the need for transfusion except in the most dire of circumstances. Furthermore, transfusion can be dangerous. The plasma volume greatly expands in the face of the severe anemia. Transfusion further increases the intravascular volume and can push a patient into congestive heart failure. The need for transfusion hinges on the patient's clinical status rather than on an arbitrary hemoglobin value. When transfusions are pursued, the procedure should be conducted slowly and with careful patient monitoring.

Oral cobalamin replacement is a delicate issue. Debate usually focuses on older people with poor absorption of food cobalamin, most often as a result of type B chronic atrophic gastritis. In theory, orally administered crystalline cobalamin should correct the deficit. However, a number of problems exist with this approach in practice. Almost no patient undergoes the food cobalamin absorption test that would definitively establish the basis of the cobalamin deficiency. Furthermore, proof that a patient absorbs crystalline cobalamin requires a modified Schilling test, which largely is unavailable. The diagnosis of food cobalamin malabsorption is usually presumptive, based on indirect evidence such as the lack of antibody to intrinsic factor. The risk of erroneous assignment is real and the consequence of error is great. Parenteral replacement is the method of choice for cobalamin deficiency irrespective of etiology.

FOLATE

Clinical Presentation of Folate Deficiency

With a few important exceptions, the clinical presentation of folate deficiency parallels that of cobalamin deficiency. Megaloblastic anemia dominates the picture. Painful glossitis occurs more commonly than with cobalamin deficiency. Painful cheilosis or angular stomatitis also arises with deficiency of the vitamin.

The most striking departure between the clinical presentations of cobalamin and folate deficiency is the lack of neurological manifestations in the latter. Patients with folate deficiency who also have the neurological manifestations seen with cobalamin deficiency must be assumed to have concomitant cobalamin deficiency until proven otherwise. The point is singularly important since folate replacement in a patient who has cobalamin deficiency can transiently ameliorate the hematological picture while irreversible neurological injury continues apace.

Diagnosis of Folate Deficiency

Demonstration of low levels of the vitamin in a clinical setting consistent with deficit is the key to the diagnosis of folate deficiency. Folate levels can be measured in the serum or in red cells.[34] Both are low in patients with untreated folate deficiency. A good meal or a folate replacement tablet raises the serum folate within a few hours, which can complicate the issue of folate status in a patient undergoing evaluation. Assessment of red cell folate can be valuable in such circumstances. Red cells contain only the folate present at the time of their release from the bone marrow. In a patient who has received partial folate replacement, the red cell folate is below normal and will remain so until the cohort of older cells is removed from the circulation.

The total serum homocysteine level increases substantially in the face of folate deficiency. Assay of this metabolite is not essential to the diagnosis of folate deficiency. However, assessment of the basis of elevated total serum homocysteine levels has assumed great importance, particularly since the demonstration that high serum homocysteine levels are a risk factor for cardiovascular disease.[35] An evaluation of cardiac risk factors that includes assay of serum tHcy levels should include simultaneous assessment of serum folate values.

Folate Biology

Folate is a water-soluble B vitamin encompassing a family of structurally related molecules that are necessary cofactors for the synthesis of purine and thymidine nucleotides as well as the conversion of homocysteine to methionine.[36] The key pteroyl residue in folate has an attached glutamate chain that varies in length between two and nine residues. In an interesting dichotomy of structure and function, the monoglutamate form of the vitamin can be transported across cell membranes but is metabolically mute. In contrast, the polyglutamates are metabolically active but cannot cross cell membranes. These facts provide an efficient way of maintaining cellular glutamate levels. Cleavage of the polyglutamate chain outside the cell to produce folate monoglutamate allows vitamin uptake followed by quick conversion back to folate polyglutamate once inside the cell (Figure 8-5). The cell thus traps the folate needed for metabolic function.

Most folate is the product of plant or microorganism metabolism, making fresh fruits and vegetables excellent sources of the vitamin. Natural folates are labile, meaning that cooked fruits and vegetables have significantly less folate than do their fresh counterparts. Liver also contains a substantial amount of folate reflecting vitamin storage by this organ.

Folate absorption occurs along the length of the small bowel, but activity is greatest in the upper jejunum. Brush border enzymes convert the folate polyglutamates to the monoglutamate form required for absorption. The vitamin is shuttled to the plasma for transport.

Two mechanisms exist for cellular uptake of plasma folate (Figure 8-5). A folate binding protein on the plasma membrane brings the vitamin within the cell by receptor-mediated endocytosis. The plasma membrane also contains a reduced

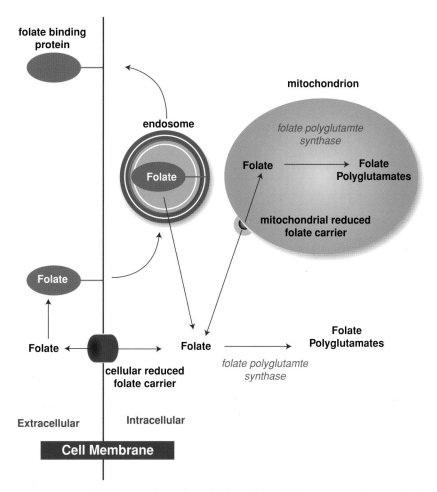

FIGURE 8–5 *Cellular uptake and metabolism of folate. Cells accumulate folate either by the folate binding protein and receptor-mediated endocytosis or a bidirectional cellular reduced folate carrier. A fraction of the vitamin enters the mitochondrion by way of a mitochondrial specific reduced folate carrier. Folate polyglutamate synthetase converts the vitamin to folate polyglutamates that are confined to the mitochondrion and participate in a host of metabolic reactions. Folate polyglutamate synthetase in the cytosol produces folate polyglutamates that are confined to this compartment and participate in a variety of metabolic functions.*

folate carrier protein that mediates bidirectional transport of the molecule. A portion of the accumulated folate makes an additional step into the mitochondrion by means of a mitochondrial reduced folate carrier. For both the cytoplasm and the mitochondrion, the enzyme folate polyglutamate synthetase traps the vitamin in the respective compartment by converting it to folate polyglutamate. The cytoplasmic and mitochondrial folate pools participate in a variety of metabolic activities and are not in equilibrium.

Most Western diets contain folate in the form of polyglutamates, with quantities of the vitamin ranging between 500 and 1500 μg. The minimum daily requirement is approximately 100 μg, meaning that a comfortable cushion normally exists with respect to folate intake. For adults, the Food and Nutrition Board of the Institute of Medicine sets the recommended daily allowance for folate at 400 μg. The 600-μg RDA during pregnancy reflects the greater folate requirement during this stage of life (see Chapter 4). Lactating women transfer a large amount of folate to their infants.[37] Transfer of folate from mother to infant in women who began the nursing process with marginal folate stores can sometimes exacerbate a vitamin deficit.[38] Furthermore, breast milk from women with a folate deficit has a lower than normal folate content, which potentially places the infant at risk of folate deficiency.[39] Consequently, the recommended daily allowance for lactating women is set at 500 μg.

For newborns, the RDA is 65 μg. The heating of milk that once was used to remove immunogenic proteins, from cow's milk particularly, also destroys folate. Megaloblastic anemia developed in some infants who received this form of sustenance. Fortification of infant formulas with folic acid has eliminated this problem. In children between 1 and 8 years, folate requirements vary between 150 and 200 μg. These quantities provide more folate on a weight basis than is the case for adults, reflecting the greater need for the vitamin during these periods of rapid growth.

A separate issue with respect to folate availability is the problems of neural tube defects that occur early in gestation. Folate is a key factor in early neural development. One of the folate receptors, folate binding protein 1, shows high levels of expression in the neural folds before neural tube closure, suggesting that it plays an important role in this stage of development. An inverse relationship exists between the frequency of neural tube defects and serum folate levels, even within the normal serum range for the vitamin. The possibility exists that low normal serum folate levels in the mother are inadequate to provide quantities of vitamin needed by the embryo for early neural tube development.

Since much of the critical embryology occurs during the first trimester before the pregnancy is appreciated, calls have been made for higher dietary folate intake by females of childbearing age. Food supplementation with folic acid is now common in the United States. The additional folate in the food supply likely will lower both the incidence of neural tube defects among newborns as well as frank folate deficiency in the population as a whole.

Folate stores in adults average approximately 5000 μg with the bulk of the vitamin found in the liver. Stores fall with a folate-deficient diet, and serum levels decline noticeably within a few weeks. Megaloblastic anemia can develop after as few as 4 months of dietary folate insufficiency. This contrasts sharply with the 2–3 year supply of cobalamin in the liver stores.

Etiology of Folate Deficiency

Table 8-4 lists some of the causes of folate deficiency. Inadequate dietary intake of the vitamin is the major culprit. Folate deficiency occurs as part of general protein/calorie malnutrition seen with inadequate availability of food. A more selective form of defi-

TABLE 8-4	CAUSES OF FOLATE DEFICIENCY

Decreased intake
  Dietary
  - General malnutrition
  - Alcoholism
  Impaired Absorption
  - Tropical sprue
  - Celiac disease

Increased requirements
  Infancy
  Pregnancy
  Lactation
  Anticonvulsant drugs
  Folate antagonist drugs
  Chronic exfoliative dermatitis

ciency arises with chronic alcoholism. In people with this disorder, the alcohol usually provides sufficient calories to prevent overall malnutrition. However, an unbalanced diet that often contains little in the way of fresh fruits and vegetables leads to severe folate deficiency. Deficits of other vitamins such as thiamine and riboflavin contribute to the overall grave clinical problems in people afflicted with alcoholism.

Disorders that impair small bowel function can also produce folate deficiency. Since folate is absorbed throughout the length of the small bowel, only disorders that produce diffuse injury and dysfunction cause folate deficiency. This contrasts with the marked disruption of cobalamin absorption that occurs with selective injury to the terminal ileum by disturbances such as Crohn's disease.

Tropical sprue, a mysterious disorder possibly caused by an infectious agent, is common in areas such as the Caribbean, Southeast Asia, and India. People from temperate zones can develop tropical sprue during visits to these regions and the disorder can last for months or even years. The manifestations vary widely, ranging from incapacitating abdominal problems to almost subclinical mildness. Abdominal pain, diarrhea, anorexia, and weight loss are typical of the problems produced by tropical sprue. Defective absorption of fats and carbohydrates lend a frothy, malodorous quality to stools. Malaise and poor food intake add to the folate deficiency produced by malabsorption. Severe megaloblastic anemia is common.

Celiac disease, or gluten-sensitive enteropathy, is an immune-mediated disorder in which proteins from wheat produces trigger a generalized inflammatory reaction in the small bowel. The clinical expression of the disorder varies tremendously. Some people with celiac disease are unaware of its presence due to its mild nature. On questioning, a history often unfolds in which the patient has come unconsciously to avoid food rich in wheat products. Folate deficiency tends to occur with more severe forms of the disease where diarrhea and steatorrhea are prominent.

Table 8-4 also lists conditions that produce folate deficiency by raising demand for the vitamin. Infancy and pregnancy top the list in accord with the earlier discussion of the higher relative need for folate during these stages of life. Lactation produces folate deficit, particularly if a problem with vitamin sufficiency existed during pregnancy.

Textbooks commonly cite hemolytic anemias as a cause of folate deficiency. The data in support of this contention largely come from studies in the early 1960s where the significance of the findings is now questionable. For instance, in retrospect, some of the bone marrow biopsies used in the evaluation of transient aplasia have morphological changes now known to represent infection with parvovirus. A more recent study evaluated the plasma MMA levels in children with sickle cell disease who did not take folic acid.[40] No significant difference existed in the MMA values from this cohort and those of normal controls, suggesting that sickle cell disease per se does not cause metabolically significant folate deficiency. Evaluation of red cell folate values in a subset of the patients likewise showed normal values. The urgency often attached to folate supplementation in patients with hemolytic anemia may not be justified.

A number of anticonvulsant drugs including phenobarbital, phenytoin, and primidone produce mild folate deficiency that occasionally includes megaloblastic anemia. The megaloblastic changes usually develop after years of use, producing a slowly progressive anemia. Folic acid supplementation easily reverses the problem.

Folate antagonist drugs can produce megaloblastic anemia by inhibiting the action of the vitamin. Such agents are used most common for cancer treatment. One drug that is more widely used and can subtly contribute to megaloblastic anemia is methotrexate, a potent inhibitor of dihydrofolate reductase. The drug is an option for treatment of conditions ranging from rheumatoid arthritis to psoriasis and exfoliative dermatitis. The high rate of cell proliferation in conditions such as psoriasis consumes abnormally large quantities of folate. The addition of methotrexate to the scenario can push some patients into a state of frank megaloblastic anemia. Vitamin supplementation easily overcomes the problem.

Treatment of Folate Deficiency

Folic acid, a stable synthetic form of the vitamin, is used most commonly for replacement. Many over-the-counter vitamin supplement tablets contain up to $600\,\mu$g of folic acid. Replacement tablets that contain more than $1000\,\mu$g of folate require prescriptions. Amounts larger than this usually are not needed over a prolonged period of time.

Parenteral preparations of folic acid that contain 5 mg of the vitamin per milliliter can be used in severely ill patients, people with malabsorption, or those who are unable to take oral medications. Use of medications at levels greatly beyond the normal level is rarely a required or wise course of action. That being said, few if any problems have been reported due to use of large quantities of folic acid.

■ ALCOHOL AND ANEMIA

Anemia associated with alcohol is a common and complex issue. The complexity derives in part from the multiple faces of alcohol use and abuse. Alcohol is a drug with primary effects on both hematopoiesis and cellular metabolism. In this sense alcohol is like isoniazid or any other chemical that affects marrow activity. The feature that distinguishes alcohol from other drugs is its interplay with a separate disease state, which is alcoholism.

Alcoholism is a disease with both physical and psychological manifestations. The interplay between the drug, alcohol, and the psychological aspects of alcoholism determine the physical manifestations of alcohol-related disorders. A powerful social component also subtends the expression of alcohol-related problems. The interaction between the physical, psychological, and social spheres creates a medical condition of singular complexity.

CLINICAL PRESENTATION

Anemia related to alcohol has wide range of presentations that depend in part on where the patient lies in the spectrum of alcohol-related illness. Obtaining a good history both from the patient and family is the key first step in the evaluation. Patients commonly downplay the extent of their alcohol consumption. Information from family members at times provides a more accurate estimate of alcohol use. The universally used term, "social drinker," is useful only when placed into a context that describes not only the quantity of alcohol consumed but the context of that consumption. A "couple of drinks a day" are more concerning when they are consumed in isolation rather than in a social context with friends. The true quantity of alcohol consumed in an isolated setting usually exceeds the reported value. Equally concerning is the fact that solitary drinking can be part of a larger picture of social isolation.

People who engage in occult excessive alcohol use often hold jobs and show high-level social function as perceived by the outside world. Overt alcohol abuse commonly erodes the ability to maintain social connections, leading to a person who functions at the margins of society. Disturbed nutrition is a major component of alcohol-related anemia. The problem is most clear in overt alcohol abusers who are socially isolated. However, poor nutrition is very common in people who show no overt signs of alcohol abuse. Alcohol supplies a substantial number of calories that often displace other food sources, particularly fresh fruits and vegetables that provide folate.[41]

People with overt intemperance often have a physical examination that shows problems related to alcohol use. Petechiae and peripheral edema are manifestations of thrombocytopenia and anemia. Ecchymoses can arise due to falls or other accidents related to alcohol overuse. Splenomegaly, hepatomegaly, spider angiomata, and jaundice point to more severe alcohol injury that affects the liver and can include hepatic fibrosis and cirrhosis.

LABORATORY FINDINGS

Mild to moderate anemia is common, with hemoglobin values often in the range of 10–11 g/dL. Macrocytosis is the most frequent feature of alcohol-related anemia. Siderocytes, red cells that Perl's Prussian blue staining shows to contain iron granules, also occur with some cases of alcohol-related anemia. Red cell size variation is common, manifested by an elevated RDW. The reticulocyte count usually is low, but can rebound to high levels following termination of alcohol consumption, which is routinely the case with hospitalized patients. Mild thrombocytopenia is common, although splenomegaly can exacerbate its severity. Neutrophil values are normal or only mildly depressed.

Megaloblastic erythroid maturation is common on bone marrow examination. This can occur even without folate deficiency and appears to reflect direct alcohol toxicity to the marrow (Table 8-5). However, megaloblastic anemia with alcohol as manifested by macroovalocytes and hypersegmented neutrophils occurs only with concomitant folate deficiency. The most striking finding in alcohol-related anemia is vacuoles in proerythroblasts (Figure 8-6). The vacuoles do not appear in latter normoblasts and are virtually diagnostic of alcohol bone marrow injury. Chloramphenicol produces very similar vacuoles but these appear at all stages of erythroblastic differentiation (see Chapter 11).

The erythroid precursors often show evidence of disturbed iron utilization manifested by iron accumulation in RE cells.[42] Ineffective erythropoiesis also contributes to iron deposition in RE cells.[43] Ring sideroblasts develop in some patients that are identical to those seen with myelodysplasia and sideroblastic anemia[44] (see Chapter 12). The sideroblastic changes often occur in association with megaloblastic erythropoiesis due to coexisting folate deficiency.[45] Termination of alcohol exposure (and folate replacement) resolves the sideroblastic anemia, distinguishing this form of sideroblastic anemia from that associated with myelodysplasia. Serum iron levels often fall with

TABLE 8-5	ALCOHOL AND ANEMIA
Cause	*Effect*
Primary	• Direct suppression of erythropoiesis • Deranged iron utilization by erythroid precursors • Ineffective erythropoiesis • Antagonism of folate action • Sideroblastic bone marrow changes
Secondary	• Iron loss (GI bleeding) • Folate deficiency • Hypersplenism • Hepatic failure

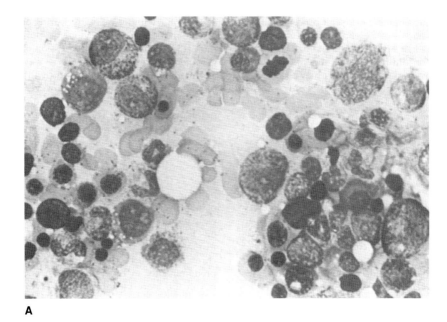

A

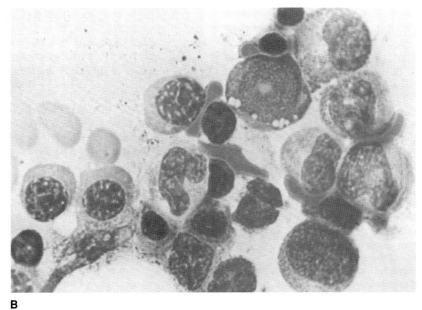

B

FIGURE 8–6   *Alcohol-induced bone marrow vacuoles. The proerythroblast in the figure has prominent cytoplasmic vacuoles that are characteristic of alcohol toxicity. Vacuoles do not appear in the latter normoblasts, which is characteristic of the phenomenon. Such vacuoles disappear several days after cessation of alcohol use. (From James H. Jandl. Blood: Textbook of Hematology. Boston: Little, Brown and Company, 1987. Figure 4-4A and B, p. 122. Used with permission of publisher.)*

TABLE 8-6	KEY DIAGNOSTIC ISSUES IN NUTRITIONAL ANEMIA

Issue	*Manifestation*	*Approach*
Clinical cobalamin deficiency with normal serum cobalamin levels	• Anemia • Macrocytosis • Hypersegmented neutrophils • Reticulocytopenia • Megaloblastic hematopoiesis	• Plasma methylmalonic acid level. An elevation would indicate functional cobalamin deficiency.
Cobalamin deficiency in infancy	• Delayed developmental progression beginning a few months after birth	• Serum cobalamin level • Family history of vegan diet by mother. • Check cobalamin level in mother. • Parenteral cobalamin to create baseline vitamin stores.
Alcohol-induced sideroblastic anemia	• Anemia • Ring sideroblasts on bone marrow examination	• Examine bone marrow for vacuoles in proerythroblasts. • Karyotype analysis to eliminate myelodysplasia. • Repeat bone marrow examination following alcohol abstinence.

termination of alcohol exposure, reflecting increased efficiency of iron utilization by the erythropoietic cells.

Alcohol possibly in concert with its metabolite, acetaldehyde, directly suppresses hematopoiesis.[46] Abstinence from alcohol reverses the changes in hematopoiesis in a matter of days.[47] Replacement of folate and other vitamins as needed speeds the recovery process. Alcohol antagonizes folate activity in hematopoiesis, meaning that people who continue to use alcohol require more of the vitamin.[48] The commonly used 1 mg folic acid tablet easily supplies enough of the vitamin, however (Tables 8-6 and 8-7).

TABLE 8-7	KEY MANAGEMENT ISSUES IN NUTRITIONAL ANEMIA
Issue	*Comment*
Neurological disturbances with cobalamin deficiency	Neurological disturbances can develop in the absence of anemia. Without early treatment the neurological deficits can become fixed. Neurocognitive abnormalities can mimic Alzheimer's disease.
Gastric cancer in pernicious anemia	Pernicious anemia increases the risk of gastric cancer to threefold over baseline. Cobalamin replacement does not lessen the cancer risk. Regular monitoring for gastric cancer is advisable.
Subclinical cobalamin deficiency	Chronic atrophic gastritis produces low cobalamin levels in about 10% of cases. Few patients have hematological or neurological manifestations of cobalamin deficiency, even when MMA levels are elevated. Cobalamin replacement is reasonable because of unknown risk of progression to clinical disease.
Resection of terminal ileum	Cobalamin deficiency occurs with a 2–3-year lag time. A monthly schedule of cobalamin replacement following the procedure avoids losing track of the issue.
Parenteral cobalamin replacement	Cobalamin replacement produces a spectacular initial hematological response. The response can unveil a previously cryptic iron deficit that requires iron replacement.
Alcohol-associated anemia	Macrocytosis without megaloblastic anemia is the most common finding. Concomitant folate deficiency often exacerbates the anemia. Alcohol abstinence reverses the anemia.

References

[1] Lindgren A, Swolin B, Nilsson O, Johansson KW, Kilander AF. 1997. Serum methylmalonic acid and total homocysteine in patients with suspected cobalamin deficiency: A clinical study based on gastrointestinal histopathological findings. Am J Hematol 56:230–238.

[2] Hvas AM, Juul S, Gerdes LU, Nexo E. 2000. The marker of cobalamin deficiency, plasma methylmalonic acid, correlates to plasma creatinine. J Intern Med 247:507–512.

[3] Moelby L, Rasmussen K, Ring T, Nielsen G. 2000. Relationship between methylmalonic acid and cobalamin in uremia. Kidney Int 57:265–273.

[4] Monsen AL, Refsum H, Markestad T, Ueland PM. 2003. Cobalamin status and its biochemical markers methylmalonic acid and homocysteine in different age groups from 4 days to 19 years. Clin Chem 49:2067–2075.

[5] Lindenbaum J, Savage DG, Stabler SP, Allen RH. 1990. Diagnosis of cobalamin deficiency. II: Relative sensitivities of serum cobalamin, methylmalonic acid, and total homocysteine concentrations. Am J Hematol 34:99–107.

[6] Clarke R, Refsum H, Birks J, et al. 2004. Screening for vitamin B-12 and folate deficiency in older persons. Am J Clin Nutr 77:1241–1247.

[7] Seetharam B, Bose S, Li N. 1999. Cellular import of cobalamin (Vitamin B-12). J Nutr 129:1761–1764.

[8] Minot GR, Murphy WP. 1983. Landmark article (JAMA 1926). Treatment of pernicious anemia by a special diet. JAMA 250:3328–3335.

[9] Zelissen PM, Bast EJ, Croughs RJ. 1995. Associated autoimmunity in Addison's disease. J Autoimmun 8:121–130.

[10] Barnadas MA, Rodriguez-Arias JM, Alomar A. 2000. Subcutaneous sarcoidosis associated with vitiligo, pernicious anaemia and autoimmune thyroiditis. Clin Exp Dermatol 25:55–56.

[11] Alkhateeb A, Fain PR, Thody A, Bennett DC, Spritz RA. 2003. Epidemiology of vitiligo and associated autoimmune diseases in Caucasian probands and their families. Pigment Cell Res 16:208–214.

[12] Stabler SP, Allen RH, Fried LP, et al. 1999. Racial differences in prevalence of cobalamin and folate deficiencies in disabled elderly women. Am J Clin Nutr 70:911–919.

[13] Clarke R, Evans JM, Schneede J, et al. 2004. Vitamin B12 and folate deficiency in later life. Age Ageing 33:34–41.

[14] Carmel R, Aurangzeb I, Qian D. 2001. Associations of food-cobalamin malabsorption with ethnic origin, age, Helicobacter pylori infection, and serum markers of gastritis. Am J Gastroenterol 96:63–70.

[15] van Asselt DZ, de Groot LC, van Staveren WA, et al. 1998. Role of cobalamin intake and atrophic gastritis in mild cobalamin deficiency in older Dutch subjects. Am J Clin Nutr 68:328–334.

[16] Lindenbaum J, Rosenberg IH, Wilson PW, Stabler SP, Allen RH. 1994. Prevalence of cobalamin deficiency in the Framingham elderly population. Am J Clin Nutr 60:2–11.

[17] Cohen H, Weinstein WM, Carmel R. 2000. Heterogeneity of gastric histology and function in food cobalamin malabsorption absence of atrophic gastritis and achlorhydria in some patients with severe malabsorption. Gut 47:638–645.

[18] Carmel R. 1996. Prevalence of undiagnosed pernicious anemia in the elderly. Arch Intern Med 156:1097–1100.

[19] Baik HW, Russell RM. 1999. Vitamin B12 deficiency in the elderly. Annu Rev Nutr 19:357–377.

[20] Summer AE, Chin MM, Abrahm JL, et al. 1996. Elevated methylmalonivc acid and total homocysteine levels show high prevalence of vitamin B12 deficiency after gastric surgery. Ann Intern Med 124:469–476.

[21] Sumner AE, Chin MM, Abrahm JL, et al. 1996. Elevated methylmalonic acid and total homocysteine levels show high prevalence of vitamin B12 deficiency after gastric surgery. Ann Intern Med 124:469–476.

[22] Monagle PT, Tauro GP. 1997. Infantile megaloblastosis secondary to maternal vitamin B12 deficiency. Clin Lab Haematol 19:23–25.

23 Fokkema MR, Woltil HA, van Beusekom CM, Schaafsma A, Dijck-Brouwer DA, Muskiet FA. 2002. Plasma total homocysteine increases from day 20 to 40 in breastfed but not formula-fed low-birthweight infants. Acta Paediatr 91:507–511.

24 Rosenblatt DS, Whitehead VM. 1999. Cobalamin and folate deficiency: Acquired and hereditary disorders in children. Semin Hematol 36:19–34.

25 Bjorke Monsen AL, Ueland PM. 2003. Homocysteine and methylmalonic acid in diagnosis and risk assessment from infancy to adolescence. Am J Clin Nutr 78:7–21.

26 Tanner SM, Aminoff M, Wright FA, et al. 2003. Amnionless, essential for mouse gastrulation, is mutated in recessive hereditary megaloblastic anemia. Nat Genet 2003 33:426–429.

27 Aminoff M, Carter JE, Chadwick RB, et al. 1999. Mutations in CUBN, encoding the intrinsic factor-vitamin B12 receptor, cubilin, cause hereditary megaloblastic anaemia 1. Nat Genet 21:309–313.

28 Fyfe JC, Madsen M, Højrup P, et al. 2004. The functional cobalamin (vitamin B12)—intrinsic factor receptor is a novel complex of cubilin and amnionless. Blood 103:1573–1579.

29 Miller DR, Bloom GE, Streiff RR, LoBuglio AF, Diamond LK. 1966. Juvenile "congenital" pernicious anemia. Clinical and immunologic studies. N Engl J Med 275:978–983.

30 Heisel MA, Siegel SE, Falk RE, et al. 1984. Congenital pernicious anemia: Report of seven patients, with studies of the extended family. J Pediatr 105:564–568.

31 Remacha AF, Sambeat MA, Barcelo MJ, Mones J, Garcia-Die J, Gimferrer E. 1992. Congenital intrinsic factor deficiency in a Spanish patient. Ann Hematol 64:202–204.

32 Levine JS, Allen RH. 1985. Intrinsic factor within parietal cells of patients with juvenile pernicious anemia. A retrospective immunohistochemical study. Gastroenterology 88(5 Pt 1):1132–1136.

33 Koury MJ, Ponka P. 2004. New insights into erythropoiesis: The roles of folate, vitamin B12, and iron. Annu Rev Nutr 24:105–131.

34 Galloway M, Rushworth L. 2003. Red cell or serum folate? Results from the National Pathology Alliance benchmarking review. J Clin Pathol 56:924–926.

35 Welch GN, Loscalzo J. 1998. Homocysteine and atherothrombosis. N Engl J Med 338:1042–1050.

36 Stover PJ. Physiology of folate and vitamin B12 in health and disease. Nutr Rev 62:S3–S12.

37 Mackey AD, Picciano MF. 1999. Maternal folate status during extended lactation and the effect of supplemental folic acid. Am J Clin Nutr 69:285–292.

38 Smith AM, Picciano MF, Deering RH. 1983. Folate supplementation during lactation: Maternal folate status, human milk folate content, and their relationship to infant folate status. J Pediatr Gastroenterol Nutr 2:622–628.

39 Cooperman JM, Dweck HS, Newman LJ, Garbarino C, Lopez R. 1982. The folate in human milk. Am J Clin Nutr 36:576–580.

40 Rodriguez-Cortes HM, Griener JC, Hyland K, et al. 1999. Plasma homocysteine levels and folate status in children with sickle cell anemia. J Pediatr Hematol Oncol 21:219–223.

41 Lindenbaum J, Roman MJ. 1980. Nutritional anemia in alcoholism. Am J Clin Nutr 33:2727–2735.

42 Boewer C. 1986. Bone marrow disturbances of iron utilisation: Cytomorphological diagnostic in chronic alcohol abuse. Acta Haematol 76:141–145.

43 Michot F, Gut J. 1987. Alcohol-induced bone marrow damage. A bone marrow study in alcohol-dependent individuals. Acta Haematol 78:252–257.

44 Pierce HI, McGuffin RG, Hillman RS. 1976. Clinical studies in alcoholic sideroblastosis. Arch Intern Med 136:283–289.

[45] Hines JD, Cowan DH. 1970. Studies on the pathogenesis of alcohol-induced sideroblastic bone-marrow abnormalities. N Engl J Med 283:441–446.

[46] Meagher RC, Sieber F, Spivak JL. 1982. Suppression of hematopoietic-progenitor-cell proliferation by ethanol and acetaldehyde. N Engl J Med 307:845–849.

[47] Sullivan LW, Herbert V. 1964. Suppression of hematopoiesis by ethanol. J Clin Invest 43:2048–2062.

[48] Savage D, Lindenbaum J. 1986. Anemia in alcoholics. Medicine (Baltimore) 65:322–338.

Hormone Deficiency

ANEMIA AND ENDOCRINE HORMONES

■ BACKGROUND

For more than a billion years, all life of Earth existed as simple single-celled organisms. The evolution of multicellular life forms was a quantum leap forward in sophistication and complexity. This giant step required the development of molecules that could coordinate the function of cells that existed both in collectives and were increasingly diverse. Hormones are signaling molecules that lash together the assorted cells of the whole organism, permitting them to function smoothly as a unit. Increased specialization likewise means that single cells from higher organisms cannot exist in isolation. A multicellular structure gives an organism flexibility and adaptability at the expense of individual cells that are functionally rigid and limited in ability. The technological breakthrough of tissue culture, which supports the growth of solitary cells from complex organisms, requires supplementation of the growth medium with a proper balance of these key hormones. Tissue culture, in essence, is a facsimile of the body's hormonal environment in a petri dish.

The best known examples of regulatory molecules that coordinate whole animal physiology are the classical endocrine hormones. These include molecules produced by the hypothalamus, pituitary, thyroid, parathyroid, and adrenal glands, as well as those synthesized by the pancreas and gonads. In order to coordinate the operation of cells and organs often separated by long distances, the endocrine hormones use the blood stream and lymphatic vessels as primary routes of transport. Peptide hormones, such as insulin, largely travel free in the circulation. In contrast, many small hormones, such as the steroids and thyroid hormones, have specific binding proteins that facilitate their intercellular movement.

Endocrine hormones mediate their effects through specific receptors that exist in key target cells and tissues. An important example is the insulin receptor expressed on adipose cells. The totality of insulin action derives from an intracellular signaling cascade triggered by insulin binding to its receptor. Advances in the understanding of hormone function led to a recognition that the influence of hormones extends far beyond the traditional target tissues. Receptors for specific hormones exist on a host of cells outside the main tissue type, meaning that hormones create a cascade of events that flow far beyond the bounds of these targets. Schematic diagrams of hormone actions often employ single arrows. However, more precise representations would resemble complex nets where the multitudinous hormonal pathways intermesh to form a powerful but sensitive control network.

Hormones produced by other tissues and glands have recently joined the classical endocrine pantheon, including erythropoietin secreted by the kidney. Early erythroid cells are the key target of this hormone. Erythropoietin acts in conjunction with a host of paracrine activators and other signaling molecules, such as stem cell factor (c-Kit ligand), to promote normal erythropoiesis. In addition to these factors that are specific to the erythroid lineage, a number of classical endocrine hormones also modulate erythropoiesis through their "ancillary" metabolic effects. The impact of classic endocrine hormones on erythropoiesis varies tremendously. Deranged hormone production has striking effects on the primary target tissues. However, hormonal imbalance can have consequences that ripple from the epicenter of impact and profoundly affect the bone marrow and hematopoiesis. Many endocrine hormones are absolutely vital to sustained, normal erythropoiesis.

ANDROGENS

Males and females differ. Anatomic evidence of this truism exists before birth and grows in magnitude with puberty. Some differences, such as the relative disparity in height, have no great significance. Others, such as the unique ability of women to bear children, have wide-ranging consequences that extend far beyond physiology and powerfully shape the social fabric of humanity. The impact of sex status on erythropoiesis falls somewhere between these extreme poles. Not surprisingly, the sex steroids are central to the disparate hemoglobin values that are characteristic of men and women, with androgens playing a lead role.

Among the striking physiological changes that accompany male puberty is a rise in blood hemoglobin concentration that averages about 2 g/dL. Puberty also witnesses a rise in serum testosterone levels from the range of 20–30 ng/dL to 300–1000 ng/dL. The logical assumption is that a causal relationship exists between the two events. Androgen-enhanced red cell production would also explain the higher mean hemoglobin levels of men relative to women.[1]

The observation that hypogonadal men have below-normal blood hemoglobin values that increase with testosterone replacement further strengthens the association between androgens and erythropoiesis. The increase in hemoglobin values in this setting usually is rapid, requiring only 2–3 months to rise from the anemic range to mid-normal values. Figure 9-1 plots the hemoglobin rise in a cohort of hypogonadal men treated with testosterone replacement therapy. The diagram shows a steep rise in values that subsequently achieve a smooth plateau.

The precise mechanism by which androgens increase erythropoiesis and serum hemoglobin values is unclear. The Leydig cells of the gonads produce about 7 mg of testosterone each day. In the plasma, the vast bulk of testosterone forms a complex

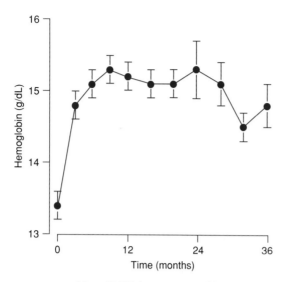

FIGURE 9–1 *Mean ($\pm SE$) hematocrit and hemoglobin values in 16 men with previously untreated hypogonadism who received replacement testosterone for 36 months. The increase in both parameters from 0 to 36 months was statistically significant (p = 0.002). (From Synder PJ, Peachey H, Berlin JA, et al. 2000. Effect of testosterone replacement in hypogonadal men. J Clin Endocrinol Metab 85:2670–2677. Figure 4. Used with permission of the publisher.)*

either with sex-hormone-binding globulin or with albumin, leaving only about 1–2% of the steroid free in the circulation.[2] This small fraction of the total plasma testosterone pool appears to be the metabolically active component.

5-α-Reductase converts testosterone to dihydrotestosterone after the molecule enters the cell. Dihydrotestosterone is the active form of the hormone that binds to and activates the intracellular androgen receptor. Within the cell nucleus, the activated androgen receptor acts as a transcriptional regulator that modulates gene expression. Androgens added to in vitro cultures of human bone marrow cells enhance the number of early erythroid precursor cells.[3] One investigation showed that bone marrow cultures of human megakaryocytes contain both estrogen receptor β and androgen receptors.[4] This work noted the presence of CD34(+) cells not of megakaryocytic lineage that were also positive for androgen receptors. Although the identity of these early progenitor cells was not further characterized, the data are consistent with androgen receptor expression in erythropoietic progenitor cells in the bone marrow.

As noted earlier, testosterone replacement in hypogonadal men evokes a rapid increase in hemoglobin levels (Table 9-1). Logically, the natural rise in androgens produced by puberty should produce a similarly coordinated rise in hemoglobin values. However, a surprising temporal dissociation exists between the rise in testosterone and the rise in hemoglobin values in this setting. The testosterone level in boys rises rapidly and relatively linearly during puberty, while hemoglobin values require a period of about 6 years to attain adult values.[5] A possible explanation for this discrepancy is a contribution to the pubertal rise in hemoglobin values in boys by the hormonal

TABLE 9-1 | **KEY DIAGNOSTIC POINTS IN ENDOCRINE ANEMIAS**

Issue	*Manifestation*	*Approach*
Anemia of hypogonadism	Low hemoglobin value, normal MCV, normal WBC, normal platelets, low serum testosterone level.	Testosterone replacement.
Anemia of hypothyroidism	Low hemoglobin value, normal or high MCV, normal WBC, normal platelets, low serum T3, T4 values.	Thyroid hormone replacement. Correction of iron deficit, if it exists.
Anemia of autoimmune thyroid disease	Low hemoglobin value, macrocytosis or microcytosis, normal WBC, normal platelets, low serum T3, T4, low serum cobalamin, low serum iron.	Replace thyroid hormone. Replace cobalamin and iron. Evaluate for autoimmune gastritis.
Anemia of anorexia nervosa	Low hemoglobin value, normal MCV, low neutrophil count, rarely low platelet count, gelatinous transformation of bone marrow.	Nutritional replacement, aiming for 1200–1500 kcal/day.

duo of growth hormone (GH) and insulin-like growth factor 1 (IGF-1), which rise in concentration during puberty and also promote erythropoiesis. Careful measurements in boys with gonadal failure who received testosterone replacement with concomitant manipulations to block the rise in GH/IGF-1 showed clearly that androgen is the primary factor responsible for the upsurge in erythropoiesis.[6] Since the GH/IGF-1 duo appears not to have a role in the process, the basis of the temporal asynchrony between testosterone rise and hemoglobin rise during puberty remains a mystery.

Although the issue is not definitively resolved, alteration in serum erythropoietin level likewise appears not to be the basis of androgen-mediated enhancement of erythropoiesis. At the other end of the erythropoietic control system, reports that androgens alter erythropoietin sensitivity of BFU-E and CFU-E[7,8] could reflect an influence of androgen receptors on the very early stages of erythroid development. Glucocorticoid receptors (GR) clearly act on erythropoiesis through metabolic changes in early committed erythroid progenitors (see below). The same might hold for androgen receptors. Additional work is required to clarify the point.

Small numbers of hematopoietic stem cells circulate in the peripheral blood. These cells appear to be in dynamic equilibrium with those in the bone marrow, which is the storehouse for the vast bulk of such cells. In fact, peripheral blood stem cells harvested by apheresis techniques have become a mainstay in hematopoietic stem cell transplantation. Assessment of these cells by clonogenic culturing assay shows significantly more circulating CFC, BFU-E, and CFU-GM cells in the peripheral blood of men than of women.[9] This observation is consistent with a higher number of early erythroid precursors in men due to higher levels of androgens.

The capacity of androgens to enhance erythropoiesis found its widest clinical use in hemodialysis patients before the advent of recombinant human erythropoietin (rHuEpo).[10] Androgen supplementation partially corrected the severe anemia in many patients on hemodialysis. With the clinical introduction of rHuEpo, androgen use in this setting virtually disappeared, although some interest remains in combined use of androgens and rHuEpo as a cost-cutting measure.[11] The side effects of androgens are a severe impediment to their use as agents to enhance erythropoiesis, however. Most of these problems center on the masculinizing properties of these agents. The rare but very serious complication of hepatic and splenic peliosis occurs only with the nondefunct 17-α-alkylated androgens and does not arise with the currently available testosterone preparations.

GLUCOCORTICOIDS

Glucocorticoids, products primarily of the adrenal glands, play an important role in regulating development, cell differentiation, and metabolic homeostasis. The hormones modulate the activity of nuclear GR, which coordinate the expression of a host of genes.[12] GR expression occurs across a wide range of cells and tissues, affecting carbohydrate, lipid, and protein metabolism. Transgenic mice bred to express no GR show an embryonic lethal phenotype that includes a failure in the development of the lungs, adrenals, and other organs.[13] This hormonal system is clearly essential not only to health but to survival itself.

The clinical impact of glucocorticoids on erythropoiesis is most apparent in patients with Addison's disease, a state of glucocorticoid deficiency. Anemia is common, although the severity is usually mild to moderate, with hemoglobin values sometimes falling to the range of 10–11 g/dL. The red cells are normochromic and normocytic, with no outstanding morphological features. The characteristically low reticulocyte count is consistent with the hypoproliferative nature of the anemia. The marked fatigue and lethargy seen with Addison's disease is a byproduct of other physiological changes associated with glucocorticoid deficit and not the low-grade anemia. Glucocorticoid replacement therapy corrects the anemia, along with the other more serious manifestations of the disorder.

Cushing's syndrome, with its overproduction of glucocorticoids, lies at the opposite end of the clinical spectrum. Hemoglobin values tend to hover in the upper normal range. Frank erythrocytosis occurs in a fraction of patients with the disorder. Shifts in electrolyte and fluid balance can complicate the interpretation of changes in simple hematocrit values in these patients. Alleviation of the glucocorticoid surfeit returns erythropoiesis to normal.

Glucocorticoids acting through GR are essential to the erythrocyte response to stresses such as hypoxia or bleeding.[14] Committed progenitor cells constantly undergo divisions that can result in either a copy (self-renewal) or a cell with a few beginning features found in the end-product cells (differentiation) (Figure 9-2). The fork leading to differentiation is an irreversible step. Excessive selection for this path would gradually deplete the pool of progenitor cells. GR activity is key to maintaining the proliferative activity of erythroid progenitors without cell movement down the path of differentiation.[15] This hovering activity of the progenitors allows expansion of their numbers in response to stress.

GR do not act in isolation in this context. In fact, activated GR alone have little biological effect on erythroid precursor cells. The molecule requires simultaneous signaling from the erythropoietin receptor (EpoR) and c-Kit, the receptor for stem cell factor. Figure 9-3 schematically displays this tripartite relationship. EpoR and c-Kit interact on the cell membrane to form a molecular signaling complex. The intercellular domains of these molecules transduce a series of signals through tyrosine kinases. These signaling pathways intersect with those of GR to produce erythroid-specific alterations in gene expression.[16] Elucidation of the precise details of the intercellular signaling cascade remains a prime focus of ongoing research.

Clinically, glucocorticoids are used in the treatment of both the patients with aplastic anemia and those with Diamond-Blackfan anemia (DBA). In aplastic anemia, the beneficial effects of glucocorticoids derive primarily from their immunosuppressive capacity in what often is a condition of deranged immune function (see Chapter 11). The clinical response does not depend on GR activation in erythroid progenitors or metabolic alterations of these cells. Rather, the removal of pathological lymphoid cells is the key to the benefit of glucocorticoids in aplastic anemia.

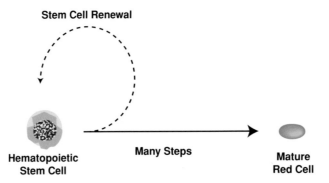

Stem Cell Renewal

Hematopoietic Stem Cell   **Many Steps**   **Mature Red Cell**

FIGURE 9-2 *Hematopoietic stem cell self-renewal versus differentiation. Stem cells must simultaneously produce mature end-product cells and renew themselves. With each cell division a stem cell can either produce a copy or produce a cell with early features of differentiation. Many hormones, cytokines, and growth factors influence this key decision fork.*

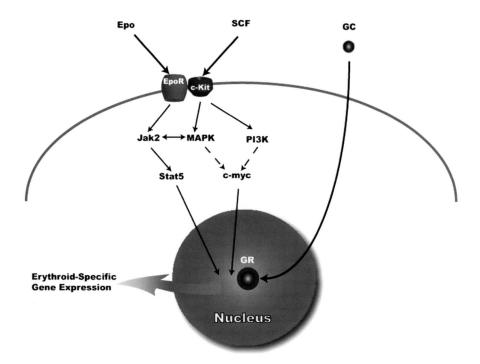

FIGURE 9-3 *Key signaling pathways in erythroid progenitor renewal. Hormonal signaling cascades that involve erythropoietin (Epo), stem cell factor (SCF), and glucocorticoids (GC) intersect to promote self-renewal of erythroid progenitors. Receptors for Epo (EpoR) and SCF (c-Kit) form a molecular complex on the cell membrane with subsequent signaling through a series of tyrosine kinases. GC activates glucocorticoid receptors (GR) that directly alter erythroid-specific gene expression in concert with STAT5 and c-myc. (Data based on Dolznig[16], 2006).*

The basis of the positive impact of glucocorticoids on anemia in up to 50% of patients with DBA has been a mystery. Equally mysterious is the etiology of this rare congenital anemia (see Chapter 11). The sole current clue to the basis of the disorder is the mutation in the gene encoding ribosomal protein S19 (RPS19) that appears in a subset of patients with DBA.[17] Although the precise role of RPS19 in erythropoiesis is unknown, experiments employing knock-down techniques to limit its expression produce severe differentiation and proliferation defects in erythroid progenitors. Glucocorticoids restore the physiology of these cells toward normal by a mechanism that is independent of RPS19.[18] The benefit of glucocorticoids in patients with DBA presumably is an in vivo reflection of this metabolic bypass event.

THYROID HORMONE

Several pathophysiologic links exist between thyroid hormone and anemia. Thyroid hormone deficiency commonly produces an anemia of mild to moderate severity, with

TABLE 9-2	KEY MANAGEMENT POINTS IN ENDOCRINE ANEMIA
Issue	*Comments*
Anemia of hypogonadism	The anemia responds well to testosterone replacement. Correction requires about 6 months.
Anemia of Addison's disease	A mild to moderate anemia exists with Addison's disease. Corticosteroid replacement corrects the problem. Note, "Addisonian anemia" is cobalamin deficiency or pernicious anemia.
Diamond-Blackfan Anemia	The basis of this congenital anemia is unknown. Between 40% and 50% of patients respond to glucocorticoid treatment, at least temporarily.
Hypothyroid, macrocytic anemia	Hypothyroidism commonly produces a mild to moderate macrocytic anemia. The MCV usually is less than 110 fL. Higher values suggest deficiency of cobalamin or folate. Liver disease is another consideration.

hemoglobin values that often hover in the range of 10–12 g/dL. More profound anemia in the setting of thyroid hormone deficiency raises the possibility of other supervening conditions. The red cells most often are macrocytic or normocytic with no morphological features of particular distinction.[19] The reticulocyte count is low, consistent with the hypoproliferative nature of the condition. Hypothyroidism is an important consideration in the differential diagnosis of macrocytic anemia in adults, along with disorders such as deficiency of folate or cobalamin and liver disease. Anemia occasionally is the sole presenting clinical feature of patients with hypothyroidism (Table 9-2).[20]

Hypothyroidism is much less frequent in children than in adults. Children affected by the condition often are anemic, however. One survey found macrocytic or normocytic anemia in two-thirds of children with hypothyroidism.[21] Anemia also is common in children with congenital hypothyroidism, even when the thyroid dysfunction is detected by neonatal screening.[22] The degree of anemia varies according to the severity of thyroid hormone deficiency and corrects over a period of months after the initiation of thyroid hormone replacement therapy.

An important connection exists between iron deficiency, hypothyroidism, and anemia. Iron deficit reduces the synthesis and activity of thyroid peroxidase, which is a heme-dependent enzyme in the thyroid hormone biosynthetic pathway.[23] Iron deficiency can tip some patients into a state of thyroid hormone deficiency, particularly if they have tenuous thyroid activity at baseline. Thyroid hormone replacement can also trigger adverse reactions in these patients.[24] Correction of iron deficiency prior to thyroid hormone replacement allows the establishment of a proper metabolic balance and avoids untoward side effects.

Plasma volume commonly is below normal in patients with hypothyroidism due to disturbances in fluid and electrolyte balance. Contraction of the intravascular space artifactually raises hematocrit values, masking the true change in hemoglobin status. Assay of red cell mass, however, shows a consistent reduction in these patients.[25] The lower red cell mass reduces the aggregate oxygen-carrying capacity of the blood. However, the dampening of metabolic activity in the hypothyroid state moderates the clinical impact of the decrease in red cell mass and the associated lower rate of tissue oxygen delivery. At one time in past, in fact, iatrogenically induced hypothyroidism was a treatment for severe coronary artery disease and cardiac ischemia. The slowed metabolic rate improved the oxygenation balance of ischemic cardiac tissue despite the lower red cell mass.

The clinical expression of anemia in people with hypothyroidism can be difficult to gauge. Anemia commonly causes tachycardia, but hypothyroidism produces a dominating bradycardia that overwhelms this tendency and dictates the cardiac picture. Hypothyroidism per se has a number of clinical manifestations, including fatigue and lethargy, which often are profound. Concomitant chronic anemia in this setting undoubtedly exacerbates these symptoms and heightens patient's disquiet. Dissecting the relative impact of the two conditions can be clinically challenging, however.

Unraveling the mechanism by which hypothyroidism produces anemia has been a thorny problem for which no satisfactory explanation currently exists. A number of investigations support the observation that L-triiodothyronine (T3), the biologically active form of thyroid hormone, promotes in vitro proliferation of erythroid progenitor cells.[26–28] Furthermore, thyroid hormone receptors exist in the nuclei of early erythroid precursor cells where they presumably modulate gene expression.[29] Attempts to create an understanding of the cell biological events that extend beyond these indirect observations have produced mixed results, however. The emergence of a more detailed understanding of the molecular and biochemical processes of thyroid hormone action has provided some insight but no major breakthrough that mechanistically links anemia and hypothyroidism.

Two thyroid hormone receptors, TR-α and TR-β, mediate the biological activities of T3.[30] TR-α, a member of the class II family of nuclear receptors, interacts with specific regions of DNA and chromatin to alter gene transcription.[31] T3 binding to TR-α modifies the conformation of the receptor, switching it between an active and an inactive state. Signal transduction from T3 through TR-α alters gene expression, which in the case of erythroid precursors appears to switch the cells between the paths of proliferation and differentiation.[32,33]

Nonetheless, the precise biochemical factors that mediate these changes remain a mystery. Interestingly, the proposed effects of T3 on the erythroid progenitor switch between proliferation and differentiation is reminiscent of the much better characterized effect of glucocorticoids in this regard. Glucocorticoids and T3 work through separate nuclear hormone receptors that belong to the same general receptor class. Each modulates gene expression by modifying chromosomal structure and interacting with transacting transcriptional regulators. A mechanistic connection between the two sets of hormones and receptors would provide an intellectually satisfying solution to the enigma. However, no interaction or exchange between the receptor systems is described in the setting of erythropoiesis.

The degree to which the known genetic and molecular effects of thyroid hormone contribute to the anemia of hypothyroidism is unclear. In aggregate, the cell biological effects of thyroid hormone are complex and pleiotropic. Other pathophysiologic alterations possibly contribute to the anemia, including altered production of erythropoietin.[34,35] The widespread effects of thyroid hormone on other cell regulatory systems, including the biochemistry of red cells themselves,[36] indicate that hypothyroidism likely has effects on red cell balance that are yet unrecognized. The important clinical point in this perplexing scenario is that thyroid hormone replacement completely alleviates the anemia in these patients.

In addition to the interplay between thyroid hormone and erythropoiesis, a profound immunological link also exists between the thyroid gland and anemia. The first notation of the common coexistence of autoimmune thyroid disease (AITD) and pernicious anemia, an archetypical autoimmune anemia, came in the early 1960s.[37–40] Approximately 2% of the patients with Grave's disease have concomitant pernicious anemia, while among patients with Hashimoto's thyroiditis the figure ranges between 4% and 12%.[41] These values exceed the prevalence of pernicious anemia in the general population by more than 10-fold.[42] The obverse clinical situation also holds true. Among patients who present with pernicious anemia, more than 10% have AITD.[43] Interestingly, the thyroid disease often is not clinically recognized until the patient is evaluated for pernicious anemia.

Autoimmune gastritis, the precursor to pernicious anemia, is even more common among patients with AITD. Fully, one-third of such patients have histologically demonstrable autoimmune gastritis with associated hypergastrinemia.[44] Eighty percent of these patients have an associated anemia. Interestingly, anti-parietal cell autoantibodies occur in only two-thirds of these individuals. Up to half of these patients are euthyroid, making anemia the initial laboratory abnormality.

Many patients have a macrocytic anemia due to cobalamin deficiency. Some, however, have a microcytic, hypochromic anemia reflecting iron deficiency. Immune-mediated damage to the gastric parietal cells ablates acid secretion, with consequent achlorhydria. Duodenal iron absorption, however, relies on relatively acidic conditions along the upper gastrointestinal track. Gastric achlorhydria raises duodenal pH and impairs iron absorption. Iron deficiency in this setting often is severe and difficult to correct.[45] Impaired production of intrinsic factor leads to slow depletion of cobalamin stores and the development of pernicious anemia in some of these patients.[46] A mixed picture of macrocytic and microcytic anemia can result from this dual pathologic defect.[47]

Patient age and gender also influence the clinical picture. Iron deficiency anemia arises more commonly in younger patients with atrophic gastritis, while anemia due to cobalamin deficiency is the more frequent finding in older patients.[48] Women have an underlying predilection for iron deficiency due in large part to physiologic iron losses related to menstruation. Furthermore, thyroid disease is common in women, with prevalence values that range between 3% and 7% when considering both overt and subclinical disease.[49] This poorly understood female predilection for thyroid dysfunction produces, for the condition, a female-to-male ratio of approximately 3:1.[50]

These modifying clinical factors are important considerations in the evaluation and treatment of patients with AITD who have concomitant autoimmune gastritis. A thorough evaluation looking for anemia is essential to the work-up. Low values for the transferrin saturation and serum ferritin indicate marginal iron stores in a patient who may not have anemia at the time of the evaluation. Adding iron supplementation to the therapeutic regimen along with thyroid hormone replacement often is a wise precaution, particularly for a young woman. In comparison to iron, cobalamin stores are harder to evaluate and to monitor over time. Close scrutiny of the patient's hematological status during subsequent follow-up sessions for the thyroid problem is a valuable adjunct to clinical management. The insidious course of onset for pernicious anemia and the severe consequences that can arise with prolonged cobalamin deficiency reinforces the importance of these measures.

Thyroid dysfunction, including AITD, is one of the most common conditions affecting people in the eighth and ninth decades of life.[51] The frequency of atrophic gastritis also increases with age. In concert, these conditions can play havoc with the health of seniors. The subtle onset of thyroid disease, particularly the manifestations of hypothyroidism, makes clinical recognition of the conditions both important and challenging.

At the other end of the age spectrum, AITD is uncommon in children. Familial disease clustering, nonetheless, often occurs when the disorder arises in children and adolescents.[52] No information exists that addresses the possibility of a connection between AITD and autoimmune gastritis in children.

AITD is multifactorial in origin.[53] As is the case with many autoimmune disorders, genetic factors appear to contribute substantially to the process,[54] but the precise mechanisms involved remain unclear. Concordant expression of Grave's disease, for instance, is 10-fold more common in monozygotic than in dizygotic twins. Cross-sectional population evaluation shows that Grave's disease and Hashimoto's thyroiditis exist in up to one-third of first- and second-degree female relatives of patients with AITD.[55]

Autoimmune gastritis and pernicious anemia also have substantial genetic influences to their expression (see Chapter 8). A single immunogen or other trigger to link the two autoimmune processes is nosologically appealing but experimentally elusive. With time, the observations of family clustering and HLA association will give way to biochemical and genetic explanations. For the moment, however, the door to that storehouse of knowledge remains firmly shut.

ANOREXIA NERVOSA

Anorexia nervosa (AN) is a serious and sometimes life-threatening eating disorder whose causes are complex and whose effects are variegating. The central feature of the condition is a fear of fat and weight gain. The result is an elaborate behavioral disturbance that focuses on measures aimed at weight loss, including determined dieting, restrictive food intake, purging, and compulsive exercising.[56,57] In some cases, binge eating occurs in association with purging. Use and misuse of laxatives and diet pills often is part of the obsessive drive to lose weight or avoid weight gain. The continued urge for weight loss despite objective evidence of what often is frank cachexia reflects a profound disturbance in body image. Emotional traits of the disorder include compulsiveness and a relentless drive for perfection.[58] Anxiety disturbances are common, as is depression.[59]

AN occurs more commonly in the industrialized world than in developing nations. The disorder affects between 0.2% and 4% of adolescent girls of all ethnic and socioeconomic groups in the United States.[60,61] Pressure from peers, family, and even cultural concepts of beauty and body image often contribute to the problem. The prevalence of AN in females is 10-fold greater than that in males, with adolescents between the ages of 15 and 18 years commonly affected.[62,63] Despite its frequent characterization as a disease of the young, AN also causes morbidity and mortality in older adults. Among all deaths from AN in Norway over a 9-year period of time, more than 40% occurred in people of age 65 years or older.[64] Reviews of other national registries, such as those involving death from AN among people in Denmark (mean age 36 years for women and 25 years for men), also showed a high mortality among adults.[65] The precise age figures differ, but the message is the same. AN must be considered in people of all age groups.

AN produces a host of medical problems that include bradycardia, cardiac arrhythmias, hypothyroidism, delayed puberty, and osteoporosis. These disturbances result from a complex, interlocking set of metabolic aberrations related to severe calorie and energy deprivation. Anemia and neutropenia are the most common hematological disturbances. As many as one-third of outpatients with AN have anemia and/or neutropenia.[66,67] The degree of anemia usually is mild to moderate with red cells that are normochromic and normocytic. Hemoglobin values in the range of 11–12 g/dL are the most common finding in anemic patients. While the red cells usually have no morphological disturbances, scattered reports exist of more severe anemia, distorted red cells, and chronic hemolysis related to lipid and metabolic imbalances in these patients.[68,69]

The hematological disturbances of AN arise in association with remarkable alterations in bone marrow composition. Bone marrow hypoplasia develops wherein a refractile, gelatinous material replaces both normal hematopoietic and stromal elements of the marrow.[70] The bone marrow transformation is related to protein-calorie deprivation as evidenced by reversal of the process with improved nutrition and weight gain. Biochemical analysis shows the gelatinous material to be depositions of hyaluronic acid.[71,72] The source of this unusual bone marrow substance is unclear as is its role in the hematologic disturbances associated with AN. Reports exist of frank bone marrow necrosis and acantholytic hemolytic anemia, but these appear to be exceptional manifestations of the disorder.[73]

MRI images of the bone marrow of these patients are often abnormal, presumably reflecting the changes in bone marrow compostion.[74,75] Imaging studies show diffuse alterations in bone marrow consistency that affects the long bones as well as the axial skeleton.[76] The few instances in which iliac crest biopsy and MR data are available show a concordance of gelatinous change and MRI. As a noninvasive technique, MR allows tracking of bone marrow changes over time with recovery from AN, a task that is otherwise extremely difficult if not impossible. In addition, MR data provide more extensive information on the degree of bone marrow alterations than is available from single and limited samples produced by bone marrow biopsy.

The discovery that adipose is an endocrine tissue by virtue of its production of leptin, a hormone newly added to the endocrine ranks, moved the hematologic disturbances of AN into the realm of endocrine anemias. Leptin is a 16-kDa nonglycosylated peptide produced primarily by white adipose tissue.[77] The hormone circulates both in a free form and as a complex with binding proteins, some of which are soluble forms of the leptin receptor.[78] Serum leptin concentrations correlate with body fat mass, with higher levels occurring with greater degrees of obesity.[79]

The primary physiological role of leptin appears to be the control of the metabolic response to energy deprivation.[80] This concept differs from the first notions of leptin physiology as a modulator of obesity that derived from the morbidly obese transgenic mice produced by knockout of the leptin gene.[81] These animals are aberrations. The preponderance of data indicates that a rapid fall in serum leptin concentrations occurs immediately in response to fasting, which signals the onset of energy deficit to the hypothalamus. The outcome is a switch of hormonal and metabolic balance into an energy conservatory mode manifested by declines in the production of thyroid hormone, insulin-like growth factor 1, and reproductive hormones. The end result is a shift toward energy homeostasis.

Leptin physiology is markedly unbalanced in people suffering from AN. Serum leptin levels are strikingly lower than those of control subjects.[82–84] Furthermore, AN markedly diminishes the normal diurnal variation in serum leptin levels.[85] Circadian variation in levels occurs commonly with hormones, such as that seen with cortisol secretion. Regular diurnal variation is as important to the normal physiologic response to hormones as is the actual serum level of these molecules. The loss of leptin circadian rhythm likely contributes significantly to the metabolic disturbances seen with AN.

An appealing concept that suggests a mechanism for the anemia in AN involves leptin physiology. Fat cells are prominent in the bone marrow stroma, and the stroma influences hematopoiesis. The proposed model for anemia in AN holds that gelatinous transformation of the marrow obliterates marrow adipocytes, removing their positive influence on hematopoiesis. In this scenario, leptin is the central source of that positive influence. Complete proof of this concept is absent, but some tantalizing data exist.

The initial information in this regard came from studies demonstrating expression of the leptin receptor in hematopoietic stem cells of both mouse and human origin.[86] Leptin receptor expression was also apparent in a number of hematopoietic cell lines in continuous culture. Further investigations suggested that leptins could stimulate proliferation and differentiation of hematopoietic cells.[87,88] Additional work showing high expression of leptin by primary cultures of human bone marrow adipocytes completed the picture of leptin activity in hematopoiesis.[89]

The synthesis of these data was a paracrine model system of hematopoietic regulation in which leptin production by local bone marrow adipocytes modulates the proliferation and development of hematopoietic cells. Leptin is a member of the cytokine family of molecules.[90] This model of leptin action would place the hormone among other members of this family that influence hematopoiesis, including erythropoietin, GM-CSF, and IL-6. Data showing that leptin not only promotes hematopoietic cell proliferation, but also works synergistically with erythropoietin and IL-3 in this regard, strengthened the idea that leptin is a vital hematopoietic cell growth factor.[91]

Gelatinous transformation of bone marrow in patients with AN disturbs this equilibrium. The transformation displaces hematopoietic marrow elements. More importantly, the change deprives surviving hematopoietic precursor cells of the growth factors needed for maturation. The AN bone marrow then is not simply one of hematopoietic cell replacement, but one of hematopoietic cell failure.

Caution is important in assessing the status of this interesting hypothesis, however. Each of the individual information packets is initiatory in nature. Additional studies that confirm and, importantly, extend the findings remain absent years after the first observations. Equally important, the details of individual reports contain a number of discrepancies and contradictions, one relative to another. Resolution of such difficulties is important before the model can be considered as being firmly established. Therefore, a role for leptin in hematopoiesis, although appealing and teleological, must at the moment be classified as tentative.

With respect to hematopoiesis in AN, the important fact is that the hematologic disturbances correct with the institution of adequate nutrition. Unfortunately, achieving this end often is extraordinarily difficult. Improving caloric intake to the recommended 1200–1500 kcal/day requires combined psychiatric and medical support.[92] Careful monitoring and support sometimes entails hospitalization with close recording of vital signs, cardiopulmonary status, and electrolyte balance. Although medications such as antidepressants can be useful adjuncts in the management of AN, support from people, including medical staff, psychiatrists, and family, is the key to recovery from this devastating illness.

References

[1] Morris FY, Loy VE, Strutz KM, Schlosser LL, Schilling RF. 1956. Hemoglobin concentrations as determined by a methemoglobin method. Am J Clin Pathol 26:1450–1455.

[2] Manni A, Parchridge WM, Cefalu W, et al. 1985. Bioavailability of albumin-bound testosterone. J Clin Endocrinol Metab 61:705–710.

[3] Claustres M, Sultan C. 1988. Androgens and erythropoiesis: Evidence for an androgen receptor in erythroblasts from human bone marrow cultures. Horm Res 29:17–22.

[4] Khetawat G, Faraday N, Nealen ML, et al. 2000. Human megakaryocytes and platelets contain the estrogen receptor β and androgen receptor (AR): Testosterone regulates AR expression. Blood 95:2289–2296.

[5] Klein KO, Marth PM, Blizzard RM, et al. 1996. A longitudinal assessment of hormonal and physical alterations during normal puberty in boys. II: Estrogen levels as determined by an ultrasensitive bioassay. J Clin Endocrinol Metab 81:3203–3207.

[6] Hero M, Wickman S, Hanhijärvi R, et al. 2005. Pubertal upregulation of erythropoiesis in boys is determined primarily by androgens. J Pediatr 146:245–252.

[7] Daniak N. 1985. The role of androgens in the treatment of anemia of chronic renal failure. Semin Nephrol 5:127–134.

8   Moriyama Y, Fisher JW. 1975. Effects of testosterone and erythropoietin on erythroid colony formation in human bone marrow cultures. Blood 45:665–670.

9   Horner S, Pasternak G, Hehlmann R. 1997. A statistically significant sex difference in the number of colony-forming cells from human peripheral blood. Ann Hematol 74:259–263.

10 Navarro JF, Mora C. 2001. Androgen therapy in elderly uremic patients. Int Urol Nephrol 32:549–557.

11 Johansen KL. 2004. Testosterone metabolism and replacement therapy in patients with end-stage renal disease. Semin Dial 17:202–208.

12 Beato M, Herrlich P, Schutz G. 1995. Steroid hormone receptors: Many actors in search of a plot. Cell 83:851–857.

13 Cole TJ, Blendy JA, Monaghan AP, et al. 1995. Targeted disruption of the glucocorticoid receptor gene blocks adrenergic chromaffin cell development and severely retards lung maturation. Genes Dev 9:1608–1621.

14 Bauer A, Tronche F, Wesseley O, et al. 1999. The glucocorticoid receptor is required for stress erythropoiesis. Genes Dev 13:2996–3002.

15 Wessely O, Deiner E-M, Beug H, et al. 1997. The glucocorticoid receptor is a key regulator of the decision between self-renewal and differentiation in erythroid progenitors. EMBO J 16:267–280.

16 Dolznig H, Grebien F, Deiner E-M, et al. 2006. Erythroid progenitor renewal versus differentiation: Genetic evidence for cell autonomous, essential functions of EpoR, Stat5 and the GR. Oncogene 25:2890–2900.

17 Draptchinskaia N, Gustavsson P, Andersson B, et al. 1999. The gene encoding ribosomal protein S19 is mutated in Diamond-Blackfan anaemia. Nat Genet 21:169–175.

18 Ebert BL, Lee MM, Pretz JL, et al. 2005. An RNA interference model of RPS19 deficiency in Diamond-Blackfan anemia recapitulates defective hematopoiesis and rescue by dexamethasone: Identification of dexamethsone-responsive genes by microarray. Blood 105:4620–4626.

19 Fein HG, Rivlin RS. 1975. Anemia in thyroid diseases. Med Clin North Am 59:1133–1145.

20 Colon-Otero G, Menke D, Hook CC. 1992. A practical approach to the differential diagnosis and evaluation of the adult patient with macrocytic anemia. Med Clin North Am 76:581–597.

21 Chu JY, Monteleone JA, Peden VH, Graviss ER, Vernava AM. 1981. Anemia in children and adolescents with hypothyroidism. Clin Pediatr (Phila) 20:696–699.

22 Franzese A, Salerno M, Argenziano A, et al. 1996. Anemia in infants with congenital hypothyroidism diagnosed by neonatal screening. J Endocrinol Invest 19:613–619.

23 Zimmermann MB, Kohrele J. 2002. The impact of iron and selenium deficiencies on iodine and thyroid metabolism: Biochemistry and relevance to public health. Thyroid 12:867–878.

24 Shakir KM, Turton D, Aprill BS, et al. 2000. Anemia: A cause of intolerance to thyroid sodium. Mayo Clin Proc 75:189–192.

25 Muldowney FP, Crooks J, Wayne FJ. 1957. The total red cell mass in thyrotoxicosis and myxoedema. Clin Sci (Oxf) 16:309–314.

26 Dainiak N, Hoffman R, Maffei LA, et al. 1978. Potentiation of human erythropoiesis in vitro by thyroid hormones. Nature 272:260–262.

27 Golde DW, Bresch N, Chopra IJ, et al. 1977. Thyroid hormones stimulate erythropoiesis in vitro. Br J Haematol 37:173–177.

28 Popovic WJ, Brown JE, Adamson JW. 1977. The influence of thyroid hormones on in vitro erythropoiesis: Mediation by a receptor with beta adrenergic properties. J Clin Invest 60:907–913.

29 Boussios T, McIntyre WR, Gordon AS, et al. 1982. Receptors specific for thyroid hormone in nuclei of mammalian erythroid cells: Involvement in erythroid cell proliferation. Br J Haematol 51:99–106.

30 Yen PM. 2001. Physiological and molecular basis of thyroid hormone action. Physiol Rev 81:1097–1142.

31 Tsai MJ, O'Malley BW. 1994. Molecular mechanisms of action of steroid/thyroid receptor superfamily members. Annu Rev Biochem 65:451–486.

32 Sainteny F, Larras-Regard E, Frindel E. 1990. Thyroid hormones induce hematopoietic pluripotent stem cell differentiation toward erythropoiesis through the production of pluripoietin-like factors. Exp Cell Res 187:174–176.

33 Bauer A, Mikulits W, Lagger G, et al. 1998. The thyroid hormone receptor functions as ligand-operated developmental switch between proliferation and differentiation of erythroid progenitors. EMBO J 17:4291–4303.

34 Fandrey J, Pagel H, Frede S, et al. 1994. Thyroid hormones enhance hypoxia-induced erythropoietin production in vitro. Exp Hematol 22:272–277.

35 Dainiak N, Sutter D, Dreczko S. 1986. L-triiodothyronine augments erythropoietic growth factor release from peripheral blood and bone marrow leukocytes. Blood 68:1289–1297.

36 Davis FB, Smith TJ, Davis PJ, et al. 1991. Sex-dependent inhibition by retinoic acid of thyroid-hormone action on rabbit reticulocyte Ca^{2+}-ATPase activity. Biochem J 273:489–492.

37 Doniach D, Roitt IM, Taylor KB. 1963. Autoimmune phenomena in pernicious anemia: Serological overlap with thyroiditis, thyrotoxicosis and systemic lupus erythematosus. BMJ 1:1374–1379.

38 Singer W, Sahey B. 1966. Myasthenia gravis, Hashimoto's thyroiditis and pernicious anaemia. BMJ 1:904–911.

39 Lee FI, Jenkins GC, Hughes DT, Kazantzis G. 1964. Pernicious anaemia, myxoedema, and hypogammaglobulinaemia—a family study. Br Med J 5383:598–602.

40 Strickland RG. 1969. Pernicious anemia and polyendocrine deficiency. Ann Intern Med 70:1001–1005.

41 Weetman AP. 2005. Non-thyroid autoantibodies in autoimmune thyroid disease. Clin Endocrinol Metab 19:17–32.

42 Jacobson DL, Gange, SJ, Rose NR, et al. 1997. Epidemiology and estimated population burden of selected autoimmune diseases in the United States. Clin Immunol Immunopathol 84:223–243.

43 Ottesen M, Feldt-Rasmussen U, Andersen J, et al. 1995. Thyroid function and autoimmunity in pernicious anemia before and during cyanocobalamin treatment. J Endocrinol Invest 18:91–97.

44 Centanni M, Marignani M, Gargano K, et al. 1999. Atrophic body gastritis with autoimmune thyroid disease: An underdiagnosed association. Arch Int Med 159:1726–1730.

45 Annibale B, Capuros G, Chistolini A, et al. 2001. Gastrointestinal causes of refractory iron deficiency anemia in patients without gastrointestinal symptoms. Am J Med 111:439–445.

46 Carmel R, Weiner JM, Johnson CS. 1987. Iron deficiency occurs frequently in patients with pernicious anemia. JAMA 257:1081–1083.

47 Marignani M, Delle Fave G, Mecarocci S, et al. 1999. High prevalence of atrophic body gastritis in patients with unexplained macrocytic and macrocytic anemia: A prospective screening study. Am J Gastroenterol 94:776–772.

48 Hershko C, Ronson A, Souroujon M, et al. 2006. Variable hematologic presentation of autoimmune gastritis: Age-related progression from iron deficiency to cobalamin depletion. Blood 107:1673–1679.

49 Wang C, Crapo LM. 1997. The epidemiology of thyroid disease and implications for screening. Endocrinol Metab Clin North Am 26:189–219.

50 Canaris GJ, Manowits NR, Mayuor G, et al. The Colorado thyroid disease prevalence study. Arch Int Med 160:526–534.

51 De Craen AJM, Gussekloo J, Teng YKO, et al. 2003. Prevalence of five common clinical abnormalities in very elderly people: Population based cross sectional study. BMJ 327:131–132.

52 Segni M, Wood J, Pucarelli I, et al. 2001. Clustering of autoimmune thyroid disease in children and adolescents: A study of 66 families. J Pediatr Endocrinol Metab 14 (Suppl 5):1297–1298.

53 Weetman AP, McGregor AM. 1994. Autoimmune thyroid disease: Further developments in our understanding. Endocr Rev 15:788–830.

54 Vaidya B, Kendall-Taylor P, Pearce SHS. 2002. Genetics of endocrine disease. The genetics of autoimmune disease. J Clin Endocrinol Metab 87:5385–5397.

55 Strieder TGA, Prummel MF, Tijssen JGP, et al. 2003. Risk factors for and prevalence of thyroid disorders in a cross-sectional study among healthy female relatives of patients with autoimmune thyroid disease. Clin Endocrinol 59:396–401.

56 Becker AE, Grinspoon SK, Klibanski A, et al. 1999. Eating disorders. N Engl J Med 340:1092–1098.

57 Yager J, Andersen AE. 2005. Anorexia nervosa. N Engl J Med 353:1481–1488.

58 Halmi KA, Sunday SR, Klump KL, et al. 2003. Obsessions and compulsions in anorexia nervosa subtypes. Int J Eat Disord 33:308–319.

59 Godart NT, Flamet MF, Curt F, et al. 2003. Anxiety disorders in subjects seeking treatment for eating disorders: A DSM-IV controlled study. Psychiatry Res 117:245–258.

60 Lucas AR, Beard CM, O'Fallon WM, et al. 1991. 50-year treads in the incidence of anorexia nervosa in Rochester, Minnesota: A population-based study. Am J Psychiatry 148:917–922.

61 Von Ranson K, Iacono W, McGue M. 2002. Disordered eating and substance abuse in an epidemiological sample. 1: Associations within individuals. Int J Eat Disord 31:389–403.

62 Halmi K, Casper R, Eckert E, et al. 1979. Unique features associated with age of onset of anorexia nervosa. Psychiatry Res 1:209–215.

63 Pope HG, Jr, Hudson JI, Yurgelun-Todd D. 1984. Prevalence of anorexia nervosa and bulimia in three student populations. Int J Eat Disord 3:45–51.

64 Reas DL, Kjelsås E, Heggestad T, et al. 2005. Characteristics of anorexia nervosa-related deaths in Norway (1992–2000): Data from the National Patient Register and Causes of Death Register. Int J Eat Disord 37:181–187.

65 Møller-Madsen S, Nysrup J, Nielsen S. 1996. Mortality in anorexia nervosa in Denmark, during the period 1970–1987. Acta Psychiatr Scand 94:454–459.

66 Misra M, Aggarwal A, Miller KK, et al. 2004. Effects of anorexia nervosa on clinical, hematologic, biochemical, and bone density parameters in community-dwelling adolescent girls. Pediatrics 114:1574–1583.

67 Miller KK, Grinspoon SK, Ciampa J, et al. 2005. Medical findings in outpatients with anorexia nervosa. Arch Int Med 165:561–566.

68 Takeshita J, Arai Y, Hirose N, et al. 2002. Abetalipoproteinemia-like lipid profile and acanthocytosis in a young woman with anorexia nervosa. Am J Med Sci 324:281–284.

69 Kaiser U, Barth N. 2001. Haemolytic anaemia in a patient with anorexia nervosa. Acta Haematol 106:133–135.

70 Pearson HA. 1967. Marrow hypoplasia in anorexia nervosa. J Pediatr 71:211–215.

71 Seaman JP, Kjeldsberg CR. 1978. Gelatinous transformation of the bone marrow. Hum Pathol 9:685–692.

72 Tavassoli M, Eastlund DT, Yam LT, et al. 1976. Gelatinous transformation of bone marrow in prolonged self-induced starvation. Scand J Haematol 16:311–319.

73 Smith RR, Spivak JL. 1985. Marrow cell necrosis in anorexia nervosa and involuntary starvation. Br J Haematol 60:525–530.

74 Vande Berg BC, Malghem J, Devuyst O, et al. 1994. Anorexia nervosa: Correlation between MR appearance of bone marrow and severity of disease. Radiology 193:859–864.

75 Vande Berg BC, Malghem J, Lecouvet FE, et al. 1996. Distribution of serous-like bone marrow changes in the lower limbs of patients with anorexia nervosa: Predominant involvement of the distal extremities. AJR 166:621–625.

76 Geiser F, Mürtz P, Lutterbey G, et al. 2001. Magnetic resonance spectroscopy and relaxometric determination of bone marrow changes in anorexia nervosa. Psychosom Med 63:631–637.

77 Mantzoros CS. 1999. The role of leptin in human obesity and disease: A review of current evidence. Ann Intern Med 130:671–680.

78 Housova J, Anderlova K, Krizova J, et al. 2005. Serum adiponectin and resistin concentrations in patients with restrictive and binge/purge form of anorexia nervosa and bulimia nervosa. J Clin Endocrinol Metab 90:1366–1370.

79 Considine RV, Singha MK, Heiman ML, et al. 1996. Serum immunoreactive-leptin concentrations in normal-weight and obese humans. N Engl J Med 334:292–295.

80 Chan JK, Mantzoros CS. 2005. Role of leptin in energy-deprivation states: Normal human physiology and clinical implications for hypothalamic amenorrhoea and anorexia nervosa. Lancet 366:74–85.

81 Zhang Y, Proenca R, Maffei M, et al. 1994. Positional cloning of the mouse obese gene and its human homologue. Nature 372:425–432.

82 Lear SA, Pauly RP, Birmingham CL. 1999. Body fat, caloric intake, and plasma leptin levels in women with anorexia nervosa. Int J Eat Disord 26:283–288.

83 Kopp W, Blum WF, Ziegler A, et al. 1998. Serum leptin and body weight in females with anorexia and bulimia nervosa. Horm Metab Res 30:272–275.

84 Grinspoon S, Gulick T, Askari H, et al. 1996. Serum leptin levels in women with anorexia nervosa. J Clin Endocrinol Metab 81:3861–3863.

85 Balligand JL, Brichard SM, Brichard V, et al. 1998. Hypoleptinemia in patients with anorexia nervosa: Loss of circadian rhythm and unresponsiveness to short-term refeeding. Eur J Endocrinol 138:415–420.

86 Cioffi JA, Shafer AW, Zapancic TJ, et al. 1996. Novel B219/OB receptor isoforms: Possible role of leptin in hematopoiesis and reproduction. Nature Med 2:585–589.

87 Gainsford T, Wilson TA, Metcalf D, et al. 1996. Leptin can induce proliferation, differentiation, and functional activation of hemopoietic cells. Proc Natl Acad Sci U S A 93:14564–14568.

88 Bennett BD, Solar GP, Yuan JQ, et al. 1996. A role for leptin and its cognate receptor in hematopoiesis. Curr Biol 6:1170–1180.

89 Laharrague P, Larrouy D, Fontanilles A-M, et al. 1998. High expression of leptin by human bone marrow adipocytes in primary culture. FASEB J 12:747–752.

90 Ouyang S, He F. 2003. Phylogeny of a growth hormone-like cytokine superfamily based on 3D structure. J Mol Evol 56:131–136.

91 Umemoto Y, Tsuji K, Yang F-C, et al. 1997. Leptin stimulates the proliferation of murine myelocytic and primitive hematopoietic progenitor cells. Blood 90:3438–3443.

92 Vitousek K, Watson S, Wilson GT. 1998. Enhancing motivation for change in treatment-resistant eating disorders. Clin Psychol Rev 18:391–420.

Stem Cell Dysfunction

PEDIATRIC BONE MARROW FAILURE SYNDROMES

A wide range of disorders that arise during infancy and childhood disrupt cell production by one or more of the three hematopoietic lines. Some of the disorders affect a single lineage while others produce pancytopenia. Some disorders, such as Fanconi's anemia (FA), commonly cause derangements in nonhematopoietic cells and tissues with the consequent finding of associated congenital anomalies. Most of the disorders present in the neonatal period or early in childhood. Improved diagnostic tools along with recognition of the variability inherent in these conditions now reveal mild manifestations or forme fruste in adolescents or even young adults. The uneven clinical texture of these conditions is a continuing challenge to clinicians.

■ FANCONI'S ANEMIA (CONGENITAL APLASTIC ANEMIA)

In 1927, Professor Guido Fanconi of Zurich, Switzerland, described several families in which there were children with striking congenital anomalies including absent radii, abnormal thumbs, short stature, and hyperpigmentation. Children with no obvious congenital anomalies have also been described. These children develop hematological abnormalities at a mean age of about 7 years; initially thrombocytopenia followed progressively by neutropenia and anemia.

FA is a heterogeneous conglomeration of disorders derived from a collection of impendent mutations involving genes on several chromosomes.[1] Cell fusion studies done in vitro show that cellular components from two unrelated patients with FA can combine to eliminate the Fanconi phenotype. In other words, cells from the two FA patients *complement* each other and correct the defect. Of the 11 currently known complementation groups, gene identification data exist for 8.[2] Three genes, *FANCA*, *FANCC*, and *FANCG*, account for 90% of FA cases. Interestingly, *FANCD1* is identical to the breast cancer susceptibility gene *BRCA2*.

The molecular details of the cellular action of the FA complementation group proteins are unclear. A number of the proteins appear to be components of a molecular complex that fosters chromosomal stability.[3,4] Absence of the FA proteins impairs the function of the complex. Deranged regulation of apoptosis in FA cells and aberrant telomere shortening could be consequences of deranged chromosome stability factors.

In the fully developed syndrome, the patients have pancytopenia and the bone marrow is hypocellular. The red cells are macrocytic with increased Hb F content that can precede marrow failure. The usual diagnostic test for FA involves culturing peripheral blood lymphocytes in the presence of a DNA cross-linking agent such as diepoxybutane (DEB). In FA, the chromosomal metaphases show DNA repair abnormalities evidenced by a high proportion of chromatid breaks, gaps, and rearrangements and endoreduplications.

Androgen therapy improves the anemia in about two-thirds of patients, but most become resistant to the treatment over time. Complications of synthetic androgen therapy include masculinization, severe acne, and hepatic damage (hepatic peliosis and liver tumors). Supportive treatment with red cell and platelet transfusions then is often required. Total bone marrow failure with consequent death within a few years of its onset is the fate of most patients.

Longer survival of some patients with FA has unveiled a high cumulative incidence of myelodysplasia and leukemia, in the range of 10% over 25 years.[5] Long-surviving patients are also 50 times more likely than normal to develop solid tumors involving particularly the esophagus and oropharynx.[6] The prognosis is dismal in such cases.

Stem cell transplantation is the only cure for FA.[7] However, because the cells of these patients cannot repair DNA damage, conditioning procedure with immunosuppressive agents and radiation must be modified with reduced intensity. Cures have been obtained using HLA-compatible stem cells from siblings, and most recently with cord blood stem cells.

■ CONGENITAL HYPOPLASTIC ANEMIA (DIAMOND-BLACKFAN ANEMIA, ERYTHROGENESIS IMPERFECTA)

In 1938, Drs. Louis K. Diamond and Kernneth Blackfan described four children with severe, aregenerative, macrocytic anemia that developed in the first year of life. The anemia was so severe that regular RBC transfusions were necessary to sustain life. The other formed elements of the blood were normal, so it was classified as a "pure red cell anemia." In the subsequent years more than 500 cases have been formally reported, but a current national registry includes more than 1000 cases.[8]

The disease appears in 2–7 per million live births. Diamond-Blackfan anemia (DBA) affects most ethnic groups, but Caucasian children predominate among the reported cases. Although repeat cases have been noted in a some families, suggesting a genetic cause, the preponderance of cases is sporadic.[9] Although the cause of DBA has not been established in most cases, about 25% of patients studied to date have mutations involving RPS19, a ubiquitously expressed ribosomal protein required for efficient translation in all cells. The mutations in DBA disrupt its normal localization in the nucleolus.[10] In vitro experiments that disrupt production of RPS19 in hematopoietic precursor cells produce a phenotype very similar to that seen in DBA.[11]

Anemia (or pallor) is noteworthy at or shortly after birth, and instances of profound intrauterine anemia causing hydrops fetalis have been described. Two-thirds of children are diagnosed by 6 months and virtually all are identified before 1 year of age. At the time of diagnosis, hemoglobin levels can be as low as 2.0 g/dL. The red cells are macrocytic with a higher than normal Hb F content. The reticulocyte count is very low (<0.1%). The remainder of the peripheral blood count is usually normal, although moderate neutropenia occurs in some patients. Erythrocyte adenosine deaminase (ADA) levels are two to three times greater than normal in most patients (Table 10-1).[12] Plasma and urinary levels of erythropoietin are elevated over baseline.

The bone marrow is normally cellular with normal complements of neutrophil precursors, megakaryocytes, and lymphocytes. However, erythroid precursors of every maturational stage are markedly reduced or absent, producing myeloid/erythroid ratios ranging from 10/1 to 200/1. Bone marrow cultures produce very few BFU-E or CFU-E.

About 25% of patients have physical abnormalities, including short stature and facial, cardiac, and renal abnormalities. A small subset of patients have tri- rather than biphalangeal thumbs (Asse syndrome). The incidence of cancer in DBA is higher than normal but lower than that seen in FA.

About two-thirds of children respond to corticosteroid therapy, maintaining normal or near normal hemoglobin levels without transfusions.[13] Corticosteroids such as oral prednisone in a dose of 2–4 mg/kg/day is the initial treatment with response heralded by a reticulocytosis in 1–2 weeks followed by a rise in hemoglobin to normal levels. At that time a gradual reduction in prednisone dose is possible, sometimes to as little as 0.5–1.0 mg/day. Some patients respond to alternate day steroids, which

TABLE 10-1	KEY DIAGNOSTIC POINTS IN PEDIATRIC BONE MARROW FAILURE	
Issue	*Manifestations*	*Approach*
DBA versus TEC	• Anemia • Normal neutrophil and platelet counts	• Normochromic red cells in TEC; macrocytic red cells in DBA • Elevated Hb F in DBA • Elevated red cell ADA in DBA
Fanconi's anemia versus aplastic anemia in older children	• Pancytopenia	• Physical examination looking for subtle features of FA • Chromosome instability test

DBA, Diamond-Blackfan anemia; TEC, transient erythroblastic anemia of childhood; ADA, adenosine deaminase; FA, Fanconi's anemia.

produce fewer side effects. Response failures sometimes occur with usual doses of steroids, but patient rescue occurs at times with higher doses. Patients who initially respond to steroids can become refractory to the treatment. Spontaneous remissions have also been described.

Children who do not respond to steroids or who need toxic doses of the drugs require regular red cell transfusions. Transfusional hemosiderosis requiring chelation therapy complicates this intervention. Children with DBA develop transfusional iron overload more slowly than do those with hemolytic anemias, probably because iron absorption is not increased. Hematopoietic stem cell transplantation can cure DBA and should be considered for transfusion-dependent children, particularly when they have an HLA-compatible sibling potential donor.[14]

Pure red cell anemia does occur in older children and adults (see Chapter 2). The condition sometimes is associated with a thymic tumor. Drugs such as chloramphenicol also occasionally induce pure red cell anemia.

■ TRANSIENT ERYTHROBLASTIC ANEMIA OF CHILDHOOD

Transient erythroblastic anemia of childhood (TEC) is a self limited, aregenerative anemia that occurs in otherwise healthy children (Table 10-2).[15] The mean age at onset is about 2 years. Pallor and symptoms of anemia are the usual presenting manifestations. TEC seems to be an autoimmune disease as indicated by the presence of circulating immunoglobulins in the patient that inhibit the growth of BFU-E and CFU-E in tissue culture. The basis of this aberrant antibody production is unknown, but it is not related to parvovirus B19 (see below).

The anemia, which may be severe, develops slowly since there is no concomitant hemolytic process. Patients often are remarkably asymptomatic given the severity

TABLE 10-2 | **KEY MANAGEMENT ISSUES IN PEDIATRIC BONE MARROW FAILURE**

Issue	*Comment*
Long-term management of DBA	Steroids should be tapered to the lowest dose that produces sufficient hematological improvement. A key goal is to avoid red cell transfusions and consequent iron overload. Stem cell transplantation should be considered in severe cases where an HLA-matched sibling exists.
Long-term management of Fanconi's anemia	Androgens improve the pancytopenia in most cases. Androgen efficacy declines over time while androgen-associated complications increase. Stem cell transplantation should be considered when an HLA-matched sibling exists.
Transient erythroblastic anemia of childhood versus parvovirus B19 infection	TEC occurs in normal children and is self-limited, usually requiring no intervention. Children with mild previously undiagnosed hemolytic anemias sometimes present due to parvovirus B19 infection. The picture can be very similar to that of TEC. These children can however develop life-threatening anemia. Serum IgM titers against parvovirus B19 clarify the diagnosis. Transfusion support may be needed until recovery.

DBA, Diamond-Blackfan anemia; TEC, transient erythroblastic anemia of childhood.

of the anemia. The reticulocyte count is very low (<0.1%). In contrast to DBA, TEC patients are older, have normocytic rather than macrocytic red cells, and the erythrocyte levels of ADA and Hb F are normal. The rest of the peripheral blood elements are usually normal, but some patients have thrombocytosis. The bone marrow is normally cellular and initially shows few red cell precursors.

Spontaneous recovery occurs within 1–2 months. In the recovery period there is a brisk reticulocytosis that may be misinterpreted as indicating a hemolytic process. The reticulocytosis ends when the hemoglobin level returns to normal. Recurrences are unusual.

■ RED CELL APLASIA ASSOCIATED WITH PARVOVIRUS B19 INFECTION

Parvovirus B19 infection often produces exaggerated anemia and reticulocytopenia (aplastic crises) in children with various kinds of hemolytic anemias. Since parvovirus infections in childhood with consequent erythema infectiosum (Fifth disease) are the norm, this complication is usually but not exclusively a pediatric problem. No parvovirus vaccine suitable for human use currently exists, although one is available for veterinary purposes.

The parvovirus directly infects the CFU-E and inhibits proliferation. A virtual cessation of red cell production ensues lasting for 1–2 weeks until host production of IgM antibodies clear the organism. In a normal child, with an erythrocyte life span of 120 days, 10 days of red cell aplasia lowers the hemoglobin level insignificantly. However, in children with hemolytic anemia, such as sickle cell disease, where red cell survival can be as short as 10–20 days, 1–2 weeks of erythroid inactivity produces profound anemia. During aplastic crises the anemia worsens and bilirubin levels decrease. Profound reticulocytopenia (<0.1%) develops. Bone marrow aspiration shows a marked decrease in erythroid precursors. Giant pronormoblasts are characteristic of this disease, and electron microscopy can demonstrate a plethora of viral particles in their cytoplasm.

The anemia can be sufficiently profound as to require red cell transfusions. Only small transfusions (5–7 mL/kg of RBC) are necessary, however, since prompt, spontaneous recovery is routine. Treatment with intravenous immunoglobulin may hasten recovery. During the recovery period, the child can still have severe anemia in association with a prodigious reticulocytosis. Children initially seen during early recovery sometimes receive an erroneous diagnosis of "hemolytic crisis."

Parvovirus infection produces lasting immunity in the immunologically intact individuals, meaning that recurrent aplastic crises do not occur. However, immunocompromised individuals who cannot mount an antibody response (e.g., HIV infection) can develop a chronic aregenerative anemia due to persistent viral infection. Periodic infusions of intravenous gamma globulin may be indicated. A mother with a primary parvovirus infection during pregnancy can transmit the virus to the fetus. Gestational infection can produce severe anemia with a mortality rate of about 10% with the occasional development of hydrops fetalis.

■ PEARSON SYNDROME

This rare syndrome is characterized by a refractory, aregenerative, macrocytic anemia that is accompanied by exocrine pancreatic dysfunction and metabolic acidosis.[16] The anemia is present in early life and is often transfusion dependent. Striking morphological abnormalities are present in the bone marrow. There is intensive vacuolization of myeloid and erythroid precursors and the presence of "ringed sideroblasts" (erythroid precursors with iron laden mitochondria in the cytoplasm) (see Chapter 12). Patients develop, and often die, of the consequence of mitochondrial dysfunction including metabolic acidosis and deranged metabolism involving oxidative phosphorylation.

The syndrome is caused by extensive deletions of mitochondrial DNA.[17,18] The inheritance of this condition is maternal, because mitochondria are present only in the ovum[19] but no familial cases have been described. Most of these children die in infancy, but a few have survived with improvement of the anemia but later developed the neurological abnormalities of Kayne-Sayres disease, another mitochondrial condition.

■ DYSKERATOSIS CONGENITA

Dyskeratosis congenita is a rare disorder in which there are striking changes of the skin and mucous membranes and frequent involvement of the bone marrow.[20] The disease is characterized by dystrophic changes of the nails, hyperpigmented mottling of the skin, and leukoplakia. Three quarters of cases are inherited as an X-linked disorder, and these boys have an abnormal gene at chromosome Xq28 that encodes the protein dyskerin. About 50% of patients develop marrow failure and pancytopenia at an average age of 15 years at onset. Various therapies aimed at the hematologic abnormalities have been used with varying degrees of effectiveness including G-CSF, androgens, and stem cell transplantation. Acute myelogenous leukemia and other malignancies have been reported in adult life. The average survival is about 30 years, most patients dying as a result of complications of pancytopenia or malignancy.

References

[1] Alter B. 1993. Fanconi's anemia: Current concepts. Am J Pediatr Hematol Oncol 14:170.

[2] Tischkowitz M, Dokal I. 2004. Fanconi anaemia and leukaemia—clinical and molecular aspects. Br J Haematol 126:176–191.

[3] Taniguchi T, Tischkowitz M, Ameziane N, et al. 2003. Disruption of the Fanconi anemia—BRCA pathway in cisplatin-sensitive ovarian tumors. Nat Med 9:568–574.

[4] Hussain S, Witt E, Huber PA, Medhurst AL, Ashworth A Mathew CG. 2003. Direct interaction of the Fanconi anaemia protein FANCG with BRCA2/FANCD1. Hum Mol Genet 12:2503–2510.

[5] Alter BP, Caruso JP, Drachtman RA, Uchida T, Velagaleti GV, Elghetany MT. 2000. Fanconi anemia. Myelodysplasia as a predictor of outcome. Cancer Genet Cytogenet 117:125–131.

[6] Alter BP, Greene MH, Velazquez I, Rosenberg PS. 2003. Cancer in Fanconi anemia. Blood 101:2072.

[7] Socie G, Devergie A, Girinski T, et al. 1998. Transplantation for Fanconi's anaemia: Longterm follow-up of fifty patients transplanted from a sibling donor after low-dose cyclophosphamide and thoraco-abdominal irradiation for conditioning. Br J Haematol 103:249–255.

[8] Vlachos A, Klein GW, Lipton JM. 2001. The Diamond Blackfan Anemia registry: Tool for investigating the epidemiology and biology of Diamond Blackfan anemia. J Pediatr Hematol Oncol 23:377–382.

[9] Orfali KA, Ohene-Abuakwa Y, Ball SE. 2004 Diamond Blackfan anaemia in the UK: Clinical and genetic heterogeneity. Br J Haematol 125:243–252.

[10] Da Costa L, Tchernia G, Gascard P, et al. 2003. Nucleolar localization of RPS19 protein in normal cells and mislocalization due to mutations in the nucleolar localization signals in 2 Diamond-Blackfan anemia patients: Potential insights into pathophysiology. Blood 101(12):5039–5045.

[11] Flygare J, Kiefer T, Miyake K, et al. 2005. Deficiency of ribosomal protein S19 in CD34+ cells generated by siRNA blocks erythroid development and mimics defects seen in Diamond-Blackfan anemia. Blood 105:4627–4634.

[12] Glader BE, Backer K. 1986. Elevated erythrocyte adenosine deaminase levels in congenital hypoplastic anemia. N Eng J Med 309:486

[13] Willig TN, Niemeyer CM, Leblanc T, et al. 1999. Identification of new prognosis factors from the clinical and epidemiologic analysis of a registry of 229 Diamond-Blackfan anemia patients. DBA group of Societe d'Hematologie et d'Immunologie Pediatrique (SHIP), Gesellshaft fur Padiatrische Onkologie und Hamatologie (GPOH), and the European Society for Pediatric Hematology and Immunology (ESPHI). Pediatr Res 46:553–561.

[14] Vlachos A, Lipton JM. Hematopoietic stem cell transplant for inherited bone marrow failure syndromes. In: Mehta P, ed. Pediatric Stem Cell Transplantation. Sudbury, MA: Jones and Bartlett; 2004:281–311.

[15] Wang NC, Mentzer WC. 1976. Differentiation of transient erythroblastopenia of childhood from congenital hypoplastic anemia. J Pediatr 88:784.

[16] Pearson HA, Lobel JS, Kocoshis SA, et al. 1979. A new syndrome of refractory sideroblastic anemia with vacuolization of marrow precursors and exocrine pancreatic dysfunction. J Pediatr 95:976–984.

[17] Cormier V, Rotig A, Quartino AR, et al. 1990. Widespread multi-tissue deletions of the mitochondrial genome in the Pearson marrow-pancreas syndrome. J Pediatr 117:599–602.

[18] Rotig A, Cormier V, Koll F, et al. 1991. Site specific deletions of the mitochondrial genome in the Pearson Marrow Pancreas Syndrome. Genomics 10:502–504.

[19] Lightowlers RN, Chinnery PF, Turnbull DM, Howell N. 1997. Mammalian mitochondrial genetics: Heredity, heteroplasmy and disease. Trends Genet 13:450–455.

[20] Drachtman RA, Alter BP. 1995. Dyskeratosis congenital. Dermatol Clin 13: 33.

ACQUIRED BONE MARROW FAILURE SYNDROMES

Normal bone marrow function is vital both to health and survival. The organ is remarkable in its ability to compensate for defects that impair the operation or function of any of the major cell lineages. Bone marrow failure produces not only anemia, but also varying degrees of thrombocytopenia and neutropenia. The clinical impact that arises from the loss of neutrophil and platelet cell lineages often determines the patient's ultimate fate with respect to bone marrow failure. Anemia often is an important but decidedly secondary factor in these events.

Table 11-1 classifies the primary causes of acquired bone marrow failure. The disorders have both similarities and differences. Placing a patient's condition specifically into one category or another at times is problematic due to the significant overlap in clinical features that characterize the several groups. Myelodysplasia has singularly important clinical characteristics that set it apart from the other three conditions in the list. Not only are chromosomal disturbances more common with myelodysplasia, the disorder has a risk of conversion into acute leukemia that substantially exceeds that associated with any of the other conditions in Table 11-1. In fact, myelodysplasia was once termed "preleukemia," a testament to its leukemic potential. The disorder is covered separately from the other conditions in Table 11-1.

■ APLASTIC ANEMIA

Aplastic anemia is a rare disorder whose incidence approximates two per million in Western countries. Paul Ehrlich introduced the concept of aplastic anemia in 1888 when he described a pregnant woman who died of bone marrow failure. In 1904,

TABLE 11-1	ACQUIRED BONE MARROW FAILURE SYNDROMES
Aplastic anemia	
Pure red cell aplasia	
Paroxysmal nocturnal hemoglobinuria	
Myelodysplasia	

Anatole Chauffard coined the term "aplastic anemia" to describe this devastating hematological syndrome. Case reports and autopsy findings in the early part of the twentieth century slowly filled in key clinical aspects of the illness and established aplastic anemia as the paradigm of bone marrow failure. A striking bimodal age distribution characterizes aplastic anemia, with the largest group of patients being adolescents or young adults. A second cohort of patients present in later adulthood, typically in the sixth or seventh decades of life.

Aplastic anemia has no ethnic or racial predilection. However, the disorder is more frequent in the developing world. Estimates vary, but the incidence in developing countries appears to exceed those in the West by between two- and fourfold. The discrepancy likely represents the impact of environmental factors that predispose to bone marrow aplasia.

CLINICAL PRESENTATION

The clinical presentation of aplastic anemia depends on where the patient stands in the evolution of the disorder. Fatigue, shortness of breath and ringing in the ears, manifestations of severe anemia, most commonly prompt the initial physician visit. Older patients sometimes have chest pains, reflecting impaired cardiac oxygen delivery in a setting of cardiac blood flow limited in part by atherosclerosis. Nearly everyone reports a recent tendency toward easy bruising that reflects the thrombocytopenia associated with bone marrow aplasia. Interestingly, complaints related to neutropenia are uncommon at presentation.

Striking pallor dominates the initial clinical impression. The manifestation is most obvious in people with relatively low levels of intrinsic skin pigmentation. Pale mucous membranes and nail beds are the key finding in people with darker skin. Jaundice typically is absent from the otherwise pasty complexion. Ecchymoses along the waistline represent bruising from clothing, including the impact of belts and supportive garments. Ecchymoses and petechiae are nearly universal on the dependent body surfaces including the pretibial surfaces, ankles, and wrists.

Direct ophthalmoscopy commonly shows pale retinae often with small areas of hemorrhage. Gingival oozing is a frequent manifestation. Although some patients spontaneously give a history of bleeding with tooth brushing, others provide this history only upon direct questioning. Poor dental hygiene and associated gingivitis increases the prominence of this finding.

Prominent manifestations on cardiac examination include tachycardia and systolic murmurs. Both findings directly reflect the enhanced cardiac activity that develops in part as compensation for the severe anemia. Bounding pulses are routine. Carotid bruits occur frequently in older patients.

Less common manifestations at presentation include folliculitis and other skin infections. Stool guaiac examination commonly is positive, but frank blood in the stool is uncommon. Women often report heavier than normal menses over the weeks or months preceding presentation. Metrorrhagia is a distinctly less common complaint. Lymphadenopathy is uncommon at presentation and prominent lymph node enlargement raises the specter of other conditions, such as lymphoma.

Pancytopenia is the hallmark of aplastic anemia. Uneven depression of hemoglobin value, platelet count, and neutrophil count often exists at presentation, particularly in the early stages in the evolution of the disorder. Aplastic anemia also varies tremendously in severity. Some people have moderate depression of all three cell lines and require little or no treatment. Other less fortunate people need immediate and sometimes heroic intervention in response to a condition of life-threatening severity. The prognosis for severe aplastic anemia is more tenebrous than that of milder disease.

The diagnosis of aplastic anemia applies to patients who show two of the following three criteria: (1) hemoglobin <10 g/dL, (2) platelets <50,000/μL, (3) neutrophils <1500/μL.[1] Bone marrow examination shows a marked reduction in the number of hematopoietic elements, with fat cells filling the vacuum. Although some of the residual hematopoietic precursors can appear aberrant, striking dysplastic features are not characteristic of aplastic anemia. Myelodysplasia is the major diagnostic consideration in patients who have marked dysplasia of the hematopoietic elements. In such diagnostic dilemmas, chromosome analysis is very useful since karyotype anomalies are hallmarks of myelodysplasia but are infrequent with aplastic anemia.

The bone marrow examination is an important step in ruling out disorders that secondarily produce peripheral blood pancytopenia and thus impersonate aplastic anemia (Table 11-2). Leukemia in which malignant cells are confined to the bone marrow produces a pancytopenia that fully mimics aplastic anemia. The occasional blast cell can evade detection on peripheral blood examination. This so-called "aleukemic leukemia" is much more of an issue in childhood acute lymphocytic leukemia than is the case with acute myelogenous leukemia.

Less commonly, marrow replacement by lymphoma cells or myeloma cells produces a peripheral blood picture consistent with aplastic anemia. Extensive bone marrow fibrosis associated with a myeloproliferative disorder, most prominently myelofibrosis with myeloid metaplasia, at times produces a bland pancytopenia. Schistocytes and other features on peripheral blood examination that point to distorted bone marrow architecture due to fibrosis are sometimes subtle. Miliary tuberculosis with extensive bone marrow involvement at times presents a peripheral blood picture that is indistinguishable from aplastic anemia.

TABLE 11-2	CONDITIONS THAT MIMIC APLASTIC ANEMIA DUE TO MARROW REPLACEMENT

Leukemia confined to the bone marrow

Lymphoma

Multiple myeloma

Myelofibrosis

Tuberculosis of the bone marrow

Metastatic neuroblastoma in children

Fat comprises up to 90% of the marrow cellularity in some patients with aplastic anemia. The fat cells do not actively replace normal marrow elements, as occurs with the fibroblasts and other stromal elements in patients with myelofibrosis. Fat cells merely fill in by default the regions of the marrow left empty by the disappearance of the hematopoietic elements. The process is general throughout the bone marrow space as shown by imaging of the vertebra with MRI or other sensitive techniques.

The severity of aplastic anemia at presentation both affects the prognosis of the condition and dictates the treatment considerations. Severe aplastic anemia as defined by the International Aplastic Anemia Study Group requires (1) bone marrow cellularity <25% of normal or 25–50% of normal with <30% residual hematopoietic cells and (2) two of the following three criteria: neutrophils <500/μL, platelets <20,000/μL, and reticulocytes <1%.[2] The prognosis is particularly dire in patients in whom the neutrophil count falls below 200 cells/μL.

ETIOLOGY

Cases of acquired aplastic anemia most commonly lack a clear cause with as many as 60% falling under the "idiopathic" rubric (Table 11-3). Table 11-3 also lists some of the conditions known to produce aplastic anemia as a secondary phenomenon. Bone marrow damage from radiation exposure can produce marrow aplasia. Radiation of sufficient intensity to produce aplastic anemia occurs only with medical treatment for cancer or in the aftermath of major disasters such as Chernobyl. Low-level environmental radiation, such as that associated with radon or other natural sources of radiation, is not a proven cause of aplastic anemia.

Chemicals and drugs figure prominently in the etiology of aplastic anemia. Some drugs produce marrow aplasia as an expected and foreseeable outcome because toxicity to proliferating cells is intrinsic to their clinical effect. Cancer chemotherapy drugs are the most obvious members of this subgroup. Benzene, one of the first industrial

TABLE 11-3	ETIOLOGY OF ACQUIRED APLASTIC ANEMIA
Cause idiopathic	Example
Radiation	• Chernobyl • Cancer irradiation
Chemicals (foreseeable)	• Cancer chemotherapy drugs • Benzene
Chemicals (idiosyncratic)	• Chloramphenicol • Gold • Penicillamine • NSAIDs • Sulphonamides • Propylthiouracil
Viruses	Hepatitis • Non-A, non-B, non-C, non-G Epstein-Barr virus • Infectious mononucleosis Human immunodeficiency virus
Immune disorders	Systemic lupus erythematosis Thymoma Transfusion-associated graft-versus-host disease Pregnancy

toxins shown to cause aplastic anemia, also directly injures hematopoietic stem cells. Controls on use and exposure to benzene as well as other organic solvents have virtually eliminated these agents as sources of aplastic anemia in Western countries. The higher incidence of aplastic anemia in many nations of the developing world likely represents unknown or unappreciated exposure to similar agents.[3] The fact that people of Asian background in the United States do not have the high incidence of aplastic anemia seen among people in their ancestral countries reinforces the fact that socioeconomic issues in these regions and not genetics dictate the expression of aplastic anemia.[4]

Some nonchemotherapy drugs, such as chloramphenicol, have a clear cause-and-effect relationship with aplastic anemia. About half the patients who take high-dose chloramphenicol develop a mild reversible suppression of erythropoiesis that clears with discontinuation of treatment. A conspicuous finding on bone marrow examination is prominent vacuoles, particularly in developing normoblasts. Chloramphenicol inhibits mRNA translation by the 70S ribosomes of prokaryotes. The drug does not affect 80S eukaryotic ribosomes. Mitochondria, key organelles for both energy production and heme biosynthesis in erythroid precursor cells, have ribosomes that are similar to prokaryotes. Chloramphenicol consequently inhibits mitochondrial protein synthesis. Chloramphenicol-induced vacuole formation in erythroid precursors and the associated anemia likely reflect this inhibition.[5]

Distinctly different is the bone marrow aplasia that develops in a small group of people following chloramphenicol exposure. In contrast to the mild suppression of erythropoiesis, this idiosyncratic reaction is severe, sustained, affects all cell lines, and does not depend on drug dose.[6] Data such as the development of aplastic anemia in identical twins treated with chloramphenicol suggest that a genetic predisposition underlies this event.[7] The basis for such a predilection to aplasia with chloramphenicol treatment remains unknown. The rare occurrence of aplastic anemia following the use of ophthalmic preparations that contain chloramphenicol emphasizes the extreme sensitivity of susceptible people.[8,9]

Establishing a cause-and-effect relationship between a specific drug and aplastic anemia often is a difficult proposition. The drugs listed in Table 11-3 only sporadically cause aplastic anemia. The devastating impact of the disorder focuses great attention on the patient and medications in the patient's history. People commonly are on more than one medication when the disorder arises, which complicates the task of making an assignment with respect to cause. In contrast to the situation with chloramphenicol where idiosyncratic aplastic anemia occurs in relatively close proximity to the start of drug use, aplastic anemia develops in some patients months or even years after they begin using the drugs (see Table 11-3). Most often, therefore, the diagnosis of drug-induced aplastic anemia is presumptive.

Viral infections often are implicated in the onset of aplastic anemia. In contrast to a history of drug or chemical exposure, objective markers in hepatitis are clear, allowing precise characterization of the post-hepatitis aplastic anemia syndrome.[10] The victims usually are young and the hepatitis almost invariably is seronegative, suggesting that a yet-undefined infectious agent is the culprit (hence, the non-A, non-B, non-C, non-G designation). Laboratory and clinical studies both support an immune component to the pathophysiology of post-hepatitis aplastic anemia. The positive response to immunosuppressive therapy both of the liver inflammation and marrow aplasia reinforces the point. Case control studies in Southeast Asia also support the strong role of an infectious etiology in aplastic anemia, identifying as risk factors low socioeconomic status, rice farming, and previous exposure to an enteric virus.[11] Aplastic anemia arises as a rare sequela of infectious mononucleosis.

Immune dysregulation is a central thread in many if not most cases of acquired aplastic anemia, both idiopathic and secondary. The seminal observation came in 1970 when Mathe and colleagues documented autologous recovery of hematopoiesis in a patient with aplastic anemia who failed to engraft after marrow transplantation.[12] The investigators proposed that the immunosuppressive regimen used for conditioning prompted recovery of the patient's endogenous hematopoietic function. Numerous subsequent studies of immunosuppressive therapy show improved marrow function in approximately 70% of patients with acquired aplastic anemia.[13] Although the identity of the inciting antigens that breach immune tolerance with subsequent autoimmunity is unknown, HLA-DR2 is overrepresented among European and American patients with aplastic anemia suggesting a role for this haplotype in the process.[14]

An expanded population of CD8 and HLA-DR$^+$ cytotoxic T lymphocytes, detectable in both the blood and bone marrow of patients with aplastic anemia, probably mediates the suppression of hematopoiesis. These cells produce cytokines such as interferon gamma and tumor necrosis factor that inhibit growth of progenitor cells in vitro. These cytokines repress hematopoiesis through effects on mitosis as well as direct cell killing through Fas-mediated apoptosis. The cytokines also induce nitric oxide synthase and nitric oxide production by marrow cells, which contributes to immune-mediated cytotoxicity and elimination of hematopoietic precursor cells.

The occasional association of aplastic anemia with immune-mediated disorders such as systemic lupus erythematosis reinforces the association of marrow aplasia with immune dysregulation. Aplastic anemia usually develops years after the onset of the primary problem, suggesting an evolution of immune disturbances associated with the underlying disorder that ultimately produce marrow aplasia. The rare association of aplastic anemia with pregnancy likely is similar to other instances of disordered immune function that can arise in pregnancy, of which postpartum deficiency of Factor VIII is a prime example. Successful pregnancy requires a reset of maternal immune function to accommodate the presence of the fetus (which de facto is a foreign body). The basis of the spectacular though thankfully rare failure in this adjustment to the immune system is a mystery.

TREATMENT OF APLASTIC ANEMIA

A number of factors impinge on treatment decisions for patients with aplastic anemia including the severity of the condition, comorbid medical conditions, and the availability of possible transplant donors. The high response rate makes immunosuppressive therapy the treatment of choice for patients whose disease does not fall into the severe category. The most common immunosuppressive regime involves treatment with antiserum against lymphoid cells derived from horse or rabbit sources. Immune suppression regimens commonly also include other drugs that modulate immune activity, such as cyclosporine. Immunosuppressive therapy also is effective in many people with severe aplastic anemia who are ineligible for the more aggressive stem cell transplantation regimen.

Hematopoietic stem cell transplantation is the approach of choice for patients with severe aplastic anemia. The age window for this treatment has gradually widened over the years, but has not disappeared. Although older people can undergo stem cell transplantation, morbidity and mortality associated with the treatment increase both with advancing age and coexisting significant medical conditions. People with significant cardiac or pulmonary disease are at particular risk of death directly related to the transplant procedure. Graft-versus-host disease is also a greater risk for older people relative to youthful victims of aplastic anemia.

The infrequency of aplastic anemia and the complexity of the treatment options mean that hematologists who specialize in the management of bone marrow failure should oversee patient care. While this is clearly the case for stem cell transplantation, the same holds for medical management using immunosuppressive drugs.

Physicians who initially see a patient with aplastic anemia must at times decide on supportive management issues before arrangements for tertiary care are complete. A patient with a hemoglobin value of 5 g/dL and signs of congestive heart failure requires immediate decisions regarding red cell transfusion and other supportive care. A key point of concern revolves around possible alloimmunization of a patient who might later prove to be a candidate for stem cell transplantation. Limited numbers of blood transfusions probably do not affect the outcome of stem cell transplantation. A few simple points allow appropriate management of the acute clinical issue without jeopardizing the long-term outcome.

Patients should receive red cell or platelet transfusions as clinically indicated. The key management point is to avoid family members as blood donors to preclude sensitization to the minor histocompatibility antigens of a potential stem cell donor.[15] Sensitization to minor histocompatibility antigens increases the risk of graft rejection following HLA-identical hematopoietic stem cell transplantation. Platelet collection by cytapheresis and leukocyte reduction by ultraviolet light or filtration techniques lowers the risk alloimmunization from transfusions. Prophylactic platelet transfusions to maintain a platelet count in excess of 10,000 cells/μL reduce the risk of catastrophic bleeds, such as intracranial hemorrhage.

■ PURE RED CELL APLASIA

Pure red cell aplasia reflects selective destruction of red cell progenitors. Manifestations of severe anemia prompt the patient to seek medical attention. With the key proviso that the neutrophil and platelet counts are normal, the presentation mirrors that of acquired aplastic anemia. Symptoms related to severe anemia exist. Patients however lack petechiae, ecchymoses, or other signs of bleeding that factor prominently in the presentation of aplastic anemia.

Severe anemia and reticulocytopenia are hallmarks of pure red cell aplasia. Absent from the peripheral blood are abnormal red cell features such as schistocytes, target cells, spherocytes, or basophilic stippling. The peripheral blood red cells are in fact remarkably insipid. One clue concerning the basis of the anemia is a modest elevation of the MCV. The mean MCV often is just over 100 fL, a value too high to be ignored and too low to indicate deficiency of folate or cobalamin.

Normal bone marrow cellularity with an overwhelming preponderance of myeloid precursors can briefly give the impression of a proliferative process involving white cells. A second look however shows the problem to be one of absent erythroid precursors rather than an excess of myeloid progenitors. The almost complete absence of late erythroid precursors is typical. Proerythroblasts sometimes exist, depending on the precise site of the block in erythroid cell maturation. Foreign elements such as fibroblasts and fibrosis are not part of the marrow picture. The profound failure of erythroid progenitors is the basis of the modest MCV elevation. Any phenomenon that severely stresses erythroid production capacity slightly increases the MCV value.

Most cases of pure red cell aplasia reflect disturbances in immune regulation that specifically suppress erythroid precursor maturation. The list of disorders associated with pure red cell aplasia is manifold, including thymoma, rheumatoid arthritis, systemic lupus erythematosis, chronic lymphocytic leukemia, and lymphoma. The fact that some of these disorders, such as systemic lupus erythematosis, are very common while pure red cell aplasia is very rare suggests that the etiology reflects an intersection with other as yet unknown factors. Particularly interesting is the association of pure red cell aplasia with large granular lymphocytic leukemia, a disorder that involves the cells of natural killer subgroup of lymphocytes.

Some patients have serum antibodies that are selectively cytotoxic for marrow erythroid cells or that are directed against erythropoietin.[16] In other instances, suppression of erythroid precursors is a cell-mediated process involving abnormal T cells.[17,18] The frequent positive response to immunosuppressive therapies, including corticosteroids and cyclosporine, in these patients stresses the immunological underpinnings of the anemia.[19]

Pure red cell aplasia at times develops in the setting of a viral infection, particularly infection with human parvovirus B19. This adeno-associated virus causes "Fifth Disease," a normally benign childhood disorder associated with fever, malaise, and a mild rash. The virus has a tropism for erythroid progenitor cells and impairs cell division for a few days during the infection. Reticulocyte counts often fall literally to zero. Normal people experience, at most, a slight drop in hematocrit since the half-life of erythrocytes in the circulation is 40–60 days. The viral infection resolves in a few days with no long-lasting problem.

The scenario differs in people who fail to clear the viral infection properly. Poor clearance sometimes reflects an underlying immune disorder, but on occasion occurs without a clear cause.[20] Persistent infection with parvovirus B19 produces pure red cell aplasia. The diagnosis of pure red cell aplasia secondary to parvovirus B19 infection is therapeutically important because these patients respond dramatically to immunoglobulin therapy.[21] Commercial immunoglobulin preparations are rich in antibodies directed against parvovirus B19 due to the high exposure rate to the virus among adults.

■ PAROXYSMAL NOCTURNAL HEMOGLOBINURIA

Paroxysmal nocturnal hemoglobinuria (PNH) is an extremely rare condition that nonetheless provides important insights into the physiology of red cells by highlighting the importance of the glycosylphosphatidylinositol (GPI) anchor that attaches many proteins to the cell membrane. The striking nature of its defining characteristic, the passage of dark urine at night, made the condition one of the first clearly described hematological disorders. The hemoglobinuria reflects the massive intravascular hemolysis that afflicts some patients with the condition. All patients with PNH have some degree of hemolysis, even those without the striking pathognomonic episodes. Although this remarkable clinical feature placed the spotlight early on the erythrocyte, significant and clinically important abnormalities exist as well in platelets and neutrophils, with marked reduction in these elements in the circulation occurring commonly. A thrombotic diathesis, particularly involving the portal and hepatic veins, is the final key clinical characteristic of the condition. The triad of hemolytic anemia, pancytopenia, and thrombosis is the defining ideograph of PNH.

To date, all cases of the disorder reflect defective synthesis of the GPI anchor due to mutations in the *PIG-A* gene (Phosphatidyl Inositol Glycan complementation group A). The gene product is part of an enzyme complex that mediates the first step in GPI synthesis. The GPI anchor couples a host of important proteins to the cell membrane, including CD59. CD59 protects cells from damage mediated by the membrane attack complex of complement (C5-C9). Deficient expression of GPI-linked proteins occurs in neutrophils and platelets as well as erythrocytes.

Hemolysis in PNH reflects erythrocyte susceptibility to complement lysis due to extreme deficiency or complete absence of red cell membrane CD59. The 1937 demonstration by Thomas H. Ham that hemolysis of PNH red cells occurs via the action of complement on abnormal red cells[22] reflected CD59 deficiency in these cells. Complement-mediated hemolysis in the setting of a low pH buffer, christened the Ham test, for many years characterized the abnormal red cells in PNH and defined the disorder.[23] Only recently has the Ham test given way to more sensitive assessment of PNH using FACS analysis to detect reduced or absent expression of GPI-linked membrane proteins.

Bone marrow failure is common in PNH and is perhaps even intrinsic to the disorder. Overlap exists between PNH and aplastic anemia and the two conditions might be different manifestations of a common pathologic process. Patients with PNH dominated by the hemolytic component often show a slow progression in bone marrow failure that eventually produces a picture virtually identical to aplastic anemia. Conversely, small clones of PNH cells exist in as many as half of the patients with aplastic anemia.[24,25]

As noted earlier, aplastic anemia is an immunological disorder resulting from the destruction of hematopoietic stem cells by aberrant T cells. Convincing evidence now shows that suppressed hematopoiesis is extremely common if not universal in PNH. This is true even in patients where hemolysis dominates the clinical picture and cell counts are otherwise normal. The last and key observation in the puzzle regarding the origin of PNH is the occurrence of small numbers of cells with a PNH phenotype in the peripheral blood of otherwise normal people.[26]

PNH appears to be a clonal acquired hematopoietic disorder that involves sequential pathological events.[27] A somatic mutation of the *PIG-A* gene produces a small clone of PNH cells in a background of otherwise normal hematopoietic precursors. The tiny PNH clone usually remains small and unimportant. Independent of the PNH mutation, some people develop an immune disorder in which T cells attack and destroy hematopoietic stem cells.[28] Part of the immunological assault is possibly directed at GPI-linked membrane proteins on the hematopoietic stem cells. The PNH clone, lacking these GPI-linked proteins, survives this component of the immune insult. This process enriches the PNH cells in the hematopoietic stem cell mix. A second mutation of the *PIG-A* gene further expands the PNH clone to the point that it dominates hematopoiesis.

TABLE 11-4	KEY DIAGNOSTIC POINTS WITH BONE MARROW FAILURE	
Issue	*Manifestation*	*Approach*
Aplastic anemia versus myelodysplasia	Anemia, thrombocytopenia, neutropenia	• Review peripheral blood for pseudo-Pelger-Huet cells and hypogranulated neutrophils. • Review bone marrow for dysplasia • Chromosome analysis looking for breaks, duplications, rearrangements.
Aplastic anemia versus "aleukemic" leukemia	Anemia, thrombocytopenia, neutropenia	• FACS analysis of peripheral blood for white cells with leukemia markers. • Bone marrow looking for blast cells.
Aplastic anemia versus myelofibrosis	Anemia, thrombocytopenia, neutropenia	• Review peripheral blood for misshapen red cells. • Bone marrow looking for fibrosis.
Aplastic anemia versus bone marrow tuberculosis	Anemia, thrombocytopenia, neutropenia	• Check PPD (tuberculosis skin test) • Bone marrow staining for acid-fast bacteria. • Bone marrow culture for mycobacteria.
Aplastic anemia versus PNH	Anemia, thrombocytopenia, neutropenia	• Ham test for red cell lysis (positive in PNH). • FACS analysis for GPI-linked membrane proteins (reduced or absent in PNH)

The demonstration that the *PIG-A* gene mutation makes CD34+ hematopoietic progenitors more resistant to apoptosis supports this model.[29,30] The close pathophysiological link between aplastic anemia and PNH led to the concept of an "aplastic anemia/PNH syndrome." The clinical character of the condition swings between the two manifestations depending on the magnitude of the immune selection and the occurrence of second mutations in the *PIG-A* gene.

The odd and still poorly understood aspect of PNH is the predilection for thrombosis. The thrombosis does not occur in the peripheral veins, as is the case with hypercoagulable states such as antithrombin III deficiency. The failure of standard anticoagulation using strategies based either on heparin or Coumadin underscores the dichotomy between thromboses seen with PNH and that associated with "routine" hypercoagulable states. This resistance to anticoagulation along with the peculiar

TABLE 11-5 | **KEY MANAGEMENT POINTS WITH BONE MARROW FAILURE**

Issue	*Comments*
Treatment of mild or moderate aplastic anemia	Some patients at the milder end of the disease spectrum require no treatment. Immunosuppressive therapy is the treatment of choice when needed because of the high response rate.
Hematopoietic stem cell transplantation (HSCT)	HSCT is used in patients with severe aplastic anemia. A full HLA-matched sibling donor is preferred. Morbidity and mortality increase with age.
Alloimmunization in transplant candidates	A limited number of transfusions do not affect transplant outcome. Family members should not provide blood for transfusion to avoid patient sensitization toward a possible donor.
Pure red cell aplasia (PRCA) secondary to parvovirus B19	PRCA is a rare complication of infection with parvovirus B19. The high response rate to immunoglobulin therapy makes important the search for parvovirus B19.

location of the thrombosis likely conveys an important biological message. Efforts at deciphering that message continue (Tables 11-4 and 11-5).

References

[1] International Agranulcytosis and Aplastic Anemia Study. 1987. Incidence of aplastic anemia: The relevance of diagnostic criteria. Blood 70:1718–1721.

[2] Camitta BM, Thomas ED, Nathan DG, et al. 1976. Severe aplastic anemia: A prospective study of the effect of early marrow transplantation on acute mortality. Blood 48:63–70.

[3] Issaragrisil S, Sriratanasatavorn C, Piankijagum A, et al. 1991. Incidence of aplastic anemia in Bangkok. The Aplastic Anemia Study Group. Blood 77:2166–2168.

[4] Issaragrisil S, Kaufman DW, Anderson TE, et al. 1995. An association of aplastic anaemia in Thailand with low socioeconomic status. Aplastic Anemia Study Group. Br J Haematol 91:80–84.

[5] Weisberger AS. 1969. Mechanisms of action of Chloramphenicol. JAMA 209:97–106.

[6] Plaut ME, Best WR. 1982. Aplastic anemia after parenteral chloramphenicol: Warning renewed. N Engl J Med 306:1486.

[7] Dameshek W. 1969. Chloramphenicol aplastic anemia in identical twins—a clue to pathogenesis.. N Engl J Med 281:42–43.

[8] Abrams SM, Degnan TJ, Vinciguerra V. 1980. Marrow aplasia following topical application of chloramphenicol eye ointment. Arch Intern Med 140:576–577.

9   McGhee CN, Anastas CN. 1996. Widespread ocular use of topical chloramphenicol: Is there justifiable concern regarding idiosyncratic aplastic anaemia? Br J Ophthalmol 80:182–184.

10 Brown KE, Tisdale J, Dunbar CE, Young NS: 1997. Hepatitis-associated aplastic anemia. N Engl J Med 336:1059–1064.

11 Issaragrisil S. 1999. Epidemiology of aplastic anemia in Thailand. Thai Aplastic Anemia Study Group. Int J Hematol 70:137–140.

12 Mathe G, Amiel JL, Schwarzenberg L, et al. 1970. Bone marrow graft in man after conditioning by antilymphocytic serum. Br Med J 2:131–136.

13 Gluckman E, Devergie A, Poros A, et al. 1982. Results of immunosuppression in 170 cases of severe aplastic anaemia. Report of the European Group of Bone Marrow Transplant (EGBMT). Br J Haematol 51:541–550.

14 Nakao S, Takamatsu H, Chuhjo T, et al. 1994. Identification of a specific HLA class II haplotype strongly associated with susceptibility to cyclosporine-dependent aplastic anemia. Blood 84:4257–4261.

15 Champlin RE, Horowitz MM, van Bekkum DW, et al. 1989. Graft failure following bone marrow transplantation for severe aplastic anemia: Risk factors and treatment results. Blood 73:606–613.

16 Tsujimura H, Sakai C, Takagi T. 1999. Pure red cell aplasia complicated by angioimmunoblastic T-cell lymphoma: Humoral factor plays a main role in the inhibition of erythropoiesis from CD34(+) progenitor cells. Am J Hematol 62:259–260.

17 Abkowitz JL, Kadin ME, Powell JS, Adamson JW. 1986. Pure red cell aplasia: Lymphocyte inhibition of erythropoiesis. Br J Haematol 63:59–67.

18 Socinski MA, Ershler WB, Tosato G, Blaese RM. 1984. Pure red blood cell aplasia associated with chronic Epstein-Barr virus infection: Evidence for T cell-mediated suppression of erythroid colony forming units. J Lab Clin Med 104:995–1006.

19 Clark DA, Dessypris EN, Krantz SB. 1984. Studies on pure red cell aplasia. XI. Results of immunosuppressive treatment of 37 patients. Blood 63:277–286.

20 Frickhofen N, Chen ZJ, Young NS, Cohen BJ, Heimpel H, Abkowitz JL. 1994. Parvovirus B19 as a cause of acquired chronic pure red cell aplasia. Br J Haematol 87:818–824.

21 Gottlieb F, Deutsch J. 1992. Red cell aplasia responsive to immunoglobulin therapy as initial manifestation of human immunodeficiency virus infection. Am J Med 92:331–333.

22 Ham TH. 1937. Chronic hemolytic anemia with paroxysmal nocturnal hemoglobinuria: Study of the mechanism of hemolysis in relation to acid-base equilibrium. N Engl J Med 217:915–918.

23 Ham TH, Shen SC, Fleming EM, Castle WB. 1948. Studies on the destruction of red blood cells. IV. Thermal Injury. Blood 3:373–403.

24 Azenishi Y, Ueda E, Machin T, et al. 1999. CD59-deficient blood cells and PIG-A gene abnormalities in Japanese patients with aplastic anaemia. Br J Haematol 101:90–93.

25 Dunn DE, Tanawattanacharoen P, Boccuni P, et al. 1999. Paroxysmal nocturnal hemoglobinuria cells in patients with bone marrow failure syndromes. Ann Intern Med 131:401–408.

26 Araten DJ, Nafa K, Pakdeesuwan K, Luzzatto L. 1999. Clonal populations of hematopoietic cells with paroxysmal nocturnal hemoglobinuria genotype and phenotype are present in normal individuals. Proc Natl Acad Sci 96:5209–5214.

27 Josten KM, Tooze JA, Borthwick-Clarke C, Gordon-Smith EC, Rutherford TR. 1991. Acquired aplastic anemia and paroxysmal nocturnal hemoglobinuria: Studies on clonality. Blood 78:3162–3167.

28 Karadimitris A, Manavalan JS, Thaler HT, et al. 2000. Abnormal T-cell repertoire is associated with immune process underlying the pathogenesis of paroxysmal nocturnal hemoglobinuria. Blood 96:2613–2620.

29 Horikawa K, Nakakuma H, Kawaguchi T, et al. 1997. Apoptosis resistance of blood cells from patients with paroxysmal nocturnal hemoglobinuria, aplastic anemia, and myelodysplastic syndrome. Blood 90:2716–2722.

30 Brodsky RA, Vala MS, Barber JP, Medof ME, Jones RJ. 1997. Resistance to apoptosis caused by PIG-A gene mutations in paroxysmal nocturnal hemoglobinuria. Proc Natl Acad Sci 94:8756–8760.

THE MYELODYSPLASTIC SYNDROMES

"Chaos" is the word that most often comes to mind with first glimpse of a bone marrow aspirate. The smear contains a dizzying array of exotic cells whose varying color, size, and shape have no obvious organizational scheme. In reality, however, the bone marrow is an organ whose delicate mosaic of well-defined cells work cooperatively to maintain a precise balance between the peripheral blood constituents. Hematologists and hematopathologists not only assess the bone marrow for the presence of foreign cells, but also appraise the character of cells indigenous to that space. Assessing the number of hematopoietic cells and their distribution between the several lineages that populate the bone marrow is an extremely important endeavor.

Equally important is the appraisal of qualitative attributes such as the stages of cell maturation and morphology. "Reading" bone marrow preparations is an area of medicine that contains as much art as science. Laboratory tests for cell surface markers or hybridization patterns of fluorescent DNA probes provide valuable data. Nonetheless, assessment of myelodysplasia remains very much in the bailiwick of "old-fashioned" light microscopists. The pattern of the bone marrow is the central spoke to which all other data are attached. An individual cell is to the bone marrow what an individual musical note is to the symphony. The whole is far greater than the sum of the parts.

The myelodysplastic disorders entail disrupted maturation and differentiation of hematopoietic precursor cells. The result is a disturbance in the quality and/or quantity of cells in the peripheral blood. Anemia is the most common abnormality at the onset of a myelodysplastic process and worsens as the derangement evolves to encompass other lineages, most particularly the myeloid and megakaryocytic lines. Myelodysplasia is not a single condition but rather is a collection of disorders whose disturbances in the peripheral blood picture have many common features. As individual members of the myelodysplasia family progress, however, they diverge dramatically in manifestations and clinical course. Consequently, the approach to myelodysplasia and the assignment of prognosis depends on the particular subcategory in question. Disturbed bone marrow function is the crux of all the conditions, however.

■ PRESENTATION

Although hereditary or congenital conditions exist, most cases of myelodysplasia are acquired. The disorder typically arises in middle age or later in life. The initial symptoms of myelodysplasia usually are insidious, making difficult any effort to mark clearly its time of onset. This fact is highlighted by instances where medical records allow retrospective analysis of the hematological profile of a person newly diagnosed with myelodysplasia. Old records sometimes show subtle but clear signs of the disorder years before the patient receives the diagnostic label. Any attempt to assess the chronology of myelodysplasia in a particular patient consequently is a difficult endeavor.

The great variation in the pathogenic mechanisms and manifestations of the myriad of myelodysplastic disorders means that no single presentation is "typical." Nonetheless, anemia most often prompts patients to seek initial medical attention (Table 12-1). On the whole the anemia associated with myelodysplasia is distinctly undistinguished. The condition most often is normochromic and normocytic at presentation. The anemia is macrocytic in some instances while a discrete minority of patients present with a microcytic anemia. Missing are concrete diagnostic markers such as those seen in disorders that produce schistocytes or sickle cells. Pappenheimer bodies exist in the erythrocytes of some patients with myelodysplasia. These fine structures are easily overlooked however and identification requires a high-quality microscope and careful examination of the blood smear. Minorities of patients display coarse basophilic stippling of erythrocytes and some have Howell-Jolly bodies.

TABLE 12-1 | **CLINICAL PRESENTATION OF MYELODYSPLASIA**

Affected Cell Line	Result	Manifestation
Erythroid	• Normochromic, normocytic anemia	Fatigue, dyspnea, dizziness
Megakaryocytic	• Thrombocytopenia • Thrombasthenia	Petechiae, bruising, minor bleeding
Myeloid	• Neutropenia • Pseudo-Pelger-Huet anomaly • Granulocyte dysfunction	Infection

Typically the anemia is mild to moderate in severity at the outset of the myelodysplastic process. Commonly, hemoglobin values are in the range of 9–11 g/dL although some people have hemoglobin levels that fall barely below the threshold of normal. The anemia usually progresses in severity over time so that most patients eventually require frequent if not routine transfusions. Concurrent medical conditions such as atherosclerotic cardiovascular disease or chronic obstructive lung disease can powerfully influence the need for transfusion. Anemia that induces angina, for instance, demands a transfusion regimen that maintains the hemoglobin level above the threshold that triggers pain. Conditions that suppress hematopoietic activity such as collagen vascular disease can also increase the need for transfusion.

The pseudo-Pelger-Huet anomaly is a neutrophil feature that points strongly to myelodysplasia as a diagnosis. These cells have a nucleus with two prominent lobes connected by a single adjoining segment, producing the so-called "pince-nez" morphology (Figure 12-1). Although 10% or more of granulocytes can exhibit the characteristic, the fraction can be low, meaning that review of several microscope fields might be necessary to confirm its presence. The neutrophils often are pale in appearance reflecting a paucity of cytoplasmic granules. The finding of pseudo-Pelger-Huet cells and granulocytes with liminal cytoplasmic granules in the setting of a normochromic, normocytic anemia speaks strongly to myelodysplasia as the underlying derangement.

Other leukocyte anomalies include peripheral blood monocytosis and basophilia. Some basophils have large, coarse granules. Others display bizarre features such as both basophilic and eosinophilic granules in the same cell. Disturbances in granulocyte number and function are often minor at the onset of myelodysplasia but usually come to dominate the clinical picture and ultimately determine the patient's fate. Some but not all cases of myelodysplasia terminate in acute myelogenous leukemia. The propensity to evolve in that direction varies enormously among the specific subcategories of myelodysplasia. Infections due to a dearth of neutrophils and impaired granulocyte function are both common and nocuous.

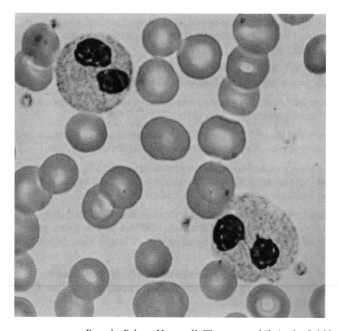

FIGURE 12–1 *Pseudo-Pelger-Huet cell. The neutrophils in the field have two prominent lobes connected by a single strand, which mimics the outline of "pince-nez" eyeglasses. While common to myelodysplasia, locating these cells often requires an extended search because of their small numbers. (From Kapff CT, Jandl JH. 1991. Blood: Atlas and Sourcebook of Hematology, 2nd edn. Boston: Little, Brown and Company. Figure 30-1, p. 71. Reproduced with permission of the publisher.)*

Platelet disturbances arise frequently and manifest most often as thrombocytopenia. Even patients whose platelet counts are in the normal range have values that cluster toward the lower end of the normal spectrum. These platelet values eventually slide into the region of frank thrombocytopenia with counts commonly in the range of 50,000–100,000 cells/μL. The platelets often have functional defects that magnify the impact of their low number. Patients occasionally develop petechiae and bruising with platelet values exceeding 100,000 cells/μL, a phenomenon not seen with functionally normal platelets. Gastrointestinal bleeding can occur, although the problem usually develops in conjunction with a structural defect of the gut such as colonic angiodysplasia. The platelets are usually morphologically unremarkable by light microscopy, although a few giant thrombocytes often are in the mix.

Routine chemistry profiles reveal high LDH values in many patients with myelodysplasia. The anomaly reflects the prominent role of ineffective erythropoiesis in the generation of myelodysplastic anemia. Hemolysis due in part to red cell fragility also contributes to the low hemoglobin values and high LDH values. More focused analysis of blood chemistry profiles frequently reveals low haptoglobin levels due to low-grade intravascular hemolysis with the release of small quantities of hemoglobin into the plasma. Gastrointestinal iron uptake is supernormal in many patients, with a consequent elevation in the plasma values for transferrin saturation and ferritin.

The relatively bland abnormalities in myelodysplasia contribute to a sometimes overly long interval between onset of symptoms and assignment of the definitive diagnosis. Some patients even receive iron supplementation during this murky phase of the disorder despite the normochromic, normocytic anemia and normal serum iron values. The anemia sometimes is attributed to coexisting disorders, the frequency of which increases with increasing age. "Old age" is blamed for some anemias despite the evidence against the existence of an anemia due solely to advancing years (see Chapter 2). As the hematological disturbances progress in severity, more disturbing findings such as peripheral blood myeloblasts usually hasten the identification of myelodysplasia as the pathological culprit.

■ DIAGNOSIS

Bone marrow examination is the key to the diagnosis of myelodysplasia. The frequently nebulous nature of the changes in bone marrow morphology can complicate the task of assigning precise subcategory labels to individual cases, however. Over the years great debates raged over the nature of myelodysplasia, particularly with respect to its relationship to acute myelogenous leukemia. In the early 1980s, a series of conferences on the subject convened by specialists from France, the United States, and the United Kingdom hammered out a consensus opinion on myelodysplasia, designated as the French-American-British (FAB) classification (Table 12-2).[1]

The widespread adoption of the FAB classification of myelodysplastic syndromes (MDSs) produced more consistent interpretations of data in studies that addressed a range of key issues including the etiology, prevalence, and treatment of these conditions. As information was complied, however, continued problems with categorization and discrepancies in interpretation indicated the need for refinement of the FAB classification.[2,3] The disorders categorized as "refractory anemia with excess blasts," "refractory anemia with excess blasts in transformation," and "acute myelogenous leukemia" appeared in many ways to comprise a disease continuum rather than discrete pathological entities.[4] Refractory anemia with excess blasts often evolved into an acute leukemia with the "in transformation" stage serving as a conduit.[5] The issue was not simply nosological since both prognostications and treatment approaches hinged on the subcategory to which a patient was assigned.

At the other end of the myelodysplastic spectrum, the conditions with anemia as the major manifestation also clearly varied within individual subcategories. Patients classified as having refractory anemia in which the sole chromosomal aberration was a deletion of the long arm of chromosome 5 [del(5q)] fared much better than those with multiple chromosomal aberrations, irrespective of the del(5q) anomaly. Similarly, refractory anemia with ringed sideroblasts appeared to have clinically important subcategories. People with ringed sideroblasts and no other dysplastic marrow changes enjoyed exceptionally stable disease courses. In particular, disturbances involving granulocytes or platelets rarely developed. In contrast, multiple dysplastic features

TABLE 12-2 | FRENCH-AMERICAN-BRITISH (FAB) CLASSIFICATION OF MYELODYSPLASTIC SYNDROMES

Category	*Characteristics*
Refractory anemia	• Cytopenia of at least one peripheral blood cell line (usually anemia). • Normocellular or hypocellular bone marrow with dysplastic changes. • Fewer than 1% blast cells in the peripheral blood; fewer than 5% blast cells in the bone marrow.
Refractory anemia with ringed sideroblasts	• Cytopenia (almost always anemia), bone marrow dysplasia and the same percentages of blood and bone marrow blast cells seen with refractory anemia. • Ringed sideroblasts accounting for more than 15% of all nucleated cells in the bone marrow.
Refractory anemia with excess blasts	• Peripheral blood cytopenia involving two or more lineages. • Bone marrow dysplastic changes of all three lineages. • Fewer than 5% blast cells in the peripheral blood and between 5% and 20% blast cells in the bone marrow.
Refractory anemia with excess blasts in transformation	• Features of refractory anemia but with more than 5% blast cells in the peripheral blood, between 21% and 30% blast cells in the bone marrow *or* Auer rods in the blasts.
Chronic myelomonocytic anemia	• Peripheral blood monocytosis (monocyte count exceeding 1×10^9 per L). • Fewer than 5% blast cells in the peripheral blood and up to 20% blast cells in the bone marrow.

in addition to ringed sideroblasts in the marrow augured a clinical course similar to "routine" refractory anemia.

Technological advances subsequent to the introduction of the FAB classification also contributed to the need for revision. Expression of the CD34 antigen, for instance, provides a new window on the issue of blast cells in myelodysplasia.[6] The International MDS Risk Analysis Workshop developed a classification that incorporated aspects other than morphology into the diagnosis of MDS. The collation of a large body of cytogenetic, morphological, and clinical data with independent risk-based prognostic systems produced the International Prognostic Scoring System for primary myelodysplasia.[7] Prognostic subdivisions included low, intermediate-1, intermediate-2, and high-risk categories, thereby providing a more global vision of patient status. This scoring system is particularly useful in assessing the impact of therapeutic interventions in myelodysplasia.

The World Health Organization (WHO) sponsored a series of conferences on myelodysplasia that included experts from around the world.[8] The result of the exhaustive process was a new classification scheme that kept the essentials of the FAB system while providing additional diagnostically and prognostically important categories (Table 12-3).[9] The WHO classification defines acute myelogenous leukemia as having 20% or more myeloblast cells in the peripheral blood. This change eliminates the commonly confusing "refractory anemia in transformation" category from the myelodysplasias.[10] The partition of refractory anemia with excess blasts into groups designated as (RAEB-1) and (RAEB-2) acknowledges the accumulated data indicating a worse prognosis when the bone marrow contains 10% or more myeloblast cells.

The subdivision of the sideroblastic anemias into "refractory anemia with ringed sideroblasts" and "refractory anemia with multilineage dysplasia and ringed sideroblasts" reflects the more benign clinical course of the former subcategory of the MDSs. Likewise, the new classification "myelodysplastic syndrome with isolated del(5q)" recognizes the relatively benign clinical course followed by this myelodysplasia subgroup. Chronic myelomonocytic leukemia, the condition that generated perhaps the greatest controversy among experts, is classified under an entirely different grouping termed *myelodysplastic/myeloproliferative diseases*. On the whole, the WHO classification of myelodysplasia provides an effective nosological framework with good predictive ability that helps clinicians manage these patients.[11]

Hematopoietic cell dysplasia manifests in many ways in people afflicted with the MDSs.[12] Table 12-4 lists some of the abnormalities that can develop. No patient shows all the changes, and in some instances the changes are few in number and subtle in nature. Subtle changes most often appear early in the course of the disorder with increasingly severe anomalies developing over time. Proper interpretation of bone marrow specimens with subtle alterations requires an experienced observer since the changes can blur with the variants of normal.

Clonal karyotype abnormalities detectable by cytopathology occur in as many as half of the patients with myelodysplasia.[13] About one-fifth of the patients have complex chromosomal changes that include deletions and translocations. In general, these patients have a more severe clinical course than do those with a single abnormality or no chromosomal abnormality. An exception involves chromosome 7 monosomy where the predilection for conversion to acute leukemia exceeds that seen with most other chromosomal aberrations.[14,15] Over time some patients acquire additional karyotype aberrations to the ones seen at diagnosis. Not surprisingly, evolving chromosomal abnormalities also bode ill.

In contrast to situations with multiple chromosomal abnormalities, an isolated del(5q) anomaly augurs a course distinctly better than is typical of other

TABLE 12-3 | **WHO CLASSIFICATION OF MYELODYSPLASTIC SYNDROMES**

Condition	Peripheral Blood	Bone Marrow
Refractory anemia	• Anemia • No or rare blast cells	• Solely erythroid dysplasia • <5% blast cells • <15% ringed sideroblasts
Refractory anemia with ringed sideroblasts	• Anemia • No blast cells	• Solely erythroid dysplasia • ≥15% ringed sideroblasts • <5% blast cells
Refractory cytopenia with multilineage dysplasia	• Multiple cytopenias • No or rare blast cells • No Auer rods • $<1 \times 10^9$/L monocytes	• Dysplasia ≥10% of cells in two or more myeloid lines • <5% marrow blast cells • No Auer rods • <15% ringed sideroblasts
Refractory cytopenia with multilineage dysplasia and ringed sideroblasts	• Multiple cytopenias • No or rare blast cells • No Auer rods • $<1 \times 10^9$/L monocytes	• Dysplasia ≥10% of cells in two or more myeloid lines • ≥15% ringed sideroblasts • <5% marrow blast cells • No Auer rods
Refractory anemia with excess blasts-1	• Multiple cytopenias • <5% blast cells • No Auer rods • $<1 \times 10^9$/L monocytes	• Single or multilineage dysplasia • 5–9% blast cells • No Auer rods
Refractory anemia with excess blasts-2	• Multiple cytopenias • <5% blast cells • No Auer rods • $<1 \times 10^9$/L monocytes	• Single or multilineage dysplasia • 10–19% blast cells • Auer rods possible
Myelodysplastic syndrome, unclassified	• Cytopenias • No or rare blast cells • No Auer rods	• Single lineage dysplasia in granulocytes or megakaryocytes • <5% blast cells • No Auer rods
Myelodysplastic syndrome associated with isolated del(5q)	• Anemia • <5% blast cells • Platelets normal or increased	• Normal to increased megakaryocytes with hypolobulated nuclei • <5% blast cells • No Auer rods • Isolated del(5q)

TABLE 12-4 | MANIFESTATIONS OF DYSPLASIA IN MYELODYSPLASTIC SYNDROMES

Cell Lineage	Bone Marrow	Peripheral Blood
Erythroid	<ul><li>Prominent erythroblast nucleoli</li><li>Irregular normoblast nuclear contour</li><li>Multiple normoblast nuclei</li><li>Cytoplasmic outpouches in normoblasts</li><li>Normoblast cytoplasmic vacuoles</li><li>Delayed normoblast hemoglobinization</li><li>Ringed sideroblasts</li><li>Karyorrhexis</li><li>Excessive numbers of myeloblasts</li></ul>	<ul><li>Basophilic stippling</li><li>Nucleated red blood cells</li><li>Macroerythrocytes</li><li>Howell-Jolly bodies</li></ul>
Myeloid	<ul><li>Prominent nucleoli in myeloblasts and promyelocytes</li><li>Irregular nuclear contour in myeloblasts and promyelocytes</li><li>Few specific granules in metamyelocytes</li><li>Mixed eosinophilic and basophilic granules in cells at the myelocyte and metamyelocyte stages</li><li>Karyorrhexis</li></ul>	<ul><li>Pseudo-Pelger-Huet cells</li><li>Hypogranulated neutrophils</li></ul>
Megakaryocytic	<ul><li>Micro-megakaryocytes</li></ul>	<ul><li>Giant platelets</li></ul>

myelodysplasia variants.[16,17] The chromosomal lesion in this subgroup of myelodysplasia involves deletion of an internal interval of the long arm of chromosome 5 that leaves the distal end intact.[18] One group of investigators reported 66 years as the mean age of onset with a projected survival exceeding 140 months.[19] Evidence exists, suggesting that multiple abnormalities involving the long arm of chromosome 5 vitiate the benefit conferred by the solitary del(5q) lesion.[20] Even when the additional chromosomal aberrations are detectable only with fluorescence in situ hybridization the effect is negation of the otherwise positive prognosis associated with the del(5q) syndrome.[21]

In addition to having low hemoglobin levels, patients with myelodysplasia on rare occasion develop patterns of abnormal hemoglobin expression that qualify as hemoglobinopathies. Acquired hemoglobin H disease is the most frequent manifestation of aberrant hemoglobin production.[22] The erythrocytes in these cases are strikingly microcytic and hypochromic with marked poikilocytosis. These small cells usually coexist with cells whose morphology is relatively normal, suggesting two populations of erythroid precursors in these patients. Supravital stains clearly show cellular inclusions consisting of precipitated clumps of hemoglobin β-chain tetramers. These pathological precipitates of hemoglobin likely increase the hemolysis associated with myelodysplasia by damaging the erythrocyte membrane. The chain synthesis ratio of α- and β-globin subunits is markedly below normal, consistent with impaired alpha chain production.[23]

The impaired alpha chain synthesis can result from deletions of chromosome 16 that remove the α-globin gene complex.[24] The result is loss of two of the four α-globin genes. For as yet unclear reasons, the clinical manifestation of the loss of two α-globin genes is more striking than occurs with hereditary two-gene deletion α-thalassemia. Other elements important to hemoglobin production could be lost as a result of the sweeping damage to chromosome 16. In some cases the acquired hemoglobin H disease of myelodysplasia results from mutations of *ATRX*, an X-linked gene encoding a chromatin-associated protein.[25] A congenital disorder derived from mutations of *ATRX* includes mild α-thalassemia as part of the syndrome complex. The basis of the more severe anemia in MDS relative to the inherited disorder is unknown.

Acquired hemoglobin H disease in myelodysplasia is not simply a disturbance of hemoglobin synthesis. The condition apparently represents advancing disease with a broad breakdown in the mechanisms that control cellular maturation and development. The higher risk of evolution to acute myelogenous leukemia associated with acquired hemoglobin H disease likely is part of the global disturbance in the biology of hematopoietic cells.[26,27] Mild elevations in fetal hemoglobin levels also occur commonly in myelodysplasia. In contrast to hemoglobin H, elevated hemoglobin F levels apparently bode a more benign course than usual for the disorder.[28,29]

High peripheral blood platelet counts with low or at most modestly elevated granulocyte counts are common features of the del(5q) form of myelodysplasia. Bone marrow histology commonly shows a hypercellular picture where often the most striking cells are megakaryocytes with few nuclei or a single nucleus.[30] Bone marrow myeloblasts are an infrequent feature in this syndrome. The known association of high bone marrow myeloblast counts with poor prognosis due to transformation into acute myelogenous leukemia fits with the relative paucity of myeloblasts in the del(5q) syndrome.

While not strictly a dysplastic change, bone marrow reticuloendothelial cells with substantial iron deposits are commonplace and easily visualized with Perl's Prussian blue staining. This finding reflects the ineffective erythropoiesis intrinsic to the disorder. Large numbers of erythroid precursors in the face of anemia are prima facie evidence of ineffective erythropoiesis. Excessive numbers of basophilic precursors are another frequent feature of myelodysplasia, along with the high numbers of circulating basophils in the peripheral blood. The granules often are coarser than normal and some precursors contain both basophilic and eosinophilic granules indicating truly confused hematopoiesis. Other patients have large numbers of dysplastic eosinophilic precursors in the bone marrow with an associated poor prognosis.[31]

Hypercellular marrows are the norm in most cases of myelodysplasia. Much less common are instances of myelodysplasia with hypocellular bone marrows.[32,33] In most such cases, the degree of marrow cellularity is in the range of 20% or 25%, values that are far below the 80% or 90% cellularity commonly seen in myelodysplasia.[34] Instances of extremely low marrow cellularity and multiple cytopenias due to myelodysplasia can pose a diagnostic dilemma vis-à-vis aplastic anemia.[35] The similarity between myelodysplasia and aplastic anemia could extend beyond surface appearance to include some common pathogenic factors.[36] For instance, some patients with myelodysplasia respond to immune suppression therapy (albeit transiently) suggesting that the disorder has an immune component.[37,38] Immunological mechanisms appear to be at the heart of many or most cases of aplastic anemia. Some subsets of the heterogeneous group of disorders that comprise myelodysplasia might overlap with aplastic anemia.

Bone marrow biopsy in myelodysplasia frequently shows a backdrop of abnormally high reticulin deposition. On rare occasions, the change in stroma is sufficiently severe to produce confusion with a myeloproliferative process.[39,40] Patients with myelodysplasia and substantial myelofibrosis lack the splenomegaly characteristic of the myeloproliferative disorders, however.[41]

■ MYELODYSPLASIA: SPECIAL CONSIDERATIONS

MYELODYSPLASIA AND LEUKEMIA

De Novo Myelodysplasia

The initial identification of myelodysplasia came with the growing recognition that some patients with what appeared to be acute myelogenous leukemia had an unusually long disease course. Instead of living for weeks or months, some survived for years. In retrospect, many of these patients had what would now be classified as refractory anemia with excess blasts (RAEB-1 or RAEB-2). The metastable nature of the condition raised questions as to whether in fact all patients with myelodysplasia were in a queue that terminated eventually in acute myelogenous leukemia. This quandary manifested in the many monikers applied to myelodysplasia prior to the FAB classification, including "smoldering leukemia" and "preleukemia."[42,43]

A tome would be required to cover adequately the enormous amount of research touching this central issue in myelodysplasia. The data can be confusing and at times frankly contradictory. Nonetheless, some key points of agreement exist among authors in the field. A close relationship exists between myelodysplasia and acute myelogenous leukemia with a substantial fraction of patients evolving from the former condition into the latter. This fate is not universal across the spectrum of the disorder, however. Some subcategories of myelodysplasia, such as refractory anemia with ringed sideroblasts, rarely convert to acute myelogenous leukemia. Larger numbers of chromosomal abnormalities generally portend a greater risk of acute leukemia. And on the whole, the larger the number of myeloblasts in the bone marrow the greater the propensity for evolution into acute myelogenous leukemia. The WHO classification removed the subgroup "refractory anemia with excess blasts in transformation" because these patients, with up to 30% marrow myeloblast cells under the FAB classification, clinically mimicked acute myelogenous leukemia.

Recently developed techniques suggest that the RAEB-1 and RAEB-2 subcategories of myelodysplasia differ biologically from de novo acute myelogenous leukemia.[44] In fact, debate continues on the relationship between the acute leukemia phenotype that develops following myelodysplasia and that seen with de novo acute myelogenous leukemia. The issue has important ramifications. Acute myelogenous leukemia can be cured by allogeneic stem cell transplantation and perhaps by aggressive chemotherapy regimens. In either case, the strategy is to eliminate the leukemic cell clone. Normal hematopoietic cells come from the donor in the case of allogeneic stem cell transplantation. Patients treated with aggressive chemotherapy regimens can realize a cure if there is a reservoir of normal hematopoietic cells to repopulate the marrow after the leukemic clone is eliminated. Some experts argue that during the evolution of myelodysplasia, the aberrant clones of hematopoietic precursors completely replace their normal counterparts. When aggressive chemotherapy eliminates the leukemic cells, no reserve of normal cells exists. If cure of the acute leukemia depends on a reservoir of normal cells, preexisting myelodysplasia would make this result unlikely. The prognosis is in fact poor in cases of acute leukemia preceded by myelodysplasia.

The response to chemotherapy or hematopoietic stem cell transplantation depends on a variety of important issues. One is the patient's age. Resiliency declines with advancing age, meaning that older people tolerate many procedures less well than do their younger counterparts. With hematopoietic stem cell transplantation, for instance, children tolerate the procedure better than do young adults who themselves fare better than older adults. Myelodysplasia largely affects older adults, meaning the room to maneuver with aggressive treatment regimens is narrow in the absence of other considerations.

An intriguing biological difference between myelodysplasia and acute myelogenous leukemia is that bone marrow cells in the former disease show a high rate of apoptosis.[45] Apoptosis is an important process in normal hematopoiesis and helps maintain the balanced cell production essential to normal marrow function.[46] The high rate of apoptosis in myelodysplasia likely contributes to the ineffective erythropoiesis that characterizes the condition.[47] Apoptosis also affects survival in myelodysplasia with higher rates of apoptosis correlating with better patient survival.[48] Apoptosis could play a role in eliminating from the bone marrow some of the more patently defective cells. The subset of myelodysplasia patients with a low rate of apoptosis could be on the path to acute leukemia where the rate of apoptosis is also low.

Analysis of subsets of bone marrow cells provides possible insight into the basis of the variable rates of apoptosis seen in subgroups of patients with myelodysplasia. Early in the disease apoptosis occurs in all bone marrow cells whereas with more advanced disease apoptosis appears confined to cells expressing the CD34 antigen.[49] The basis for the differences in apoptotic characteristics between subgroups of patients with myelodysplasia is unknown.[50,51] Differential rates of apoptosis within cohorts of bone marrow cells could restructure the cell population into one that fits the criteria for acute myelogenous leukemia.

Although acute myelogenous leukemia dominates discussions of the clinical course of myelodysplasia, other complications dominate the clinical fate of the patients. Many people with myelodysplasia succumb to infections resulting from neutropenia, neutrophil dysfunction, or both. In contrast to anemia where transfusions can partially reverse the hemoglobin deficit, no means exists to supply allogeneic granulocytes. Recombinant human granulocyte colony-stimulating factor (rHuGCSF) can enhance production and release of neutrophils from the bone marrow. The response to the drug often is poor, however. Bleeding due to thrombocytopenia or platelet dysfunction is another serious complication of myelodysplasia. Whether acute myelogenous leukemia would arise in all patients if they survived long enough is an unanswered question. However, the impact of the cytopenias on the morbidity and mortality associated with myelodysplasia makes the term "preleukemia" a misnomer.

Therapy-Related Myelodysplasia

Therapy-related myelodysplasia is a particularly virulent form of the disorder.[52] The rate of devolution to acute myelogenous leukemia is high with a shorter time course to conversion than occurs with spontaneous myelodysplasia. Drugs are the most common cause of therapy-related myelodysplasia, with alkylating agents and inhibitors of topoisomerase II dominating the field.[53] Myelodysplasia sometimes develops after radiation therapy particularly if the treatment involves large fields that include hematopoietically active marrow in the pelvis and central skeleton. Table 12-5 lists some of the agents specifically implicated in secondary myelodysplasia. The WHO classification combines alkylating agent treatment and radiation as one subgroup of therapy-related myelodysplasia based on similarities in secondary cytogenetic abnormalities. Therapy-related myelodysplasia arising from treatment with topoisomerase II inhibitors forms a second group.[54]

DNA damage is the common feature linking drug-induced myelodysplasia to that deriving from radiation exposure. Alkylating agents and topoisomerase II inhibitors create covalent DNA adducts that interfere with cell division. Radiation generates

TABLE 12-5	**TREATMENT-RELATED MYELODYSPLASIA**	
Category	*Groups*	*Examples*
Drugs	Alkylating agents	Busulfan, cyclophosphamide, melphalan, nitrogen mustard
	Topoisomerase II inhibitors	Etoposide, teniposide, doxorubicin, daunorubicin
	Antimetabolites	Fluorouracil, methotrexate, cytarabine
	Antitubulin agents	Vincristine, paclitaxel, docetaxel
Radiation		Broad field irradiation including pelvis and central skeleton

highly reactive free radical species that form cross-links with DNA and also impair cell division. Malignancy most commonly justifies use of these power treatment modalities. The risk of secondary myelodysplasia is on the order of 5% over 5 years.[55] The interval between treatment and development of myelodysplasia tends to be shorter for topoisomerase II inhibitors than is the case with alkylating agent treatment or radiation therapy.[56] While concerning, the risk of myelodysplasia is clearly worth running given inexorably fatal course of the underlying cancer.

Hematological malignancies such as Hodgkin's disease have a greater predilection for therapy-related myelodysplasia than do solid tumors.[57–59] While the basis of the difference is unclear, the phenomenon could reflect a deficit in bone marrow cells that might also have produced the primary hematological malignancy. The initial hematological disorder could reflect either hematopoietic cell injury or an impaired ability to repress malignant cell clones. The treatment suppresses or cures the primary hematological disorder but damages the bone marrow further, setting the stage for myelodysplasia. A few disorders that do not technically qualify as malignancies are nonetheless pernicious to the point that alkylating agents are necessary for their control. Therapy-related myelodysplasia is less frequent when patients are treated for conditions such as aggressive rheumatoid arthritis than is the case for cancer. The lower doses of chemotherapy agents used for nonmalignant conditions might account for this difference.

Complex and sometimes bizarre chromosomal anomalies occur in more than 90% of therapy-related myelodysplasias.[60] A pattern exists in these karyotypic abnormalities with deletions involving chromosomes 5 and 7 arising commonly following treatment with alkylating agents or radiation therapy.[61] The topoisomerase II inhibitors sometimes produce balanced translocations often involving chromosome bands 11q23 or 21q22.[62] These chromosomal changes profoundly alter expression of genes that are important to cell maturation and development. *AML1*, a 260-kb gene that maps to chromosome 21q22, encodes a binding protein that associates with other subunits to form a transcription factor complex important to hematopoiesis. Missense mutations, splicing defects, and truncations involving the gene are common in therapy-related myelodysplasia.[63] These mutations disrupt *AML1* function as manifested by poor heterodimerization of the AML1 protein product with its partner in the transcriptional control complex, impaired in vitro DNA binding, and low rates of DNA transcription by the defective transcription regulation complex.[64]

The prognosis is gloomy for therapy-related myelodysplasia.[65] The conversion rate to acute myelogenous leukemia is high and the response of the leukemia to subsequent treatment is poor. Most patients succumb to therapy-related myelodysplasia within a year of diagnosis.

PEDIATRIC MYELODYSPLASIA

Pediatric myelodysplasia is a rare group of heterogeneous disorders that accounts for perhaps 1% of childhood malignancies.[66] The infrequency of the condition complicates analysis since many reports are retrospective data compilations from multiple institutions. Also, a number of congenital conditions can produce dysplastic bone marrow morphology and must be separated from primary myelodysplasia. These include Down's syndrome, neurofibromatosis type 1, Fanconi's anemia, and Schwachman syndrome. The mitochondrial cytopathies, such as Pearson's syndrome, have unusual bone marrow features that include ringed sideroblasts and must also be differentiated from idiopathic myelodysplasia. Occasionally, children develop marrow dysplasia due to infection, immunodeficiency, or even nutritional deficiency, further complicating the diagnosis of pediatric myelodysplasia.

Children with primary myelodysplasia present with neutropenia or thrombocytopenia more often than do adults.[67] Red cells tend to be macrocytic even when age-adjusted parameters are used. Some reports suggest that fetal hemoglobin levels are also high. This point deserves caution since fetal hemoglobin levels can be naturally high in infants. Furthermore, fetal hemoglobin levels tend to rise with bone marrow stress, such as that produced by transient virally mediated aplasia, for instance. Consequently, separating primary and secondary changes in fetal hemoglobin levels can be a challenge.

Hypocellular bone marrows exist in more than one-third of children at the time of diagnosis, a number strikingly higher than for adults. The question of whether a particular case is "myelodysplasia" or "aplastic anemia" is sometimes problematic with severely hypoplastic bone marrows. Some children with myelodysplasia and bone marrow hypoplasia progress to a condition that is indistinguishable from aplastic anemia. The opposite sequence also occurs where children with acquired aplastic anemia later develop myelodysplasia, raising the possibility of a close relationship between the two disorders.[68]

Clonal karyotype abnormalities exist at the time of diagnosis in as many as half of the children with myelodysplasia. Monosomy 7 is the most frequent aberration either alone or in conjunction with other chromosomal abnormalities.[69] Anomalies involving chromosome 8 are also common, including trisomy 8. The poor prognosis conferred by monosomy 7 in adult hematological disorders might not hold for pediatric myelodysplasia.[70,71] The relatively small number of patients in most reports and the retrospective nature of the work limits the scope of their interpretation, however.[72]

Children with myelodysplasia fare poorly on the whole.[73] As many as one-third of the patients develop acute myelogenous leukemia within 2 years of diagnosis.[74] A lower rate of remission occurs in pediatric myelodysplasias that convert to acute leukemia relative to de novo cases of leukemia, and the duration of remission is shorter.[75] Hematopoietic stem cell transplant shows reasonable success in these children and should be considered as a high-priority option when a suitable donor exists.[76] Limited information on matched unrelated donor transplants currently precludes statements on the utility of this intervention for these children.

■ **SIDEROBLASTIC ANEMIA**

The sideroblastic anemias are a singularly instructive set of disorders with respect to the physiology and pathophysiology of erythropoiesis. Some sideroblastic anemias fall under the rubric of myelodysplasia while others do not. The presence of ringed

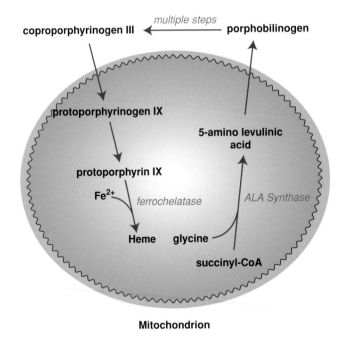

FIGURE 12-2 *Simplified schema of heme biosynthesis. Heme biosynthesis begins in the mitochondrion with the condensation of succinyl-CoA and glycine to form 5-aminolevulinic acid (δ-aminolevulinic acid). Biosynthesis moves to the cytosol where multiple enzymatic steps produce coproporphyrinogen III. This molecule enters the mitochondrion for the final steps of heme biosynthesis.*

sideroblasts (abnormal erythroblasts with excessive mitochondrial iron deposition) in the bone marrow is the phenotypic expression of a heterogeneous group of disorders whose unifying feature is deranged heme biosynthesis. Unraveling of the biochemistry and genetics of sideroblastic anemia provides unique insight into heme and iron metabolism along with an expanded understanding of erythropoiesis. Center stage in this drama features the heme molecule.

Figure 12-2 is a simplified schema of heme biosynthesis. The process begins in the mitochondrion with the condensation of glycine and succinyl-CoA to form δ-aminolevulinic acid (ALA) with pyridoxal phosphate as a cofactor.[77] The processing of ALA then moves to the cytoplasm where serial enzymatic transformations produce coproporphyrinogen III. This molecule enters the mitochondrion where additional modifications, including the insertion of iron into the protoporphyrin IX ring by ferrochelatase, produce heme.

Numerous studies involving various subtypes of sideroblastic anemias demonstrate impaired heme production.[78–80] Most commonly, the sideroblastic anemias are classified as hereditary or acquired conditions (Table 12-6). The hereditary forms are primarily X-linked, although some families display autosomal dominant or autosomal

TABLE 12-6 | **CATEGORIES OF SIDEROBLASTIC ANEMIA**

Category	Groups	Etiology
Hereditary	X-linked	• ALAS-2 mutations
		• *hABC7* gene
	Autosomal dominant	Unknown
	Autosomal recessive	Unknown
	Mitochondrial cytopathy	mtDNA deletions
	Wolfram syndrome	Mutations in *WFS1/wolframin*[a]
Acquired	Myelodysplasia	mtDNA point mutations, and unknown
	Drugs	Ethanol, INH, chloramphenicol, cycloserine
	Toxins	Zinc
	Nutritional	• Pyridoxine deficiency (animals)
		• Copper deficiency
	Other	Hypothermia
Congenital	Sporadic	Unknown

[a] Additional undiscovered defects may exist in the subset of Wolfram patients with sideroblastic anemia as *WFS1/wolframin* mutations alone do not produce the hematological anomaly.

recessive modes of transmission.[81] Isolated cases of congenital sideroblastic anemia often defy classification as they lack the well-documented pedigrees needed to firmly establish the modes of transmission.[82] The heterogeneity of the hereditary sideroblastic anemias can produce cases with mild or moderate anemia and varying degrees of iron overload.[83] While hereditary sideroblastic anemias most often have striking phenotypes that manifest in childhood or infancy, mild cases sometimes evade detection until adulthood.

The acquired sideroblastic anemias are far more common than the hereditary forms of the disorder. Sideroblastic anemias secondary to drugs and toxins dominate this category, propelled largely by the high frequency of alcohol abuse in many societies.[84,85] The next largest subgroup, refractory anemia with ring sideroblasts, is itself a subset of the myelodysplastic disorders.[86] Hypothermia is a rare antecedent of sideroblastic anemia.[87] In contrast to the hereditary conditions, the acquired sideroblastic anemias, particularly those associated with myelodysplasia, nearly always occur in older adults.

The exact mechanism by which disturbed heme metabolism produces sideroblastic anemias is problematic. Heme is an essential component of many mitochondrial enzymes (e.g., cytochromes b, c_1, c, a, a_3) as well as cytosolic enzymes such as catalase.[88–90] The molecule also is an integral component of hemoglobin where it has both structural and functional roles. Heme modulates translation of globin mRNA, stabilizes the globin protein chains, and mediates reversible oxygen binding.

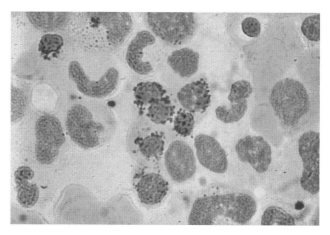

FIGURE 12-3   *Ring sideroblasts. The Perl's Prussian blue stain of this marrow aspirate highlights the small granules that circle the nucleus in some of the normoblasts. These cells are the pathognomonic ring sideroblasts.*

5-Aminolevulinic acid synthase (ALAS) is both the first and rate-limiting enzyme in heme biosynthesis (Figure 12-2). Heme modulates its activity through feedback inhibition. The gene that encodes ALAS-1 (also called ALAS-n) resides on chromosome 3 (3p21).[91] This ubiquitous enzyme is particularly abundant in the liver. ALAS-1, which provides the basal heme production needed by all cells, maintains a relatively stable level. The central importance of the enzyme to cell viability belies the epithet "housekeeping" that it sometimes receives.

The enzyme directly relevant to sideroblastic anemia is ALAS-2 or ALAS-e (erythroid). The gene encoding this enzyme resides on the X chromosome (Xp11.21). Expression of ALAS-2 is restricted to the erythroid lineage.[92,93] ALAS-2 activity lacks known feedback regulation by heme. The enzyme is, however, a member of a small family of genes whose expression is modulated by iron.[94–96]

The cardinal feature of sideroblastic anemia is mitochondrial iron deposition.[97] Normal erythroid precursors stained for iron with Perl's Prussian blue often show two or three bluish green inclusions called siderosomes. The cells that contain these iron granules are called sideroblasts. In sideroblastic anemia, the iron-containing particles are larger and more numerous than normal. Many erythroblasts contain six or more blue-green particles that circle the nucleus, creating the pathognomonic "ringed sideroblasts" (Figure 12-3). While ringed sideroblasts commonly comprise between 15% and 50% of erythroblasts, some bone marrows display ringed sideroblasts exclusively. Electron microscopy shows crystalline iron deposits between cristae in the mitochondrial matrix.[98,99] The basis of this phenomenon is unknown.

Mitochondrial iron deposits could be more than histological curiosities. Iron catalyzes the formation of reactive oxygen species through Fenton chemistry.[100] Oxidation reactions that occur in proximity to iron produce highly reactive molecules such as the hydroxyl radical ($\cdot$OH).[101] The oxidative metabolic machinery of the mitochondrion creates an ideal environment for the generation of reactive oxygen species. The primary damage in sideroblastic anemia that produces iron-laden mitochondria could establish a feedback loop with escalating levels of mitochondrial injury. The hydroxyl radical, for instance, promotes lipid and protein peroxidation as well as cross-links in DNA strands.[102,103] The latter phenomenon could be particularly injurious given the paucity of DNA repair enzymes in mitochondria.[104]

Sideroblastic bone marrows often show erythroid hyperplasia, consistent with the ineffective erythropoiesis characteristic of this condition. The bone marrow's plethora of erythroid precursors fails to produce sufficient numbers of mature erythrocytes, making erythropoiesis ineffective by definition. Ineffective erythropoiesis increases gastrointestinal iron absorption. Therefore, patients with even mild sideroblastic anemia can develop substantial iron overload.[105]

X-LINKED SIDEROBLASTIC ANEMIA

In 1945, Thomas Cooley described the first cases of X-linked sideroblastic anemia in two brothers from a large family where the inheritance of the disease was documented through six generations.[106] Although rare, this disorder nonetheless is the most common of the hereditary sideroblastic anemias. Defects involving at least two independent genes on the X-chromosome produce X-linked sideroblastic anemia. The more common of the two derives from mutations of the gene encoding ALAS-2.[107]

Missense mutations of the *ALAS-2* gene produce most cases of X-linked sideroblastic anemia.[108–111] Years after their initial evaluation, investigators located several members of the pedigree originally described by Cooley and analyzed their DNA using current techniques in molecular biology.[112] These family members did indeed have missense mutations involving the *ALAS-2* gene. Through a combination of acumen and meticulous observation, Cooley correctly categorized a complex new disorder 50 years before confirmatory scientific tools existed.

Mutations of the *ALAS-2* gene can be classified according to their effects on the enzyme product: low affinity for pyridoxal phosphate, structural instability, abnormal catalytic site, or increased susceptibility to mitochondrial proteases. Any of these abnormalities decrease the biosynthesis and/or steady-state level of ALAS and consequently lower production of protoporphyrin and heme. The degree of anemia can improve with pyridoxine supplementation when the mutation disrupts the catalytic association between ALAS-2 and pyridoxal phosphate.[113] Rounding out the documented causes of aberrant ALAS-2 activity and sideroblastic anemia is the report of a mutation in the gene promoter that reduces enzyme production.[114]

Hereditary X-linked sideroblastic anemia occurs almost exclusively in males, of course. The rare cases involving females in a family derive most probably from skewed lyonization patterns in the affected girls.[115–118] Proof of unbalanced lyonization is difficult to produce, unfortunately. Some women in affected families have developed sideroblastic anemia later in life due to progressive stochastic inactivation over time of the X-chromosome bearing the normal ALAS-2 gene.[119]

A second group of hereditary X-linked sideroblastic anemias derive from the defects involving a different gene on the X-chromosome and manifest a strikingly different phenotype. The syndrome produces a severe congenital ataxia, in addition to sideroblastic anemia. The causal gene encodes an ATP-binding cassette (ABC) protein now designated as hABC7.[120] The gene localizes to chromosome Xq13.1-q13.3.[121] ABC proteins generally mediate transmembrane transport of various small molecules. *hABC7* is an ortholog of the yeast *ATMl* gene whose product localizes to the inner mitochondrial membrane.[122]

A family with X-linked sideroblastic anemia and ataxia displayed a mutation in the *hABC7* gene that segregated with the affected males in the kindred and was absent in controls.[123] The *hABC7* gene in another family contained a single missense mutation that reduced the protein's functional activity by half as assessed by complementation studies using yeast with a deleted *ATMl* gene.[124] The complementation assay assesses maturation of proteins containing an iron–sulfur (Fe/S) cluster. The investigators hypothesized that impaired production of Fe/S cluster proteins in erythroid precursors could produce sideroblastic anemia. The ataxia could reflect dysfunction of cytoplasmic proteins crucial to spinocerebellar development. Evidence in other fields points to an important role for Fe/S cluster proteins in neuropathology.[125] The production of both sideroblastic anemia and neuropathology due to defects in Fe/S cluster proteins is plausible.

The two well-characterized forms of X-linked sideroblastic anemia reinforce the importance of mitochondrial function in the syndrome. Despite radically different genetic alterations, the overlapping similarity between "traditional" X-linked sideroblastic anemias and the hABC7 cases are proteins that functionally localize to the mitochondrion. Sideroblastic anemias due to defects of other mitochondrial proteins or enzymes undoubtedly exist. Future discoveries in this area will certainly provide new vistas into mitochondrial metabolism and erythropoiesis.

MITOCHONDRIAL CYTOPATHIES

Oxidative phosphorylation within mitochondria generates most of the ATP produced by eukaryotic cells. The mature erythrocyte is the sole mammalian cell devoid of mitochondria, with consequent total reliance on glycolysis for energy. Most cells contain between 100 and 300 mitochondria.[126] These semiautonomous organelles likely developed from freestanding prokaryotes that invaded eukaryotic cells more than a billion years ago.[127] The intruders eventually evolved a symbiotic relationship with their eukaryotic hosts. The whilom prokaryotes lost the capacity for independent existence, but became indispensable sources of energy for their eukaryotic hosts.

Mitochondria retain vestiges of their erstwhile independent existence. Most importantly the organelles have a small DNA genome (about 16 kb) and replicate independently of host cell mitosis. Mitochondrial DNA retains many features of a prokaryotic genome, including a circular structure lacking introns.[128] The mitochondrial genome encodes a small number of proteins as well as several transfer RNA molecules. Mitochondrial DNA lacks chromatin and the organelles have limited DNA repair capacity.[129] Consequently, mutations in the mitochondrial genome that produce sideroblastic anemia likely remain uncorrected.

Mitochondria replicate independently of the nuclear genome. When cells undergo mitosis, the organelles distribute randomly to the daughter cells. Acquired mitochondrial defects therefore pass unevenly to the daughter cells.[130] This property imparts interesting and unusual attributes to the hereditary mitochondrial disorders that produce sideroblastic anemia.

The mitochondrial cytopathies are a heterogeneous group of disorders produced by deletions in the mitochondrial genome.[131,132] Some deletions encompass as much as 30% of the 16-kb mitochondrial genome. Two factors contribute to the peculiar inheritance patterns in these disorders. First, independent mitochondrial replication combined with random segregation into the daughter cells at cell division means that by pure chance newly produced cells can have more or fewer defective mitochondria.[133] Second, mitochondrial cytopathies are maternally transmitted because ova are the sole source of an embryo's mitochondria. A mother with mild manifestations of a syndrome can thus have one child who is unaffected and another who has extremely severe disease (mitochondrial heteroplasmy).[134]

Pearson and colleagues made the seminal observation that children from several unrelated families manifested sideroblastic anemia and exocrine pancreatic dysfunction.[135] Subsequent cases of what is now called Pearson's syndrome also had varying degrees of lactic acidosis and hepatic and renal failure. Bone marrow examination showed, in addition to prominent ringed sideroblasts, large vacuoles in the erythroid and myeloid precursors. Few of the probands survived past early childhood.

The disorder results from mitochondrial DNA deletions that often are as large as 4 kb.[136] Southern blots of mitochondrial DNA show genomes of normal size along with the truncated DNA. Variation in the intensity of the two bands reflects mitochondrial heteroplasmy in cells from the mother and offspring.[137] These deletions impair biosynthesis of various components of the mitochondrial respiratory chain critical to mitochondrial function. Other disorders result from deletions of different portions of the mitochondrial genome [e.g., myopathy, encephalopathy, ragged red fibers (in muscles), and lactic acidosis, or MERRL].[138] Although sideroblastic anemia is not part of the clinical spectrum of most such syndromes, exceptions exist.[139]

Wolfram syndrome is an instructive condition that could shed additional light on the interplay between nuclear genes and mitochondria.[140] The condition results from large deletions of the mitochondrial genome. The heteroplasmic nature of the mitochondrial defect in Wolfram syndrome is typical of a mitochondrial cytopathy. The defining characteristics of the disorder are diabetes insipidus, diabetes mellitus, optic atrophy, and deafness (DIDMOAD). Sideroblastic anemia in association with mitochondrial deletions occurs in a subset of these patients.[141] Wolfram syndrome differs from other mitochondrial cytopathies by way of its autosomal inheritance pattern.[142]

Mutations in the gene designated *WFS1/wolframin* produce the DIDMOAD constellation of defects.[143,144] The gene product is a transmembrane protein of undetermined function.[145] Patients with defects in the *WFS1/wolframin* gene do not invariably develop sideroblastic anemia in addition to the DIDMOAD anomalies.[146] Mutations in *WSF1/wolframin* could be necessary but not sufficient to produce sideroblastic anemia. The rarity both of Wolfram syndrome and mitochondrial cytopathy makes coincidence unlikely in the subset of Wolfram patients who develop sideroblastic anemia. Clearly, Wolfram syndrome is a fertile ground in the search for links between the function of nuclear genes and the mitochondrion.

ACQUIRED SIDEROBLASTIC ANEMIAS

Acquired sideroblastic anemias substantially exceed hereditary forms in frequency. The disorder sometimes surfaces in the context of an MDS. Other instances of acquired sideroblastic anemias reflect exposure to toxins or deficiencies of nutritional factors. Because the heterogeneity of hereditary sideroblastic anemias produces cases with mild or moderate anemia, some affected individuals evade detection until adulthood. Such patients can be misclassified as having acquired sideroblastic anemia. The all-important family history (and, if necessary, family examination) quickly reveals the hereditary nature of these cases. In contrast, the acquired sideroblastic anemias, particularly those associated with myelodysplasia, arise randomly and almost exclusively in older adults.

Damaged hematopoietic stem cells with disturbed function are the fulcrum of the MDSs. Extensive stem cell damage, manifested most clearly by multiple chromosomal aberrations, produces severely dysfunctional cells with a proclivity toward acute leukemia (e.g., RAEB-1, RAEB-2). More restricted stem cell injury produces a narrower range of deficits. The "refractory anemia with ringed sideroblasts" of the WHO classification is a case in point. Sharply focused injury produces anomalies mimicking the point mutations of the X-linked sideroblastic anemias. As the range of stem cell injury broadens so does the range of hematopoietic cell dysfunction. The resulting conditions retain the ringed sideroblast phenotype but acquire other anomalies. This subgroup is the "refractory cytopenia with multilineage dysplasia and ringed sideroblasts" category.

The ringed sideroblasts associated with MDSs manifest in both the early and late erythroid precursors. This contrasts with the hereditary X-linked conditions in which prominent sideroblastic rings generally appear in the more differentiated normoblasts. While helpful, the distinction is not diagnostically definitive.

DRUG- AND TOXIN-INDUCED SIDEROBLASTIC ANEMIA

Drugs and toxins are important causes of sideroblastic anemias, and Table 12-6 lists some of the etiological agents. The compounds most commonly implicated inhibit steps in the heme biosynthetic pathway. Eliminating the offending agent usually corrects the sideroblastic anemia. Ethanol is the most frequent cause of toxin-induced sideroblastic anemia.[147,148] The complication is uncommon, but the use (and misuse) of the agent is widespread. Ethanol probably causes sideroblastic anemia by two mechanisms: direct antagonism to pyridoxal phosphate and/or associated dietary deficiency of this compound.[149–151] The bone marrow changes associated with ethanol toxicity include vacuoles in the normoblasts in addition to ringed sideroblasts. Interestingly, chloramphenicol commonly produces vacuoles in the normoblasts and likewise can induce sideroblastic anemia.[152]

Chloramphenicol inhibits mRNA translation by the 70S ribosomes of prokaryotes. The drug does not affect 80S eukaryotic ribosomes. Most mitochondrial proteins are encoded by nuclear DNA and are imported into the organelles from the cytosol where they are synthesized. Mitochondria retain the capacity to translate a few proteins encoded by the mitochondrial genome using endogenous ribosomes. True to their prokaryotic heritage, mitochondrial ribosomes are similar to those of bacteria, meaning that chloramphenicol inhibits mitochondrial protein synthesis. Chloramphenicol-induced sideroblastic anemia likely reflects this inhibition. Animal studies document diminished ALAS and ferrochelatase activity in cases of sideroblastic anemia secondary to chloramphenicol intoxication.[153]

Isoniazid frequently causes sideroblastic anemia.[154] Pyridoxine prophylaxis as part of treatment regimens involving the drug aims at preventing this complication. Isoniazid-induced sideroblastic likely reflects inhibition of ALAS activity.[155,156]

Lead intoxication is a particularly insidious cause of anemia.[157] Although lead toxicity is commonly mentioned as a cause of sideroblastic anemia, no well-documented case exists in the literature.[158] The assertion that lead produces sideroblastic anemia appears to be preserved in the literature by reference to indirect sources. Concomitant pyridoxine deficiency might have been the basis of erroneous reports. Lead contamination of homemade distilled liquors once was a prevalent problem. Lead might have been blamed for cases of sideroblastic anemia that were due in reality to a combination of pyridoxine deficiency and ethanol abuse.[159]

■ TREATMENT OF MYELODYSPLASIA

Supportive therapy is the mainstay of care for patients with myelodysplasia. Morbidity and mortality derive primarily from the multiple cytopenias that characterize the condition. With the exception of erythropoietin and rHuGCSF, interventions that aim at improving the underlying marrow dysfunction are investigational and should be performed by experienced practitioners, optimally in the setting of a clinical trial.

STANDARD SUPPORTIVE CARE

Transfusions correct the anemia that characterizes most cases of myelodysplasia. Since patients usually require indefinite transfusion support, a number of management issues must be addressed early in the course of the illness to avoid long-term complications. Alloimmunization against minor red cell antigens is a cumulative problem for patients with myelodysplasia whose severity can be tempered with proper care. Limited phenotype matching can slow the appearance of alloantibodies against minor antigens. Once antibodies are formed, management becomes extremely difficult. Finding compatible units of blood becomes increasingly difficult and sometimes places patients at risk for anemia of life-threatening severity.

Patients with myelodysplasia often have fragile skin and veins related to age that are easily ruptured. Care is needed with each transfusion in order to preserve the integrity of the veins. Following the infusion of blood, prolonged pressure should be applied to the wound to prevent leakage into the subcutaneous tissues.

Thrombocytopenia heightens the danger in these patients since hemostasis is delayed. Loss of peripheral infusion sites is a significant problem to be avoided, if possible.

The combined use of erythropoietin and rHuGCSF raises hemoglobin levels significantly in about one-third of patients with myelodysplasia. Patients whose serum erythropoietin levels are low (i.e., less than 500 mU/mL) and those with ringed sideroblasts are particularly favored in this regard.[160] The dose of erythropoietin required for response is much higher than is required in renal insufficiency. Some treatment regimens call for erythropoietin administration at a level of 20,000 units three times per week. A high initial dose of erythropoietin can be lowered over time if the patient responses to the drug. Weekly doses of erythropoietin (40,000 units) appear to be an effective alternative treatment for these patients.[161] Daily injections of rHuGCSF accompany the erythropoietin therapy.

With sideroblastic anemia, a trial of pyridoxine (100 mg/day orally) is reasonable since the drug has few drawbacks and is an enormous benefit in responsive cases.[162] The few reported instances of side effects have involved patients taking 1000 or more milligrams of pyridoxine daily. Complete responses to pyridoxine occur most often in cases due to ethanol abuse or the use of pyridoxine antagonists. Cessation of the offending agent hastens recovery. Some patients with hereditary, X-linked sideroblastic anemia also respond to pyridoxine.[110] Improvement with pyridoxine is uncommon for sideroblastic anemias of other etiologies.

Iron overload is inevitable with chronic transfusions since no physiological means of iron excretion exists. Iron overload eventually produces a host of problems, with hepatic and heart damage being among the most prominent issues. Desferrioxamine is an excellent iron chelator that prevents the problems produced by excessive iron loading. Unfortunately, delivery of the drug is cumbersome, requiring a portable pump for subcutaneous infusion over 12 hours per day for at least 5 days per week. This rigorous regimen is a problem for all patients. Oral iron chelators are increasingly available, creating possible treatment alternatives to desferrioxamine.

Platelet issues are the second major burden shouldered by people with myelodysplasia. Although platelet transfusions are possible, they are less effective at correcting thrombocytopenia than red cell transfusions are at correcting anemia. Platelet counts rise for mere hours following transfusion. Consequently, platelet infusions are most efficacious in the setting of an acute bleeding episode. Prophylactic platelet transfusion is a judicious strategy in the setting of a defined period of high bleeding risk, such as the perioperative setting. Alloimmunization against platelets occurs frequently and all too often early in the course of this treatment approach making patients refractory to treatment.

Platelets are available either as pooled products from up to 10 donors or as material obtained by pheresis from a single donor. The pooled product is preferable for people who have developed platelet alloimmunization and refractoriness. The degree of antibody reactivity against the 10 pools of platelets in the mixture will vary, meaning that some of the infused platelets might escape rapid clearance and provide some hemostatic benefit in the interim. The platelets in a pheresis unit by contrast are cleared uniformly, which can be a serious problem if this occurs rapidly in a setting that requires hemostatic control.

Neutropenia is the thorniest of the cytopenias associated with myelodysplasia. Granulocyte transfusion is not an option, making antibiotics the mainstay of infection control. Antibiotics alone cannot eliminate infection, however. While antibiotics can temporarily hold the fort, neutrophils are the sole mediators of cure in cases of infection. Early in the course of myelodysplasia the number of neutrophils often is sufficient to resolve infectious complications. As the disorder progresses, the neutrophil count often declines. Poor neutrophil function exacerbates an already dire situation. Over time, infection treatment involves longer courses of more potent antibiotics in an effort to parry growing bacterial resistance to antimicrobial agents. Ultimately infection gains the upper hand.

Although rHuGCSF can increase neutrophil production in people with normal bone marrow function, the intervention is not effective in cases of myelodysplasia with its defective bone marrow. The ability to respond effectively to the cytokine simply does not exist. The gesture is made even more futile by the fact that any increase in circulating granulocytes often is made up of cells with poor antimicrobial function.

AGGRESSIVE THERAPY FOR MYELODYSPLASIA

Supportive care works well in the management of the anemia that accompanies myelodysplasia. Serious problems that defy conservative approaches develop in the two other arms of the trilineage hematopoietic cell dysfunction that plagues these patients, however. This is the field on which the battle to control myelodysplasia is either won or lost.

The clear relationship between myelodysplasia, particularly RAEB, and leukemia made treatment regimens for acute myelogenous leukemia an early area of exploration in myelodysplasia management. Response rates were uniformly lower for myelodysplasia than for de novo acute myelogenous leukemia. Newer drug combinations have not improved the overall poor response rate of myelodysplasia to intensive chemotherapy.[163] Intensive chemotherapy is an option that should be reserved for patients with good performance status who have aggressive subtypes of myelodysplasia, such as RAEB-2.

Hematopoietic stem cell transplantation can cure a variety of hematological disorders, including acute myelogenous leukemia. Myelodysplasia throws a number of hurtles in the path of this modality. The higher mean age of the patients with myelodysplasia places them at higher risk for complications related to transplantation. Many people affected by myelodysplasia have significant comorbid conditions that reduce the chances of a good outcome with transplantation.[164] Younger patients and those with a good performance status are most likely to benefit from hematopoietic stem cell transplantation.

Biological response modifiers have been used in an attempt to moderate the severity of deranged hematopoietic cell function in myelodysplasia. One intriguing approach uses drugs such as 5-azacytidine to enhance cell differentiation. Exposure to 5-azacytidine promotes DNA hypomethylation in cultured cells, a phenomenon that reverses gene inactivation produced by methylation of cytosine residues. The driving hypothesis behind this approach is that deranged cell maturation in myelodysplasia reflects loss of expression of genes important to differentiation. A significant fraction of patients respond to 5-azacytidine, but the positive effects are transient.[165]

Immunosuppressive agents such as antithymocyte immune globulin and cyclosporin have also been used in trials involving patients with myelodysplasia. These agents are often successful in the management of aplastic anemia where an immune component is clear. Some overlap might exist between myelodysplasia and aplastic anemia with respect to immune mechanisms of etiology. Reports exist of good responses to immunosuppressive agents in myelodysplasia.[166] More information is needed to know where this approach fits in the therapeutic armamentarium (Tables 12-7 and 12-8).

TABLE 12-7 | **KEY DIAGNOSTIC ISSUES IN MYELODYSPLASIA**

Issue	*Manifestation*	*Approach*
Myelodysplastic syndrome versus aplastic anemia	• Anemia • Neutropenia • Thrombocytopenia • Bone marrow aplasia	• Review peripheral blood for pseudo-Pelger-Huet neutrophil anomaly • Review bone marrow for dysplastic features • Bone marrow karyotype analysis for anomalies associated with myelodysplasia • Bone marrow iron stain for ring sideroblasts
Pure sideroblastic anemia	• Anemia • No neutropenia or thrombocytopenia • Favorable clinical course	• Bone marrow iron stain for ring sideroblasts • Bone marrow karyotype analysis for anomalies associated with myelodysplasia
Myelodysplastic syndrome versus myeloproliferative disorder	• Anemia	• Peripheral blood examination for schistocytes associated with myeloproliferative disorders • Peripheral blood examination for pseudo-Pelger-Huet cells associated with myelodysplasia • Reticulin stain of bone marrow • Karyotype analysis • Assess spleen size and texture (enlarged with myeloproliferative disorder)

TABLE 12-8	KEY MANAGEMENT ISSUES IN MYELODYSPLASIA
Issue	*Comment*
Pure sideroblastic anemia	Pure sideroblastic anemia follows a course dominated by anemia with infrequent disturbances of neutrophils and platelets. Evolution into acute leukemia is rare. Management is transfusion support.
Del5(q) myelodysplasia	This subset follows a relatively benign course with anemia as the primary manifestation. Management is transfusion support.
Monosomy 7 myelodysplasia	Monosomy 7 bodes ill with conversion to acute leukemia as an early and common event. Early, aggressive therapy is reasonable.
Anemia	Transfusion support is basic. Erythropoietin, G-CSF and biological response modifiers sometimes dampen the severity of the anemia. Iron overload is a common complication.
Thrombocytopenia	Bleeding in myelodysplasia reflects both low platelet number and poor platelet function. Petechia and ecchymoses are common. GI bleeding often is associated with a gut structural defect. Platelet alloimmunization following repeated transfusions is common.
Neutropenia	Infection is a leading cause of death in myelodysplasia. Responses to growth factors such as G-CSF are poor and often transient.

G-CSF, granulocyte colony-stimulating factor.

References

[1] Bennett J, Catovsky D, Daniel M, et al. 1982. Proposals for the classification of the myelodysplastic syndromes. Br J Haematol 51:189–199.
[2] Heaney M, Golde D. 1999. Myelodysplasia. N Engl J Med 340:1649–1660.
[3] Aul C, Gattermann N, Heyll A, Germing U, Derigs G, Schneider W. 1992. Primary myelodysplastic syndromes: Analysis of prognostic factors in 235 patients and proposals for an improved scoring system. Leukemia 6:52–59.

[4]   van Lom K, Hagemeijer A, Vandekerckhove F, Smit E, Lowenberg B. 1996. Cytoge-
      netic clonality analysis: Typical patterns in myelodysplastic syndrome and acute myeloid
      leukaemia. Br J Haematol 93:594–600.

[5]   Ghaddar H, Stass S, Pierce S, Estey E. 1994. Cytogenetic evolution following the transfor-
      mation of myelodysplastic syndrome to acute myelogenous leukemia: Implications on the
      overlap between the two diseases. Leukemia 8:1649–1653.

[6]   Ogata K, Nakamura K, Yokose N, et al. 2002. Clinical significance of phenotypic features
      of blasts in patients with myelodysplastic syndrome. Blood 100:3887–3896.

[7]   Greenberg P, Cox C, LeBeau M, et al. 1997. International scoring system for evaluating
      prognosis in myelodysplastic syndromes. Blood 89:2079–2088.

[8]   Harris NL, Jaffe ES, Diebold J, et al. 1999. World Health Organization classification of neo-
      plastic diseases of the hematopoietic and lymphoid tissues: Report of the Clinical Advisory
      Committee meeting—Airlie House, Virginia, November 1997. J Clin Oncol 17:3835–3849.

[9]   Vardiman J, Harris N, Brunning R. 2002. The World Health Organization (WHO) classifi-
      cation of the myeloid neoplasms. Blood 100:2292–2302.

[10] Scoazec JY, Imbert M, Crofts M, et al. 1985. Myelodysplastic syndrome or acute myeloid
      leukemia? A study of 28 cases presenting with borderline features. Cancer 55:2390–2394.

[11] Howe R, Porwit-MacDonald A, Wanat R, Tehranchi R, Hellstrom-Lindberg E. 2004. The
      WHO classification of MDS does make a difference. Blood 103:3265–3270.

[12] Rios A, Canizo M, Sanz M, et al. 1990. Bone marrow biopsy in myelodysplastic syndromes:
      Morphological characteristics and contribution to the study of prognostic factors. Br J
      Haematol 75:26–33.

[13] Haase D, Fonatsch C, Freund M, et al. 1995. Cytogenetic findings in 179 patients with
      myelodysplastic syndromes. Ann Hematol 70:171–187.

[14] Velloso E, Michaux L, Ferrant A, et al. 1996. Deletions of the long arm of chromosome 7 in
      myeloid disorders: Loss of band 7q32 implies worst prognosis. Br J Haematol 92:574–581.

[15] Wheatley K, Burnett AK, Goldstone AH, et al. 1999. A simple, robust, validated and highly
      predictive index for the determination of risk-directed therapy in acute myeloid leukaemia
      derived from the MRC AML 10 trial. Br J Haematol 107:69–79.

[16] Mathew P, Tefferi A, Dewald G, et al. 1993. The 5q-syndrome: A single-institution study
      of 43 consecutive patients. Blood 81:1040–1045.

[17] Boultwood J, Lewis S, Wainscoat JS. 1994. The 5q-syndrome. Blood 84:3253–3260.

[18] Van Den Berghe H, Cassiman JJ, David G, Fryns JP, Michaux JL, Sokal G. 1974. Distinct
      haematological disorder with deletion of long arm of No. 5 chromosome. Nature 251:437–
      438.

[19] Giagounidis A, Germing U, Haase S, et al. 2004. Clinical, morphological, cytogenetic,
      and prognostic features of patients with myelodysplastic syndromes and del(5q) including
      band q31. Leukemia 18:113–119.

[20] Lewis S, Oscier D, Boultwood J, et al. 1995. Hematological features of patients with
      myelodysplastic syndromes associated with a chromosome 5q deletion. Am J Hematol
      49:194–200.

[21] Cermak J, Michalova K, Brezinova J, Zemanova Z. 2003. A prognostic impact of separa-
      tion of refractory cytopenia with multilineage dysplasia and 5q-syndrome from refractory
      anemia in primary myelodysplastic syndrome. Leuk Res 27:221–229.

[22] Higgs DR, Wood WG, Barton C, Weatherall DJ. 1983. Clinical features and molecular
      analysis of acquired hemoglobin H disease. Am J Med 75:181–191.

[23] Yoo D, Schechter G, Amigable A, Nienhuis A. 1980. Myeloproliferative syndrome with
      sideroblastic anemia and acquired hemoglobin H disease. Cancer 45:78–83.

24 Steensma D, Viprakasit V, Hendrick A, et al. 2004. Deletion of the alpha-globin gene cluster as a cause of acquired alpha-thalassemia in myelodysplastic syndrome. Blood 103:1518–1520.

25 Gibbons R, Pellagatti A, Garrick D, et al. 2003. Identification of acquired somatic mutations in the gene encoding chromatin-remodeling factor ATRX in the a-thalassemia myelodysplasia syndrome (ATMDS). Nat Genet 34:446–449.

26 Boehme W, Piira T, Kurnick J, Bethlenfalvay N. 1978. Acquired hemoglobin H in refractory sideroblastic anemia. A preleukemic marker. Arch Intern Med 138:603–606.

27 Annino L, Di Giovanni S, Tentori L, Jr, et al. 1984. Acquired hemoglobin H disease in a case of refractory anemia with excess of blasts (RAEB) evolving into acute nonlymphoid leukemia. Acta Haematol 72:41–44.

28 Reinhardt D, Haase D, Schoch C, et al. 1998. Hemoglobin F in myelodysplastic syndrome. Ann Hematol 76:135–138.

29 Mendek-Czajokska E, Slomkowski M, et al. 2003. Hemoglobin F in primary myelofibrosis and in myelodysplasia. Clin Lab Haematol 25:289–292.

30 Washington L, Doherty D, Glassman A, Martins J, Ibrahim S, Lai R. 2002. Myeloid disorders with deletion of 5q as the sole karyotypic abnormality: The clinical and pathologic spectrum. Leuk Lymphoma 43:761–765.

31 Matsushima T, Murakami H, Tsuchiya J. 1994. Myelodysplastic syndrome with bone marrow eosinophilia: Clinical and cytogenetic features. Leuk Lymphoma 15:491–497.

32 Nand S, Godwin J. 1988. Hypoplastic myelodysplastic syndrome. Cancer 62:958–964.

33 Maschek H, Kaloutsi V, Rodriguez-Kaiser M, et al. 1993. Hypoplastic myelodysplastic syndrome: Incidence, morphology, cytogenetics, and prognosis. Ann Hematol 66:117–122.

34 Tuzuner N, Cox C, Rowe J, Watrous D, Bennett J. 1995. Hypocellular myelodysplastic syndromes (MDS): New proposals. Br J Haematol 91:612–617.

35 Kearns W, Sutton J, Maciejewski J, Young N, Liu J. 2004. Genomic instability in bone marrow failure syndromes. Am J Hematol 76:220–224.

36 Barrett AJ, Saunthararajah Y, Molldrem J. 2000. Myelodysplastic syndrome and aplastic anemia: Distinct entities or diseases linked by a common pathophysiology? Semin Hematol 37:15–29.

37 Biesma DH, van den Tweel JG, Verdonck LF. 1997. Immunosuppressive therapy for hypoplastic myelodysplastic syndrome. Cancer 79:1548–1551.

38 Molldrem J, Caples M, Mavroudis D, Plante M, Young NS, Barrett AJ. 1997. Antithymocyte globulin (ATG) abrogates cytopenias in patients with myelodysplastic syndrome. Br J Haematol 99:699–705.

39 Butler W, Taylor H, Viswanathan U. 1982. Idiopathic acquired sideroblastic anemia terminating in acute myelosclerosis. Cancer 49:2497–2499.

40 Bested A, Cheng G, Pinkerton P, Kassim O, Senn J. 1984. Idiopathic acquired sideroblastic anaemia transforming to acute myelosclerosis. J Clin Pathol 37:1032–1034.

41 Lambertenghi-Deliliers G, Orazi A, Luksch R, Annaloro C, Soligo D. 1991. Myelodysplastic syndrome with increased marrow fibrosis: A distinct clinico-pathological entity. Br J Haematol 78:161–166.

42 Hoagland HC. 1995. Myelodysplastic (preleukemia) syndromes: The bone marrow factory failure problem. Mayo Clin Proc 70:673–676.

43 Greenberg PL. 1983. The smouldering myeloid leukemic states: Clinical and biologic features. Blood 61:1035–1044.

44 Albitar M, Manshouri T, Shen Y, et al. 2002. Myelodysplastic syndrome is not merely "preleukemia." Blood 100:791–798.

[45] Raza A, Grezer S, Mundle S, et al. 1995. Apoptosis in bone marrow biopsy samples involving stromal and hematopoietic cells in 50 patients with myelodysplastic syndromes. Blood 86:268–276.

[46] Testa U. 2004. Apoptotic mechanisms in the control of erythropoiesis. Leukemia 18:1176–1199.

[47] Raza A, Mundle S, Iftikhar A, et al. 1995. Simultaneous assessment of cell kinetics and programmed cell death in bone marrow biopsies of myelodysplastics reveals extensive apoptosis as the probable basis for ineffective hematopoiesis. Am J Hematol 48:143–154.

[48] Shimazaki K, Ohshima K, Suzumiya J, Kawasaki C, Kikuchi M. 2000. Evaluation of apoptosis as a prognostic factor in myelodysplastic syndromes. Br J Haematol 110:584–590.

[49] Tsoplou P, Kouraklis-Symeonidis A, Thanopoulou E, Zikos P, Orphanos V, Zoumbos N. 1999. Apoptosis in patients with myelodysplastic syndromes: Differential involvement of marrow cells in 'good' versus 'poor' prognosis patients and correlation with apoptosis-related genes. Leukemia 13:1554–15563.

[50] Lin C, Manshouri T, Jilani I, et al. 2002. Proliferation and apoptosis in acute and chronic leukemias and myelodysplastic syndrome. Leuk Res 26:551–559.

[51] Pecci A, Travaglino E, Klersy C, Invernizzi R. 2003. Apoptosis in relation to CD34 antigen expression in normal and myelodysplastic bone marrow. Acta Haematol 109:29–34.

[52] Pedersen-Bjergaard J. 1995. Therapy-related myelodysplasia and acute leukemia. Leuk Lymphoma 15:11–12.

[53] Bernard-Marty C, Mano M, Paesmans M, et al. 2003. Second malignancies following adjuvant chemotherapy: 6-Year results from a Belgian randomized study comparing cyclophosphamide, methotrexate and 5-fluorouracil (CMF) with an anthracycline-based regimen in adjuvant treatment of node-positive breast cancer patients. Ann Oncol 14:693–698.

[54] Pedersen-Bjergaard J, Andersen M, Christiansen D, Nerlov C. 2002. Genetic pathways in therapy-related myelodysplasia and acute myeloid leukemia. Blood 99:1909–1912.

[55] Michels S, McKenna R, Arthur D, Brunning R. 1985. Therapy-related acute myeloid leukemia and myelodysplastic syndrome: A clinical and morphologic study of 65 cases. Blood 65:1364–1372.

[56] Takeyama K, Seto M, Uike N, et al. 2000. Therapy-related leukemia and myelodysplastic syndrome: A large-scale Japanese study of clinical and cytogenetic features as well as prognostic factors. Int J Hematol 71:144–152.

[57] Pedersen-Bjergaard J, Larsen SO. 1982. Incidence of acute nonlymphocytic leukemia, preleukemia, and acute myeloproliferative syndrome up to 10 years after treatment of Hodgkin's disease. N Engl J Med 307:965–971.

[58] Henry-Amar M, Joly F. 1996. Late complications after Hodgkin's disease. Ann Oncol 7(Suppl 4):115–126.

[59] Smith R. 2003. Risk for the development of treatment-related acute myelocytic leukemia and myelodysplastic syndrome among patients with breast cancer: Review of the literature and the National Surgical Adjuvant Breast and Bowel Project experience. Clin Breast Cancer 4:273–279.

[60] Pedersen-Bjergaard J, Philip P, Larsen S, Jensen G, Byrsting K. 1990. Chromosome aberrations and prognostic factors in therapy-related myelodysplasia and acute nonlymphocytic leukemia. Blood 76:1083–1091.

[61] Mauritzson N, Albin M, Rylander L, et al. 2002. Pooled analysis of clinical and cytogenetic features in treatment-related and de novo adult acute myeloid leukemia and myelodysplastic

syndromes based on a consecutive series of 761 patients analyzed 1976–1993 and on 5098 unselected cases reported in the literature 1974–2001. Leukemia 16:2366–7238.

[62] Smith S, Le Beau M, Huo D, et al. 2003. Clinical-cytogenetic associations in 306 patients with therapy-related myelodysplasia and myeloid leukemia: The University of Chicago series. Blood 102:43–52.

[63] Nucifora G, Begy CR, Kobayashi H, et al. 1994. Consistent intergenic splicing and production of multiple transcripts between AML1 at 21q22 and unrelated genes at 3q26 in (3;21)(q26;q22) translocations. Proc Natl Acad Sci U S A 91:4004–4008.

[64] Harada H, Harada Y, Tanaka H, Kimura A, Inaba T. 2003. Implications of somatic mutations in the AML1 gene in radiation-associated and therapy-related myelodysplastic syndrome/acute myeloid leukemia. Blood 101:673–680.

[65] Rund D, Ben-Yehuda D. 2004. Therapy-related leukemia and myelodysplasia: Evolving concepts of pathogenesis and treatment. Hematology 9:179–187.

[66] Jackson GH, Carey PJ, Cant AJ, Bown NP, Reid MM. 1993. Myelodysplastic syndromes in children. Br J Haematol 84:185–186.

[67] Kardos G, Baumann I, Passmore S, et al. 2003. Refractory anemia in childhood: A retrospective analysis of 67 patients with particular reference to monosomy 7. Blood 102:1997–2003.

[68] Ohara A, Kojima S, Hamajima N, et al. 1997. Myelodysplastic syndrome and acute myelogenous leukemia as a late clonal complication in children with acquired aplastic anemia. Blood 90:1009–1013.

[69] Luna-Fineman S, Shannon KM, Lange BJ. 1995. Childhood monosomy 7: Epidemiology, biology, and mechanistic implications. Blood 85:1985–1999.

[70] Hasle H, Arico M, Basso G, et al. 1999. Myelodysplastic syndrome, juvenile myelomonocytic leukemia, and acute myeloid leukemia associated with complete or partial monosomy 7. Leukemia 13:376–385.

[71] Webb D, Passmore S, Hann I, Harrison G, Wheatley K, Chessells J. 2002. Results of treatment of children with refractory anaemia with excess blasts (RAEB) and RAEB in transformation (RAEBt) in Great Britain 1990–99. Br J Haematol 117:33–39.

[72] Bader-Meunier B, Mielot F, Tchernia G, et al. 1996. Myelodysplastic syndromes in childhood: Report of 49 patients from a French multicentre study. Br J Haematol 92:344–350.

[73] Creutzig U, Cantu-Rajnoldi A, Ritter J, et al. 1987. Myelodysplastic syndromes in childhood. Report of 21 patients from Italy and West Germany. Am J Pediatr Hematol Oncol 9:324–330.

[74] Luna-Fineman S, Shannon K, Atwater S, et al. 1999. Myelodysplastic and myeloproliferative disorders of childhood: A study of 167 patients. Blood 93 (2):459.

[75] Chan G, Wang W, Raimondi S, et al. 1997. Myelodysplastic syndrome in children: Differentiation from acute myeloid leukemia with a low blast count. Leukemia 11:206–211.

[76] Yusuf U, Frangoul H, Gooley T, et al. 2004. Allogeneic bone marrow transplantation in children with myelodysplastic syndrome or juvenile myelomonocytic leukemia: The Seattle experience. Bone Marrow Transplant 33:805–814.

[77] Bottomley SS, Muller-Eberhard U. 1988. Pathophysiology of heme synthesis. Semin Hematol 25:282–302.

[78] Vogler WR, Mingioli ES. 1968. Porphyrin synthesis and heme synthetase activity in pyridoxine-responsive anemia. Blood 32:979–988.

[79] Konopka L, Hoffbrand AV. 1979. Haem synthesis in sideroblastic anaemia. Br J Haematol 42(1):73–83.

[80] Pasanen AV, Eklof M, Tenhunen R. 1985. Coproporphyrinogen oxidase activity and porphyrin concentrations in peripheral red blood cells in hereditary sideroblastic anaemia. Scand J Haematol 34:235–237.

81 Amos RJ, Miller AL, Amess JA. 1988. Autosomal inheritance of sideroblastic anaemia. Clin Lab Haematol 10:347–353.

82 Dolan, G, Reid, MM. 1991. Congenital sideroblastic anaemia in two girls. J Clin Pathol 44:464–465.

83 Fitzcharles MA, Kirwan JR, Colvin BT, Currey HL. 1982. Sideroblastic anaemia with iron overload presenting as an arthropathy. Ann Rheum 41:97–99.

84 Pierce HI, McGuffin RG, Hillman RS. 1976. Clinical studies in alcoholic sideroblastosis. Arch Intern Med 136:283–289.

85 Larkin EC, Watson-Williams EJ. 1984. Alcohol and the blood. Med Clin North Am 68:105–120.

86 Hast R. 1986. Sideroblasts in myelodysplasia: Their nature and clinical significance. Scand J Haematol Suppl 45:53–55.

87 O'Brien H, Amess JA, Mollin DL. 1982. Recurrent thrombocytopenia, erythroid hypoplasia and sideroblastic anaemia associated with hypothermia. Br J Haematol 51:451–456.

88 Barros MH, Carlson CG, Glerum DM, Tzagoloff A. 2001. Involvement of mitochondrial ferredoxin and Cox15p in hydroxylation of heme O. FEBS Lett 492:133–138.

89 Matsuno-Yagi A, Hatefi Y. 2001. Ubiquinol: cytochrome c oxidoreductase (complex III). Effect of inhibitors on cytochrome b reduction in submitochondrial particles and the role of ubiquinone in complex III. J Biol Chem 276:19006–19011.

90 Verkhovsky MI, Morgan JE, Puustinen A, Wikstrom M. 1996. The "ferrous-oxy" intermediate in the reaction of dioxygen with fully reduced cytochromes aa3 and bo3. Biochemistry 35:16241–16246.

91 Bishop DF, Henderson AS, Astrin KH. 1990. Human delta-aminolevulinate synthase: Assignment of the housekeeping gene to 3p21 and erythroid-specific gene to the X chromosome. Genomics 7:207–214.

92 Cox TC, Bawden MJ, Abraham NG, et al. 1990. Erythroid 5-aminolevulinate synthase is located on the X chromosome. Am J Hum Genet 46:107–111.

93 Cotter PD, Willard HF, Gorski JL, Bishop DF. 1992. Assignment of human erythroid delta-aminolevulinate synthase (ALAS2) to a distal subregion of band Xp11.21 by PCR analysis of somatic cell hybrids containing X; autosome translocations. Genomics 13:211–212.

94 Cox TC, Bawden MJ, Martin A, May BK. 1991. Human erythroid 5'-aminolevulinate synthase: Promoter analysis and identification of an iron-responsive element in the mRNA. EMBO J 10:1891–1902.

95 Bhasker CR, Burgiel G, Neupert B, Emery-Goodman A, Kuhn LC, May BK. 1993. The putative iron-responsive element in the human erythroid 5-aminolevulinate synthase mRNA mediates translational control. J Biol 268:12699–12705.

96 Melefors O, Goossen B, Johansson HE, Stripecke R, Gray NK, Hentze MW. 1993. Translational control of 5-aminolevulinate synthase mRNA by iron-responsive elements in erythroid cells. J Biol Chem 268:5974–5978.

97 Koc S, Harris JW. 1998. Sideroblastic anemias: Variations on imprecision in diagnostic criteria, proposal for an extended classification of sideroblastic anemias. Am J Hematol 57:1–6.

98 Grasso JA, Hines JD. 1969. A comparative electron microscopic study of refractory and alcoholic sideroblastic anaemia. Br J Haematol 17:35–44.

99 Maldonado JE, Maigne J, Lecoq D. 1976. Comparative electron-microscopic study of the erythrocytic line in refractory anemia (preleukemia) and myelomonocytic leukemia. Blood Cells 2:167–185.

100 Liochev SI, Fridovich I. 1994. The role of O_2^- in the production of ·OH: In vitro and in vivo. Free Radic Biol Med 16:29–33.

[101] Gutteridge JMC, Rowley DA, Halliwell B. 1981. Superoxide-dependent formation of hydroxyl radicals in the presence of iron salts. Biochem J 199:263–265.

[102] Park JW, Floyd RA. 1992. Lipid peroxidation products mediate the formation of 8-hydroxydeoxyguanosine in DNA. Free Radic Biol Med 12:245–250.

[103] Thomas JP, Geiger PG, Girotti AW. 1993. Lethal damage to endothelial cells by oxidized low density lipoprotein: Role of selenoperoxidases in cytoprotection against lipid hydroperoxide- and iron-mediated reactions. J Lipid Res 34:479–490.

[104] Boore JL. 1999. Animal mitochondrial genomes. Nucleic Acids Res 27:767–780.

[105] Peto TE, Pippard MJ, Weatherall DJ. 1983. Iron overload in mild sideroblastic anaemias. Lancet 8321:375–378.

[106] Cooley TB. 1945. A severe type of hereditary anemia with elliptocytosis. Am J Med Sci 209:561–569.

[107] Bottomley SS, May BK, Cox TC, Cotter PD, Bishop DF. 1995. Molecular defects of erythroid 5-aminolevulinate synthase in X-linked sideroblastic anemia. J Bioenerg Biomembr 27:161–168.

[108] Bottomley SS, Healy HM, Brandenburg MA, May BK. 1992. 5-Aminolevulinate synthase in sideroblastic anemia: mRNA and enzyme activity levels in bone marrow cells. Am J Hematol 41:76–83.

[109] Cotter PD, Baumann M, Bishop DF. 1992. Enzymatic defect in "X-linked" sideroblastic anemia: Molecular evidence for erythroid delta-aminolevulinate synthase deficiency. Proc Natl Acad Sci U S A 89:4028–4032.

[110] Edgar AJ, Losowsky MS, Noble JS, Wickramasinghe SN. 1997. Identification of an arginine452 to histidine substitution in the erythroid 5-aminolaevulinate synthetase gene in a large pedigree with X-linked hereditary sideroblastic anaemia. Eur J Haematol 58:1–4.

[111] Cox TC, Kozman HM, Raskind WH, May BK, Mulley JC. 1992. Identification of a highly polymorphic marker within intron 7 of the ALAS2 gene and suggestion of at least two loci for X-linked sideroblastic anemia. Hum Mol Genet 1:639–641.

[112] Cotter PD, Rucknagel DL, Bishop DF. 1994. X-linked sideroblastic anemia: Identification of the mutation in the erythroid-specific delta-aminolevulinate synthase gene (ALAS2) in the original family described by Cooley. Blood 84:3915–3924.

[113] Cox TC, Bottomley SS, Wiley JS, Bawden MJ, Matthews CS, May BK. 1994. X-linked pyridoxine-responsive sideroblastic anemia due to a Thr388-to-Ser substitution in erythroid 5-aminolevulinate synthase. N Engl J Med 330:675–679.

[114] Bekri S, May A, Cotter P, et al. 2003. A promoter mutation in the erythroid-specific 5-aminolevulinate synthase (ALAS2) gene causes X-linked sideroblastic anemia. Blood 102:698–704.

[115] Seip M, Gjessing LR, Lie SO. 1971. Congenital sideroblastic anaemia in a girl. Scand J Haematol 8:505–512.

[116] Buchanan GR, Bottomley SS, Nitchke R. 1980. Bone marrow δ-aminolevulinic acid synthetase deficiency in a female with congenital sideroblastic anemia. Blood 55:109–115.

[117] Dolan G, Reid MM. 1991. Congenital sideroblastic anaemia in two girls. J Clin Pathol 44:464–465.

[118] Seto S, Furusho K, Aoki YA. 1982. Study of a female with congenital sideroblastic anemia. Am J Hematol 12:63–67.

[119] Cazzola M, May A, Bergamaschi G, Cerani P, Rosti V, Bishop DF. 2000. Familial-skewed X-chromosome inactivation as a predisposing factor for late-onset X-linked sideroblastic anemia in carrier females. Blood 96:4363–5.

[120] Shimada Y, Okuno S, Kawai A, et al. 1998. Cloning and chromosomal mapping of a novel ABC transporter gene (hABC7), a candidate for X-linked sideroblastic anemia with spinocerebellar ataxia. J Hum Genet 43:115–122.

[121] Raskind WH, Wijsman E, Pagon RA, et al. 1991. X-linked sideroblastic anemia and ataxia: Linkage to phosphoglycerate kinase at Xq13. Am J Hum Genet 48:335–341.

[122] Csere P, Lill R, Kispal G. 1998. Identification of a human mitochondrial ABC transporter, the functional orthologue of yeast Atm1p. FEBS Lett 441:266–270.

[123] Allikmets R, Raskind WH, Hutchinson A, Schueck ND, Dean M, Koeller DM. 1999. Mutation of a putative mitochondrial iron transporter gene (ABC7) in X-linked sideroblastic anemia and ataxia (XLSA/A). Hum Mol Genet 8:743–749.

[124] Bekri S, Kispal G, Lange H, et al. 2000. Human ABC7 transporter: Gene structure and mutation causing X-linked sideroblastic anemia with ataxia with disruption of cytosolic iron-sulfur protein maturation. Blood 96:3256–3264.

[125] Huang X, Moir RD, Tanzi RE, Bush AI, Rogers JT. 2004. Redox-active metals, oxidative stress, Alzheimer's disease pathology. Ann N Y Acad Sci 1012:153–163.

[126] Jaussi R. 1995. Homologous nuclear-encoded mitochondrial and cytosolic isoproteins. A review of structure, biosynthesis and genes. Eur J Biochem 228:551–561.

[127] Jansen RP. 2000. Origin and persistence of the mitochondrial genome. Hum Reprod 15(Suppl 2):1–10.

[128] Saccone C, Gissi C, Lanave C, Larizza A, Pesole G, Reyes A. 2000. Evolution of the mitochondrial genetic system: An overview. Gene 261:153–159.

[129] Higuchi Y, Linn S. 1995. Purification of all forms of Hela cell mitochondrial DNA and assessment of damage to it caused by hydrogen peroxide treatment of mitochondria or cells. J Biol Chem 270:7950–7956.

[130] Lightowlers RN, Chinnery PF, Turnbull DM, Howell N. 1997. Mammalian mitochondrial genetics: Heredity, heteroplasmy and disease. Trends Genet 13:450–455.

[131] Wallace DC. 1992. Diseases of the mitochondrial DNA. Annu Rev Biochem 61:1175–1212.

[132] Kitano A, Nishiyama S, Miike T, Hattori S, Ohtani Y, Matsuda I. 1986. Mitochondrial cytopathy with lactic acidosis, carnitine deficiency and DeToni-Fanconi-Debre syndrome. Brain Dev 8:289–295.

[133] Chinnery PF, Samuels DC. 1999. Relaxed replication of mtDNA: A model with implications for the expression of disease. Am J Hum Genet 64:1158–1165.

[134] Larsson NG, Clayton DA. 1995. Molecular genetic aspects of human mitochondrial disorders. Annu Rev Genet 29:151–178.

[135] Pearson HA, Lobel JS, Kocoshis SA, et al. 1979. A new syndrome of refractory sideroblastic anemia with vacuolization of marrow precursors and exocrine pancreatic dysfunction. J Pediatr 95:976–984.

[136] Cormier V, Rotig A, Quartino AR, et al. 1990. Widespread multi-tissue deletions of the mitochondrial genome in the Pearson marrow-pancreas syndrome. J Pediatr 117:599–602.

[137] Bernes SM, Bacino C, Prezant TR, et al. 1993. Identical mitochondrial DNA deletion in mother with progressive external ophthalmoplegia and son with Pearson marrow-pancreas syndrome. J Pediatr 123:598–602.

[138] Egger J, Lake BD, Wilson J. 1981. Mitochondrial cytopathy. A multisystem disorder with ragged red fibres on muscle biopsy. Arch Dis Child 56:741–752.

[139] Inbal A, Avissar N, Shaklai M, et al. 1995. Myopathy, lactic acidosis, and sideroblastic anemia: A new syndrome. Am J Med Genet 55:372–378.

[140] Borgna-Pignatti C, Marradi P, Pinelli L, Monetti N, Patrini C. 1989. Thiamine-responsive anemia in DIDMOAD syndrome. J Pediatr 114:405–410.

[141] Rotig A, Cormier V, Chatelain P, et al. 1993. Deletion of mitochondrial DNA in a case of early-onset diabetes mellitus, optic atrophy, and deafness (Wolfram syndrome, MIM 222300). J Clin Invest 91:1095–1098.

[142] Barrientos A, Volpini V, Casademont J, et al. 1996. A nuclear defect in the 4p16 region predisposes to multiple mitochondrial DNA deletions in families with Wolfram syndrome. J Clin Invest 97:1570–1576.

[143] Inoue H, Tanizawa Y, Wasson J, et al. 1998. A gene encoding a transmembrane protein is mutated in patients with diabetes mellitus and optic atrophy (Wolfram syndrome). Nat Genet 20:143–148.

[144] Strom TM, Hortnagel K, Hofmann S, et al. 1998. Diabetes insipidus, diabetes mellitus, optic atrophy and deafness (DIDMOAD) caused by mutations in a novel gene (wolframin) coding for a predicted transmembrane protein. Hum Mol Genet 7:2021–2028.

[145] Takeda K, Inoue H, Tanizawa Y, et al. 2001. WFS1 (Wolfram syndrome 1) gene product: Predominant subcellular localization to endoplasmic reticulum in cultured cells and neuronal expression in rat brain. Hum Mol Genet 10:477–484.

[146] Hardy C, Khanim F, Torres R, et al. 1999. Clinical and molecular genetic analysis of 19 Wolfram syndrome kindreds demonstrating a wide spectrum of mutations in WFS1. Am J Hum Genet 65:1279–1290.

[147] Lindenbaum J, Roman MJ. 1980. Nutritional anemia in alcoholism. Am J Clin Nutr 33:2727–2735.

[148] Larkin EC, Watson-Williams EJ. 1984. Alcohol and the blood. Med Clin North Am 68:105–120.

[149] McColl KE, Thompson GG, Moore MR, Goldberg A. 1980. Acute ethanol ingestion and haem biosynthesis in healthy subjects. Eur J Clin Invest 10(2 Pt 1):107–112.

[150] Middleton HM, 3rd. 1986. Intestinal hydrolysis of pyridoxal 5′-phosphate in vitro and in vivo in the rat: Effect of ethanol. Am J Clin Nutr 43:374–381.

[151] Leibman D, Furth-Walker D, Smolen TN, Smolen A. 1990. Pyridoxal 5′-phosphate and pyridoxamine 5′-phosphate concentrations in blood and tissues of mice fed ethanol-containing liquid diets. Alcohol 7:61–68.

[152] Beck EA, Ziegler G, Schmid R, Ludin H. 1967. Reversible sideroblastic anemia caused by chloramphenicol. Acta Haematol 38:1–10.

[153] Rosenberg A, Marcus O. 1974. Effect of chloramphenicol on reticulocyte delta-aminolaevulinic acid synthetase in rabbits. Br J Haematol 26:79–83.

[154] Sharp RA, Lowe JG, Johnston RN. 1990. Anti-tuberculous drugs and sideroblastic anaemia. Br J Clin Pract 44:706–707.

[155] Haden HT. 1967. Pyridoxine-responsive sideroblastic anemia due to antituberculous drugs. Arch Intern Med 120:602–606.

[156] Yunis AA, Salem Z. 1980. Drug-induced mitochondrial damage and sideroblastic change. Clin Haematol 9:607–619.

[157] Vivier P, Hogan J, Simon P, Leddy P, Dansereau L, Alario A. 2001. A statewide assessment of lead screening histories of preschool children enrolled in a medicaid managed care program. Pediatrics 108:e29.

[158] Goyer RA. 1993. Lead toxicity: Current concerns. Environ Health Perspect 100:177–187.

[159] Hines JD, Cowan DH. 1970. Studies on the pathogenesis of alcohol-induced sideroblastic bone-marrow abnormalities. N Engl J Med 283:441–446.

[160] Blinder VS, Roboz GJ. 2003. Hematopoietic growth factors in myelodysplastic syndromes. Curr Hematol Rep 2:453–458.

[161] Musto P, Falcone A, Sanpaolo G, et al. 2003. Efficacy of a single, weekly dose of recombinant erythropoietin in myelodysplastic syndromes. Br J Haematol 122:269–271.

[162] Murakami R, Takumi T, Gouji J, Nakamura H, Kondou M. 1991. Sideroblastic anemia showing unique response to pyridoxine. Am J Pediatr Hematol 13:345–350.

[163] Estey E, Thall P, Cortes J, et al. 2001. Comparison of idarubicin + ara-C-, fludarabine + ara-C-, and topotecan + ara-C-based regimens in treatment of newly diagnosed acute myeloid leukemia, refractory anemia with excess blasts in transformation, or refractory anemia with excess blasts. Blood 98:3575–3583.

[164] Jurado M, Deeg H, Storer B, et al. 2002. Hematopoietic stem cell transplantation for advanced myelodysplastic syndrome after conditioning with busulfan and fractionated total body irradiation is associated with low relapse rate but considerable nonrelapse mortality. Biol Blood Marrow Transplant 8:161–169.

[165] Silverman L, Demakos E, Peterson B, et al. 2002. Randomized controlled trial of azacitidine in patients with the myelodysplastic syndrome: A study of the cancer and leukemia group B. J Clin Oncol 20:2429–2440.

[166] Molldrem J, Leifer E, Bahceci E, et al. 2002. Antithymocyte globulin for treatment of the bone marrow failure associated with myelodysplastic syndromes. Ann Intern Med 137:156–163.

Hemoglobin Disorders

SICKLE CELL DISEASE

In the opening days of the twentieth century, a young graduate student from Grenada troubled by chronic fatigue and lethargy called on Dr. James Herrick at Cook County Hospital in Chicago for evaluation of these increasingly troublesome symptoms. Dr. Herrick's history revealed the additional issue of intermittent joint aches persisting over a number of years that were punctuated by episodes of more generalized and severe pain. The patient's examination was remarkable only for mild scleral icterus. The most striking aspect of the evaluation was the presence on peripheral blood smear of abnormal red cells that were shaped like crescents or sickles. Dr. Herrick summarized his findings in a 1910 report that provided the first description of sickle cell disease in the medical literature.[1]

A number of important observations over the ensuing 40 years clarified important aspects of the pathophysiology of sickle cell disease. The landmark report came in 1949 when Linus Pauling, Harvey Itano and colleagues used the recently developed analytical technique of protein electrophoresis to show that patients with sickle cell disease have a physically different hemoglobin from that found in normal people.[2] The investigators speculated that this hemoglobin difference caused sickle cell disease. In 1956, Vernon Ingram, then at the MRC in the UK, reported on his successful hemoglobin sequencing that established a substitution of valine for glutamic acid at the 6th amino acid position in the β-globin chain as the basis for the difference between sickle and normal hemoglobin.[3] Sickle cell disease thus became the first disorder characterized at a molecular level. The challenge of the twenty-first century is finally to convert this basic science information into effective clinical interventions.

Sickle cell disease remains one of the most challenging disorders in medicine. The condition affects about 80,000 people in the US, making it the most common basis of serious anemia in the country. Worldwide, sickle cell disease is extremely prevalent in sub-Saharan Africa and India, a consequence of the protection against falciparum malaria afforded by sickle cell trait (see Chapter 6). Few other disorders present such a striking contrast between knowledge of the molecular basis of a disease and the ability to convert that knowledge into effective therapy. Some of the complexity arises from the fact that sickle cell disease is not a single disorder. Rather, it is a collection of related genetic syndromes involving the β-globin gene with overlapping traits and manifestations. Furthermore, sickle cell disease is a condition whose nature changes over time, placing additional burdens on the patient and physician.

■ SICKLE CELL SYNDROMES

Hb S is the central character in the sickle syndromes. Hb C, which derives from an amino acid substitution of lysine for glutamic acid at the 6th position of the β-globin chain, is a prominent co-star. Homozygous Hb C disease is a mild condition characterized by low-grade hemolysis, mild splenomegaly and occasionally symptomatic cholecystitis. Hemoglobin C trait produces no symptoms. In contrast, Hb SC disease, the compound heterozygous state for hemglobins S and C, produces a clinical condition that often is indistinguishable from homozygous Hb SS.

The abandonment of the name *sickle cell anemia* in favor of the term *sickle cell disease* reflects the evolving appreciation of the complex nature of the disorder. The sickle cell diseases are a group of disorders in which most (>50%) of the hemoglobin within the red cell is Hb S. Although anemia is an integral part of these disorders, low hemoglobin values are relatively minor considerations with respect to the overall impact of the disease. The four most common sickle cell disease states are Hb SS, Hb S β^0-thalassemia, Hb SC and Hb S β^+-thalassemia (Table 13-1). The ordering of the syndromes reflects a decreasing degree of clinical and hematological severity. Hb SS disease and Hb S β^0-thalassemia are the most severe and are associated with hemoglobin values of 7 or 8 g/dL, vaso-occlusive (painful) crises, long term organ damage and decreased survival. In Hb SC disease, hemoglobin values of 9–11 gm/dL are usual. Painful episodes are usually less prominent than in Hb SS disease, but a

TABLE 13-1 | **SICKLE CELL DISEASE SYNDROMES**

Disorder	β-Globin Genes	Typical Hemoglobin Content	Disease Severity
Homozygous hemoglobin S	• Two hemoglobin S genes	• Hb S—99% • Hb A—0% • Hb A2—1% • Hb F—1%	Moderate to severe
Sickle β^0-thalassemia	• One hemoglobin S gene • One gene producing no β-subunit	• Hb S—91% • Hb A—0% • Hb A2—5% • Hb F—4%	Moderate to severe
Sickle β^+-thalassemia	• One hemoglobin S gene • One gene producing reduced quantities of β-subunit	• Hb S—71% • Hb A—20% • Hb A2—5% • Hb F—4%	Mild to moderate
Hemoglobin SC disease	• Hemoglobin S gene • Hemoglobin C gene	• Hb S—53% • Hb A—0% • Hb A2—1% • Hb C—46 • Hb F—0%	Mild to severe

wide spectrum exists in that regard. Long-term complications such as retinopathy and avascular necrosis of the femur tend to occur more frequently. Hb S β^+-thalassemia can be relatively mild, but again a range of severity exists.

The truly malevolent impact of sickle cell disease stems from the complications of impaired blood flow through the microcirculation with consequent local tissue hypoxia. Until recently, the distorted erythrocytes produced by polymerization of deoxygenated sickle hemoglobin received primary blame for this problem. Now, however, prominent attention goes to the contributions of other factors such as red cell adhesion to the endothelium and the local effects of inflammatory cytokines. Sickle cell disease has a single initiation point for its pathology, the abnormal properties of Hb S within the red cell. However, the stream quickly branches into a myriad of sluices and rivulets of dizzying complexity.

■ CHALLENGES OF SICKLE CELL DISEASE

Sickle cell diseases are determined at the time of conception when an affected infant inherits an abnormal β-globin gene from each parent. Prenatal diagnosis of sickle cell disease can be made by analysis of DNA obtained by chorionic villus biopsy as early as 10–12 weeks of gestation.[4] Because of the predominant production of Hb F during fetal life, newborn infants with Hb SS disease are healthy and have normal birth weights and normal hemoglobin levels. Anemia and hemolysis are not usually evident until after 4–6 months of age. Today, the diagnosis of sickle cell disease are usually made by newborn screening of blood by hemoglobin electrophoresis or high pressure liquid chromatography which is currently performed routinely in 47 states of the US and the District of Columbia.[5] Approximately 1/500 African/Carribean American newborns have a major sickle cell disease. Table 13-2 summarizes the readout of newborn screening tests. The letters list the detected hemoglobins beginning with the most highly represented form.

ACUTE CLINICAL ISSUES IN CHILDREN

In sickle cell disease, clinical manifestations are usually not seen in the first 6–9 months of age because of high levels of Hb F in the red cells inhibit sickling.[6] The first clinical manifestation is often sickle cell dactylitis an acute, symmetrical painful swelling of the hands and feet. The so-called "hand-foot syndrome" occurs in about a third of infants. After the second and third year of age, painful episodes involving the extremities, back and abdomen may occur, although considerable patient-to-patient variation in frequency exists. This variability in the clinical character of sickle cell disease presents great challenges to physicians who care for these patients. The management style must be customized for every patient. One tot who comes to the office has a visit that differs little from the typical well child visit. With another youngster, the visit can be dominated by the problems associated with recurrent vaso-occlusive pain episodes or intractable problems such as chronic leg ulcers.

TABLE 13-2	INTERPRETATION OF NEWBORN SCREEN RESULTS
Hemoglobins Detected in Order of Proportion	**Probable Genotype**
FA	Normal; β-thalassemia trait cannot be excluded.
FAS	Sickle cell trait; Hb G and D traits must be excluded
FSA	Hb S β^+-thalassemia
FS	Hb SS disease; Hb S β^0-thalassemia and S-HPFH must be excluded.
FSC	Hb SC disease
FAC	Hb C trait
FCA	Hb C β^+-thalassemia
FC	Hb CC disease; Hb C β^0-thalassemia must be excluded
FAE	Hb E trait
FE	Hb EE diseae; Hb E β^0-thalassemia must be excluded
FEA	Hb E β^+-thalassemia
FF	Homozyous β-thalassemia; homozygous HPFH must be excluded.

The presence of small amount of Hb Bart's indicates α-thalassemia that can be present with any of the above hemoglobin patterns.

Adapted from Frempong K. 2003. Abnormalities of hemoglobin structure and function. In: Rudolph CD, Rudolph AM, Hostetter MK, Siegel, NJ, eds. *Rudolph's Pediatrics*, 21st edn. New York: McGraw-Hill. Chapter 19.4, p. 1531–1536.

Sickle cell disease tends to follow a particularly severe course in children with the clinical triad of (a) acute dactylitis prior to 1 year of age, (b) a hemoglobin level of less than 7 g/dL before 2 years of age, and (c) persistent leucocytosis in the absence of infection.[7] Close monitoring and support of these children is vital to the goal of avoiding complications. This clinical triad also opens the door to exploring early management options that might prevent long-term end organ injury and death. For instance, a child with this ominous combination who has an HLA-matched sibling might be considered for hematopoietic stem cell transplantation early in the clinical course.

In the past, young children with sickle cell disease were at high risk of developing severe and often fatal Streptococcal or *Hemophilus influenzae* (HIB) sepsis and meningitis. This susceptibility in large measure reflected reduced splenic function (functional hyposplenia) that arises in these children during the first 12–18 months of life. These infectious complications, which occurred in 10–15% of children, have been markedly reduced by neonatal diagnosis coupled with comprehensive follow up of affected infants that includes prophylactic penicillin therapy and immunization with conjugated pneumococcal and HIB vaccines.[8,9]

A second serious pediatric complication of sickle cell disease is acute splenic sequestration in which the spleen becomes acutely engorged with large amount of blood sequestered from the circulating blood volume resulting in hypotension and shock and very severe anemia (Hb as low as 2–4 gm/dL) and death in some cases. Fluid therapy and blood transfusion to correct anemia and hypovolemic shock are indicated. Because these events may be repetitive, splenectomy often is advocated.[10]

A third serious pediatric complication is the aplastic crisis assocciated with parvovirus B19 infection—a pediatric infection called "Fifth Disease."[11] This virus invades early red cell precursors in the bone marrow, essentially shutting off red cell production. Because of the only 10–15 days survival of Hb SS red cells, profound anemia develops quickly with hemoglobin levels of 2–3 g/dL and 0.0% reticulocytes. After about 10–14 days the child begins to make IgM antibodies that clear the virus from the bone marrow permitting restoration of RBC production and spontaneous recovery. RBC transfusions are often necessary to sustain the child until spontaneous recovery occurs. One bout of this disease confers long lasting immunity, so there are no recurrences of the syndrome.

Sickle cell disease in children also produces significant systemic problems. The chronic and vigorous production and destruction of red cells creates a tremendous energy demand. These children tend to be thin and short of stature. A 2–3 year delay in the onset of puberty is common. The rapid red cell turnover and high bilirubin production can produce pigmented gallstones in children as young as 5 years of age.

One of the most serious consequences of sickle cell disease in childhood is damage to the central nervous system. Clinically apparent vaso-occlusive strokes occur in about 10% of children between 3 and 12 years of age and these tend to be repetitive.[12] Up to 20% of children have abnormal brain magnetic resonance images, suggesting subclinical infarction.[13] A chronic red cell transfusion program designed to maintain the proportion of circulating Hb S at below 30–40% of the total hemoglobin is the only effective intervention to prevent stroke recurrence.[14]

These CNS complications reflect obstructive lesions in the major intracerebral blood vessels. Transcranial dopler (TCD) flow assessment combined with magnetic resonance angiography identifies areas of stenosis of the major cerebral vessels and assesses the risk of vaso-occlusion.[15] Children with Hb SS and Hb S β^0-thalassemia should have regular TCD studies during the first 12 years of age. Chronic transfusions be should be started if significant stenosis exists.[16]

The variable nature of sickle cell disease expression is a major challenge in management. Sickle cell disease sometimes produces few problems and these can be mild in nature. Occasionally, a person with sickle cell disease escapes detection until adulthood. Some of the variability in expression stems from differences in the genetic makeup of the disorder. Hb SS disease is more severe on average than is the compound heterozygous condition, Hb SC disease. Even within a single genotype, however, great variation exists in phenotypic expression.

Another confounding aspect of sickle cell disease is a change in severity that commonly occurs with puberty or late in adolescence. Most often, the change is from relatively mild disease to a condition of severe character. For instance, a youngster who had few problems during childhood can begin to suffer from frequent and severe vaso-occlusion pain episodes. The problem of a child who goes from a serious but relatively tractable medical condition to one that is recalcitrant often to the most aggressive interventions is extremely disconcerting to patient and family.

Over time, however, the repeated episodes of tissue hypoxia produced by vaso-occlusion produce regions of chronic organ injury. Such chronic organ damage begins to dominate the clinical picture during adolescence and adulthood. Chronic injury can affect nearly every organ in the body. In most cases, the capacity to reverse the chronic damage is limited. Therefore, prevention is key to the management of many problems experienced during and after adolescence. Optimal care in sickle cell disease revolves around knowledge of the problems that can develop and implementation of preventative measures where possible.

ACUTE CLINICAL ISSUES IN ADULTS

Pain is the central problem in sickle cell disease that spans pediatric and adult care. Vaso-occlusive pain episodes vary tremendously in frequency and severity. The co-operative study of the natural history of sickle cell disease showed that about 5% of patients accounted for one-third of hospital days devoted to pain control.[17] To complicate matters further, the pattern of pain varies over time, so that a patient who has particularly severe problems one year might later have a prolonged period characterized by only minor discomfort.

Sickle cell pain episodes also vary in pattern. Patients can develop agonizingly severe pain in as little as 15 minutes without prevenient problems. In other cases, the pain gradually evolves over hours or even days. Patients manage most episodes of pain at home. Oral analgesics along with rest and fluids often allow people to "ride out" the pain episode. Some patients report that warm baths or warm compresses applied to aching joints ameliorate the severity of the pain.

A question commonly posed to patients is "what triggered the pain?" The most common reply is "nothing that I can recall." Patients and providers constantly seek triggers to the problem in an often futile quest to understand the basic mystery of what produces vaso-occlusive episodes. Common instigators include viral upper respiratory infections and significant dehydration. Esoteric triggers include trips to high altitudes, such as a ski resort in Steamboat Springs, Colorado. Most often, however, the sickle cell pain episode comes "out of the blue." Outdoor Swimming followed by coming out of the water into cool air produced an "epidemic" of painful crises at the Hole-in-the-Wall-Gang Camp in Connecticut. Heating the pool to 85°F and provision of a poolside warming compartment eliminated the problem.

The sites affected in acute painful episodes vary. Pain occurs commonly in the extremities, thorax, abdomen, and back. Pain tends to recur at the same site for a particular person, however. For each patient, the quality of the vaso-occlusive pain is usually similar from one episode to another. *During the evaluation, the provider should inquire as to whether the pain feels like "typical" sickle cell pain.* Most patients can distinguish back pain due to pyelonephritis or abdominal pain due to cholecystitis, for instance, from their typical sickle cell pain. If the quality of the pain is not typical of their sickle cell disease, other causes should be investigated before ascribing the event to vaso-occlusion.

No reliable objective index of pain exists. The provider depends solely on the patient's report. One of the most difficult problems faced by patients with sickle cell disease is seeking treatment for pain in a setting in which they are unknown. Some providers mistakenly believe that the number of deformed sickle cells on the peripheral blood smear reflects the degree of patient pain. Others look to parameters such as blood pressure and heart rate. Although the latter measures provide more information than the peripheral smear, neither is an accurate gauge of pain severity. Trust in the patient report is key to the management of sickle cell pain episodes.

Acute chest syndrome (ACS) can be difficult to diagnose because its etiology varies and its manifestations are variegated.[18] Key characteristics include fever, dyspnea, cough, and pulmonary infiltrates. The infiltrates can have a lobar distribution, but often are bilateral. Sometimes, the pulmonary picture is one of diffuse, hazy opacities that resemble acute respiratory distress syndrome. In other cases, ACS mimics a simple pneumonia. This problem in diagnosis is aggravated by the fact that infectious agents such as viruses, bacteria, and mycoplasma can trigger the syndrome.[19] Bone marrow infarction with secondary pulmonary fat emboli also can trigger the ACS. In most instances, the etiology of ACS is a mystery.

The arterial blood oxygen saturation is key to the diagnosis of ACS. Values commonly fall to a greater degree than occurs with a simple pneumonia of the same magnitude. Patients with ACS often have progressive pulmonary infiltrates despite treatment with antibiotics. Infection can set off a wave of local ischemia that produces focal sickling, deoxygenation and additional sickling.

The microcirculatory vessels in the lung tend to constrict with hypoxia rather than dilate, as occurs with vessels in other parts of the body. Regions of vascular constriction can worsen microcirculatory occlusion. Consequently, bronchodilators are important components of the treatment regimen. Unchecked, ACS can produce cardiovascular collapse and death. ACS occurs more commonly in children than adults. People who survive an episode of ACS have a high propensity for future attacks. Patients who suffer recurrent episodes of ACS can develop chronic pulmonary insufficiency.

The most important step in the treatment of ACS is to recognize the disorder. Potential pneumonia in sickle cell patients should be treated with appropriate antibiotics. When symptoms progress, particularly in concert with falling arterial oxygen saturation and worsening of the chest roentgenogram, ACS must be considered. Blood gases are vital. Pulse oximetry provides limited information and in particular lacks crucial data on blood carbon dioxide levels and pH. A relentless decline in arterial oxygenation is a harbinger of ill with ACS and demands urgent action.

Transfusion is key to the treatment of ACS. Exchange transfusion is one option.[20] The procedure involves exchange of the total blood volume and is done most efficiently using a pheresis machine. When a pheresis setup is not available, sequential transfusion/phlebotomy can be performed. A hemoglobin electrophoresis should be sent prior to the exchange transfusion. A second should be sent after the procedure. The object is to ensure that the exchange has reduced the percentage of Hb S cells to below 30%. Patients can improve substantially within hours of an exchange. Simple transfusion works as well, particularly with low starting hemoglobin values, which commonly exist. In this circumstance, simple transfusion alone decreases the fraction of sickle cells in the circulation.[21]

Rising arterial oxygenation and decreasing dyspnea usually presage recovery. The chest roentgenogram typically lags behind the clinical status. Since a bacterial pneumonia rarely can be excluded in these patients, most receive concomitant broad-spectrum antibiotics. Blood cultures are vital since a positive culture provides valuable guidance to antibiotic therapy.

Delayed transfusion reaction is a serious potential problem with exchange transfusion.[22] Most patients with sickle cell disease are of African ancestry. Most of the blood available for transfusion in the US comes from people of European descent. A number of minor red cell antigens are expressed at different frequencies in these two groups. Repeated transfusion of any African-American can induce antibodies directed against these minor antigens.[23] Transfusion with blood containing an offending antigen often rekindles formerly undetectable antibody production.

With exchange transfusion, a large fraction of the circulating red cells can be destroyed in a deadly delayed transfusion reaction. Antibody screening should be repeated three to four weeks after the exchange transfusion to look for new alloantibodies to minor antigens. The results of testing for alloantibodies should have a prominent place in the medical record. Computerized records in transfusion services further reduce the chance of error producing a serious delayed hemolytic transfusion reaction.

Acute bone marrow necrosis is now recognized more often as a complication of sickle cell disease, in part due to improved methods of detection. Magnetic resonance imaging (MRI) techniques are most important in this regard.[24] Bone marrow should have the density of other body tissues on MRI scans. With bone marrow necrosis, marrow liquefaction on scan is obvious (Figure 13-1). The very severe pain produced by acute bone marrow necrosis leaves most patients unable

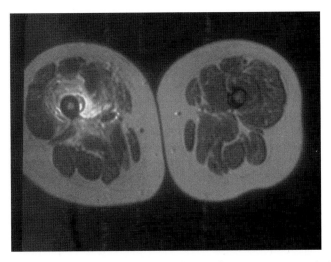

FIGURE 13–1 *MRI in a patient with acute bone marrow necrosis. The scan was performed 3 days after hospitalization for excruciating pain in the lower extremities controlled only by epidural infusion of opioid analgesics. The light region along the length of the right femur is bone marrow that was liquefied during the acute necrosis event.*

to cooperate with the MRI procedure. MRI scans therefore are used most often for retrospective confirmation of the diagnosis.

Acute bone marrow necrosis produces excruciatingly severe pain. Some patients require drastic measures, such as epidural anesthesia to control wrenchingly intense pain. Acute bone marrow necrosis frequently involves marrow of the ribs, femur or tibia and often produces "the worst pain I've ever experienced." This simple statement should place acute bone marrow necrosis at the forefront of the differential diagnosis.

A declining hemoglobin level due to marrow injury and explosive release of immature cells into the circulation, including a plethora of nucleated red blood cells, are key findings in episodes of acute bone marrow necrosis. Exchange transfusion has been used with success in some patients. The experience is anecdotal, since the ability to document bone marrow necrosis is a relatively recent development. Pulmonary fat emboli can complicate episodes of acute bone marrow necrosis. Fat emboli can trigger respiratory insufficiency or even ACS.[25] Fortunately, acute bone marrow necrosis is self-limiting. Proper support with transfusion, analgesics and oxygen allow patients to weather the horrific storm.

Hepatic sequestration crisis occurs when sickled cells lodge in the liver obstructing blood flow through the organ. The result is painful hepatic enlargement accompanying rising plasma levels of hepatic synthetic enzymes (e.g., ALT, AST). The serum bilirubin levels often skyrocket to values in the range of 30–40 mg/dL. Acute hepatic failure can ensue. Fluids, oxygen and analgesia are the management interventions commonly undertaken. The benefit of more aggressive measures such as exchange transfusion is unknown.

Multiorgan failure syndrome is one of the most deadly complications of sickle cell disease, occurring both in children and adults.[26] Pain commonly brings the victim to immediate attention where clinical events quickly highlight the gravity of the situation vis-à-vis "ordinary" vaso-occlusive sickle cell disease episodes.[27] Declining arterial oxygen saturation accompanied by patchy lung opacities shows the condition to be more akin to ACS. Falling hemoglobin values are both typical and ominous. Declining renal function manifested by rising BUN and serum creatinine values along with oliguria bodes ill for the patient. Mental status changes manifested as somnolence and confusion often punctuate this dire clinical condition. Exchange transfusion along with other supportive measures such as ventilator assistance and antibiotics early in the course sometimes reverses an otherwise grim scenario.

Priapism is a serious problem for many boys and young men with sickle cell disease.[28] The condition is believed to result from impaired blood egress from the corpus spongiosum of the penis, leading to prolonged painful erections. The affliction often occurs in association with spontaneous nocturnal erections. Episodes of priapism range in duration from several hours to several days. Stuttering priapism refers to episodes that occur over one or two hours for several consecutive days. These episodes often presage prolonged attacks. Priapism often coincides with or triggers generalized vaso-occlusive pain episodes. One group of investigators reported a 90% actuarial probability of at least one episode of priapism by age 21 years.[29] Many patients are too embarrassed to spontaneously raise the subject of priapism. Therefore, direct questioning on the issue is important.

Parenteral analgesics can diminish the generalized vaso-occlusive pain associated with priapism. Unfortunately, these drugs do little to relieve penile pain that often is excruciating. The intervention most commonly used in the past specifically to address priapism was irrigation of the ventral vein of the penis by a urologist in an attempt to alleviate blocked blood flow.[30] The results of this approach generally were poor since the problem is one of microvascular occlusion. The more recently introduced exchange transfusion has produced mixed results. Vasodilators such as pseudoephedrine (Sudafed®) or etilefrine hydrochloride (Effortil®) sometimes help young men with subacute episodes of priapism.[31] These drugs can be useful interventions with stuttering priapism. No overall consensus exists on a treatment algorithm for this debilitating complication of sickle cell disease.

CHRONIC CLINICAL ISSUES IN ADULTS

Avascular necrosis of bone is a common and debilitating complication of sickle cell disease. This problem differs totally from the acute bone marrow necrosis discussed earlier. Acute bone marrow necrosis involves damage to hematopoietic elements *within* the bone marrow cavity. Avascular necrosis of bone involves injury to the bone proper.

Bone is living tissue that can die due to poor blood circulation within the wall of the bone itself. The areas of bone most frequently affected are the acetabulum and the head of the humerus. The etiology of avascular necrosis of bone is unknown. One hypothesis posits that marrow hyperplasia in the femoral head crowds tissue and secondarily reduces blood flow outward into bony trabeculae that provide the bone's blood supply.

The quality of the pain associated with avascular bone necrosis differs substantially from vaso-occlusive sickle cell pain. The articular cartilage thins and often disappears as the process progresses. The joints can deteriorate producing a bone-on-bone interface. Movement then becomes wrenchingly painful. Nonsteroidal anti-inflammatory agents can be useful early in the process. With more severe situations corticosteroid injection into the joint articular space can relieve symptoms. While sometimes helpful for hip pain, this treatment works best for avascular necrosis of the shoulder. Opioid analgesics partially relieve severe pain, but can open the Pandora's box associated with chronic use of these drugs. Finally, some orthopedic surgeons attempt decompression of the marrow tissue in the head of the humerus or the head of the femur. This invasive procedure should be reserved for patients with more advanced avascular necrosis. Unfortunately, no definitive data address the efficacy of the intervention.

Measures that are literally supportive can help limit the rate at which avascular necrosis progresses. Minimizing weight bearing by the hip is valuable. Possible interventions range from complete elimination of weight bearing using wheel chairs to measures such as canes or walkers. The first option often is impractical. The impact of the latter two is modest at best. Patients should certainly avoid long periods of standing.

These interventions slow osteonecrosis without halting the process. Avascular necrosis can necessitate joint replacement. Some patients with sickle syndromes tolerate prosthetic joints poorly. As many as one-third of patients require a second surgery within 4 years of joint replacement. Also, these patients, for unclear reasons, are vulnerable to infections involving their orthopedic hardware. The unfortunate result can be a destroyed articular interface and a flail joint that, in the case of the femur, produces wheelchair confinement.

MRI imaging is a promising addition to the diagnostic armamentarium that exceeds the sensitivity of plain bone films in detecting avascular necrosis. The technique highlights very early evidence of damage.[32] The previously mentioned conservative support measures might have a greater impact if begun earlier in the process of bone degeneration.

Renal injury is also a long-term issue in sickle cell disease.[33] The most common renal defect is impaired urine concentrating ability (hyposthenuria) that often appears by 2 or 3 years of age. The condition can produce bedwetting in children or embarrassing wetting in public places like classrooms. Hyposthenuria also occurs with compound heterozygous states (e.g., sickle β-thalassemia). The extremely high osmolality in the distal tubule produces renal medullary sickling even in people with sickle trait. Consequently, hyposthenuria is the most common abnormality associated with sickle cell trait.

Medullary ischemia and papillary necrosis occur commonly. Sometimes, the necrotic papillae slough into the collecting system, obstructing the outflow tract. No effective specific intervention exists for this problem. Rising BUN and creatinine values herald sickle glomerulonephropathy. Proteinuria is an early and common manifestation of glomerular injury.[34] The most important intervention is limiting protein consumption, as is recommended for many types of renal dysfunction including that associated with diabetic nephropathy. One report suggested that angiotensin converting enzyme inhibitors (e.g., Nifedipine®) might retard nephropathy progression in sickle cell disease.[35] Unfortunately, confirmatory studies addressing this important issue were never conducted.

A fact not commonly appreciated is that patients with sickle cell disease usually have *low* serum creatinine and BUN levels. This reflects the high glomerular filtration rate along with a high rate of creatinine secretion in the distal tubule. BUN values of 7 mg/dL and creatinine values of 0.5 mg/dL are typical for patients with sickle cell disease. Creatinine clearance often exceeds 150 cc/min/1.73 m^2 surface area. A formal evaluation of glomerular filtration should be considered for patients in whom the serum creatinine rises above the level of about 1.0 mg/dL.

Limited experience exists on the efficacy of dialysis with sickle cell disease. Reports that hemodialysis is problematic in patients with sickle cell disease are anecdotal. Every effort should be undertaken to prevent renal deterioration. Microscopic hematuria is common with sickle cell disease. Hematuria per se requires no intervention unless blood loss is massive. Some patients with sickle cell disease and renal failure have successfully received renal allografts.[36]

Sickle cell trait is benign, but on rare occasion and for unknown reasons can produce massive hematuria. Interestingly, the bleeding often comes from the left kidney. Hydration and alkalization of the urine are commonly used interventions. Anecdotal reports of the use of desmopressin (DDAVP®) in this situation are encouraging. Epsilon amino caproic acid (Amicar®) has been used in some patients with refractory bleeding from the kidney. Bleeding can continue for weeks. Iron replacement may be necessary as treatment interventions continue. Nephrectomy has been performed but this frightful intervention should be a last-ditch approach to a life-threatening situation.

Pulmonary hypertension is a problem of increasing concern in adults with sickle cell disease.[37] Repeat episodes of ACS clearly promotes long-term injury to the lung, including pulmonary hypertension. There is growing recognition that pulmonary hypertension is not confined to patients with histories of dramatic episodes of lung injury. Recurrent injury to the lung due to small areas of ischemia and infarction of lung tissue could be at fault. Small aggregates of sickled cells that escape the peripheral microcirculation can occlude small areas of the pulmonary microcirculation before the higher oxygen tension allows a return to their normal shape. The resulting injury to the pulmonary circulatory system and parenchymal would be slow but steady.

The manifestations of pulmonary hypertension are insidious. Right-sided pulmonary hypertension produces disproportionate enlargement of the right atrium. Patients begin to experience edema of the lower extremities, particularly with intravenous hydration. As the condition progresses, hepatic congestion leads to hepatomegaly and ascites at times. Treatment of this serious problem is currently supportive. Specific interventions are currently in trials and might provide alternatives in the future.

Retinopathy is an often devastating problem that affects 10–20% of people with sickle cell disease.[38] The peak onset is during the third decade. For unknown reasons, the condition occurs more commonly in patients with Hb SC disease than in those with homozygous hemoglobin S disease. The problem bears striking resemblence to diabetic retinopathy both clinically and pathologically with retinal thinning and neovascularization as common manifestations.

The areas affected, at least initially, are in the periphery of the retina and require indirect opthalmoscopy for detection. The delicate vessels of the neovascular tangles are prone to rupture with consequent retinal hemorrhage. The initial hemorrhage often is beyond the region of primary visual acuity of the retina and escapes notice. As the blood clots, organizes and begins to contract, the lesions can rip segments of retina away from the posterior surface of the eye producing sudden vision loss. Some patients notice flashes of light in their visual field, leading them to seek medical help.

Laser photocoagulation has been used in an effort to prevent retinal hemorrhage.[39] A retina specialist is the preferred opalmologic provider, particularly if diabetic retinopathy is a practice focus. Annual evaluation is key to early detection of lesions and prevention of complications. Retinopathy has no correlation with the sickle cell disease pain profile. *All patients must have regular retinal examinations irrespective of clinical status.*

PREGNANCY IN SICKLE CELL DISEASE

A mistaken belief common to the medical community is that sickle cell disease precludes pregancy. While concern is justifiable, the proscription of pregnancy for women with sickle cell disease is not. Women with sickle cell disease can successfully carry pregnancies to term.[40] While the process sometimes is complicated, appropriate care and anticipation allow successful management of issues that might arise. High-risk obstetrical specialists best manage these patients. The frequency of painful crises commonly increases during pregnancy.[41] Women who have painful crises during pregnancy should receive analgesics as necessary, including opioid drugs. The new-borns with intrauterine drug exposure must undergo opioid withdrawal. Warned of this issue, neonatologists can easily manage the problem. Routine transfusion is not indicated during pregnancy.

■ PERIPHERAL BLOOD SMEAR

The peripheral blood smear is strikingly abnormal in sickle cell disease. The smear is similar in three of the major sickle syndromes listed in Table 13-1, namely homozygous hemoglobin S disease, sickle β^+-thalassemia and sickle β^0-thalassemia. Hemoglobin SC disease has interesting characteristics not seen with the other three conditions.

The most striking feature of the erythrocytes in sickle cell disease is bizarre red cell distortion (Figure 13-2). Irregular crenated cells are common along with small, distorted cells that appear almost as erythrocyte fragments. Some cells have multiple membrane projections giving them a star-like appearance. In the midst of this mix are cells that have the sickle shape portrayed in most drawings and captured in most illustrative photomicrographs. These cells are in fact a minority among the cohort of abnormal cells in sickle cell disease. Target cells are common in both sickle β^0-thalassemia and sickle β^+-thalassemia and help distinguish these two compound heterozygous conditions from homozygous hemoglobin S disease.

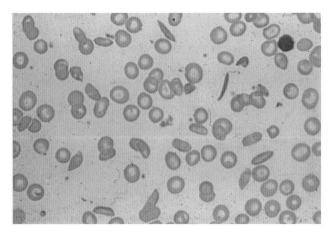

FIGURE 13–2 *Peripheral blood in Sickle β°-thalassemia. The marked variation in cell size is typical of sickle cell disease. The irregular sickle-shaped cells on the smear are irreversibly sickled cells (smears are done at ambient oxygen tension allowing shape reversion of cells that can do so).*

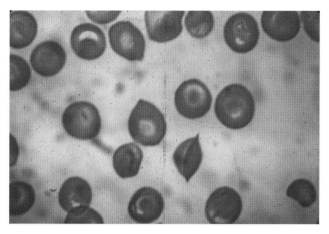

FIGURE 13-3 *Peripheral blood in Hb SC disease. Target cells are typical of Hb SC disease. Many of the cells appear to have folded edges, which is typical of Hb SC disease.*

Target cells are also prominent with hemoglobin SC disease (Figure 13-3). Bizarre cells exist on the smear but are much less marked than with the three other main sickle cell syndromes. Many of the cells appear to have edges that fold over onto them, creating a cymbiform appearance.

A host of intracellular inclusions exist in the cells. Howell-Jolly bodies are a common feature. Basophilic stippling is prominent in many of the cells. Pappenheimer bodies exist in the cells of some patients, particularly those with iron overload due to repeated transfusions. Nucleated red cells are common. Some patients show only a few such cells per low power microscopic field. Others show enormous numbers of nucleated red cells. Bone marrow stress, such as that produced by a severe infection, can induce a massive outpouring of nucleated red cells.

Large polychromatophilic erythrocytes are common. These cells usually are reticulocytes. Supravital staining with an agent such as new methylene blue definitively identifies the cells as reticulocytes.

The neutrophils are qualitatively normal in sickle cell disease. Close observation often leaves the correct impression that their number is greater than normal. Platelets in sickle cell disease also are qualitatively normal in size and appearance. However, the number of platelets often appears to be higher than normal on examination of the peripheral smear.

■ LABORATORY VALUES

Low hemoglobin and hematocrit values are invariable components of sickle cell disease. The degree of the depression varies greatly, modulated in some cases by factors such as high hemoglobin F values or coexistent α-thalassemia. Hemoglobin values of 7 or 8 g/dL are common. Exceptional patients routinely have values as low as 5 g/dL or as high as 10 g/dL. The hemoglobin value is usually higher in patients with hemoglobin SC disease. Here values commonly range between 9 and 11 g/dL.

The MCV provides a valuable clue to the genotype of patients with sickle cell disease. The values for this parameter are normal in homozygous hemoglobin S disease. The MCV sometimes is as low as 70 fL in cases of sickle β-thalassemia. The distinction is muddled however at times by instances of homozygous hemoglobin S disease with coinheritance of α-thalassemia, where the α-thalassemia produces modest microcytosis. The MCV is low with hemoglobin SC disease reflecting the cellular dehydration of erythrocytes characteristic of this condition.

All of the sickle cell syndromes have elevated RDW values consistent with the marked variation in cell size seen on the peripheral smear. Values are commonly as high as 25 with homozygous hemoglobin S disease. The RDW tends to be only moderately elevated with hemoglobin SC disease. The erythrocyte sedimentation rate is low in sickle cell disease. The test therefore is less useful as a screen for inflammation than in the general population.

Reticulocytosis is the norm in patients with homozygous hemoglobin S disease and the sickle β-thalassemia syndromes. Baseline percentages can be as low as 4% or 5% in some patients while others average values as high as 15%. The absolute reticulocyte count can be as low as 100,000 cells/μL or as high as 400,000 cells/μL. The reticulocyte count tends to remain relatively stable for individual patients. Deviation from the personal norm is cause for concern. Patients with hemoglobin SC disease typically have normal reticulocyte values.

The WBC in patients with sickle cell disease often exceeds normal limits. Values in the range of 12,000–14,000 cells/μL are common. Neutrophilia is part of this pattern of leukocytosis. A question sometimes arises as to whether a patient with a WBC of, for instance, 13,000 cells/μL has an underlying infection. The best approach to the issue is to review prior counts because the WBC is steady for individuals. A value of 13,000 cells/μL might not be cause for concern in a patient who routinely runs a count of 12,000 cells/μL. The same value sounds an alarm in a patient who normally has only 6000 cells/μL.

In the absence of information on prior white counts, a higher than normal WBC in a patient with sickle cell disease cannot be simply attributed to the sickle cell disease. People with sickle cell disease respond normally to infections and inflammatory stimuli manifesting brisk leukocytosis. A patient with sickle cell disease who develops pneumonia might, for instance, show a rise in the WBC from the personal routine of 8,000 to a value of 13,000 cells/μL. In the absence of historical information, data regarding the white count must be interpreted cautiously with a constant eye to the clinical setting.

An important point regarding the WBC in sickle cell disease is that the white cell distribution is normal in the absence of inflammation or infection. Bands on the peripheral smear are evidence of infection as with any patient. Metamyelocytes in the circulation means that the patient has an infection until proven otherwise.

The platelet count in sickle cell disease typically falls within the normal range. Some patients display modest thrombocytosis, however.

TABLE 13-3 | **IDENTIFICATION OF THE HEMOGLOBINS COMMON IN THE SICKLE CELL SYNDROMES**

Technique	Positives	Negatives	Direct Quantification	Time	Use/ Availability
Cellulose acetate electrophoresis	Separates A, S, F, C	Not acceptable for A2. Poor F, A, S separation	No	60 min	High
Citrate agar electrophoresis	Clear separation of F from A, S	Not acceptable for A2	No	60 min	High
Isoelectric focusing	Clear separation of F, A, S, C	Not acceptable for A2	Yes	45 min	Low
HPLC	Identifies A, S, C, F, A2	None	Yes	5 min	Moderate
PCR	Identifies all common Hb variants; useful for prenatal screening	Relatively expensive	Yes	30 min	Low

■ DIAGNOSIS OF SICKLE CELL DISEASE

The amino acid substitutions in hemoglobin S and hemoglobin C change the charge characteristics of the molecules so that they migrate differently in an electric field than does hemoglobin A. Hemoglobin F and hemoglobin A2 each has different migration patterns from hemoglobin A, S, and C because of their structural differences. Nonetheless, the various hemoglobins overlap in pattern depending on the electrophoretic technique. No single approach can provide complete identification of aberrant and normal hemoglobin in one fell swoop. The most commonly used approach to identification of aberrant hemoglobins is cellulose acetate electrophoresis (at alkaline pH) followed by citrate agar electrophoresis at acid pH, when necessary. Table 13-3 summarizes this information.

The amino acid substitutions in hemoglobin S and C also change size and biophysical characteristics of the molecules. High performance liquid chromatography (HPLC) takes advantage of these differences to separate the hemoglobin variants from hemoglobin A. The technique requires a very small amount of blood and much less time than the electrophoretic approaches. In contrast to electrophoresis, HPLC also gives a quantitative readout of the relative hemoglobin content of a sample. HPLC is slowly displacing electrophoresis for the identification of common aberrant hemoglobins.

The representative values for the hemoglobin distributions of the four primary sickle cell syndromes in Table 13-1 derive from this type of analysis. Homozygous hemoglobin S disease shows almost exclusive expression of hemoglobin S with no hemoglobin A. Typically the electrophoresis shows small amounts of hemoglobin A2 and hemoglobin F. With sickle β^0-thalassemia, hemoglobin S is again the preponderant subunit on electrophoresis. With this syndrome, however, the values for hemoglobin A2 and hemoglobin F are above normal, reflecting the thalassemic nature of the second β-chain of this compound heterozygous hemoglobin.

Sickle β^+-thalassemia has a substantial amount of hemoglobin A on electrophoresis. The quantity of hemoglobin A is always far less than that of hemoglobin S, as shown in Table 13-1. Misinterpretation of the hemoglobin electrophoresis on rare occasion leads to people with this hemoglobin electrophoretic pattern receiving the erroneous designation of "sickle cell trait." The electrophoretic pattern with sickle cell trait, however, always shows more hemoglobin A than hemoglobin S. A more common cause of error is transfusion before the procedure, which floods the system with Hb A and confounds the interpretation of the electrophoresis.

Hemoglobin SC disease shows slightly more hemoglobin S than hemoglobin C on electrophoresis. No hemoglobin A exists while levels are low for both Hb A2 and Hb F.

■ PATHOLOGICAL BASIS OF SICKLE CELL DISEASE

RED CELL PROBLEM

Sickle hemoglobin derives from the glutamic acid to valine substitution at position 6 in the β subunit of hemoglobin. With a few minor exceptions, people with one hemoglobin S gene are phenotypically normal (sickle trait). People who inherit two hemoglobin S genes have homozygous hemoglobin S disease. The ultimate expression of the pathology in sickle cell disease reflects a complex and to some degree confusing set of effects that are "down stream" from this simple amino acid substitution. Some of the factors that contribute to sickle cell disease expression and progression do not in fact involve the red cell at all. The change at the 6th position of the β subunit is without question the trigger from which flows all other pathologic events in sickle cell disease.

The central event is the polymerization of deoxygenated sickle hemoglobin. Hemoglobin S binds and releases oxygen normally. Oxygenated hemoglobin S in the red cell behaves identically to oxygenated hemoglobin A. In contrast, deoxygenated hemoglobin S molecules tend to adhere one to the other forming long strands. The slight change in quaternary structure that accompanies the shift from oxygenated to deoxygenated hemoglobin exposes "sticky" patches on the β subunits brought about by the aberrant valine residue at position 6. The forces that promote the adhesive interaction between any two hemoglobin molecules are quite weak. The key to the creation of stable hemoglobin polymers is the formation of an ordered structure with a twisting α-helical orientation involving 14 hemoglobin strands. Multiple interactions exist across the hemoglobin molecules that reinforce polymer stability.

Electronmicrographic images show that the polymers grow out from a central nidus, often call the crystallization point, that is the focus of polymerization. Multiple branching structures represent the crisscrossing of polymers that have grown out from different foci. The growing polymers eventually reach a size such that they stretch and distort the erythrocyte membrane. The result is the spectrum of distorted red cells that are pathognomonic of sickle cell disease. The cells are not only misshapen. The regions of distorted membrane are stiff and inflexible. This change in the erythrocytes is the nexus of the problem in sickle cell disease.

With a rise in ambient oxygen tension to levels typical of the pulmonary circulation, the hemoglobin S molecules return to the oxygenated state. The molecules resume the conformation typical of oxygenated hemoglobin with the consequent breakdown of the hemoglobin polymer. The "melting" of the hemoglobin polymer allows the red cells to resume their normal biconcave shape. Most importantly, the erythrocytes resume the deformable, flexible characteristics typical of normal red cells.

Red cells in the arterial circulation pass through vessels of progressively smaller bore as they travel to the peripheral tissues to fulfil their task of oxygen delivery. The capillaries are the smallest conduits with a diameter smaller than the average size of an erythrocyte. The inherent flexibility of the red cells allows them pass through these small channels. Video microscopy of erythrocytes passing through capillaries shows these cells stretching and often forming elongated structures before popping through the stricture.

The release of oxygen to tissues deprives erythrocytes containing hemoglobin S of the flexibility needed to pass through the capillaries. The hemoglobin polymerization does not occur instantly. A veritable race against time occurs. If the hemoglobin S erythrocytes can complete the journey through the microcirculation and enter the larger venules before gross cell distortion occurs, they have a change of returning to the high oxygen tension realm of the lungs where the hemoglobin S polymer melts and the cells reassume a normal shape.

Should significant cellular distortion set in while the red cells are still in the microcirculation, the erythrocytes can become wedged and block flow through the vessels (Figure 13-4). Oxygen delivery to the peripheral tissue beyond the occlusion halts, leading to tissue ischemia and damage. The pain, chronic organ damage and myriad of other characteristic problems of sickle cell disease derive from this interruption in blood flow.

The repeated episodes of erythrocyte distortion by hemoglobin polymers formed with each circuit through the peripheral vasculature damages the cell membrane and impairs its integrity. One of the important consequences is oxidative membrane damage characterized by cross-links involving both membrane proteins and lipids.[42] Heme molecules dislocate from the hemoglobin subunits and attach to the membrane. These structures, called hemichromes, promote further oxidant damage since the iron in these complexes catalyzes the formation of injurious reactive oxygen species.[43] The damaged membranes become permanently rigid, failing to resume their normal shape even in the absence of hemoglobin S polymer. These are the irreversibly sickled cells seen on routine Wright Geimsa stain of peripheral blood.

Red cells in the circulation move effortlessly through vessels and rarely adhere to the endothelial cells that line these conduits. The erythrocyte membrane damage that occurs with repetitive cycles of hemoglobin S polymerization eventually produce subtle membrane alterations enhance red cell adhesion to the endothelium.[44] Blockade of blood flow promotes vaso-occlusive tissue injury.

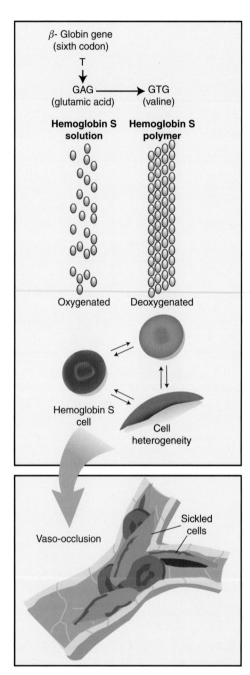

FIGURE 13–4   *Vaso-occlusion in sickle cell disease. Deoxygenation of sickle red cells leads to the formation of Hb S polymer that distorts the cells and damages the membrane. The distorted cells occlude the microcirculation leading to local ischemia and tissue injury. (From Steinberg M. 1999. Management of sickle cell disease. N Engl J Med 340:1021–1130. Figure 1.)*

COCONSPIRATORS

Other cells in the circulation probably moderate the vaso-occlusion process in sickle cell disease and thereby affect disease manifestation. Neutrophils appear to be important role in this regard.[45] These cells tend naturally to adhere to the endothelium. In the circulation they appear almost to bounce along the vessel lining due to brief episodes of adhesion with endothelial cells. In sickle cell disease these neutrophils probably interfere with the smooth flow of blood through smaller vessels thereby increasing the chance that distorted erythrocytes will block flow. The fact that high neutrophil counts correlate with a worse prognosis in sickle cell disease attests to the importance of these cells to the pathology of the disorder.

Elevated neutrophils counts at steady state correlates with early mortality and disease adverse outcome, ACS, and stroke. During vaso-occlusive episodes most patients develop leukocytosis and evidence of neutrophil activation.[46] Moreover, rapid, marked elevation of the neutrophil count by growth factor administration can precipitate a vaso-occlusive episode.[47] Anti-inflammatory therapy, potentially targeting neutrophils, benefits painful vaso-occlusive crisis and ACS. Finally, some of the benefit to hydroxyurea treatment might reflect its effect on the neutrophil count.[48]

Platelets are circulating cells with the greatest adhesive capacity since their normal function is to attach to regions of vascular injury help seal breaches in these conduits. Platelets might well contribute to impaired blood flow in sickle cell disease. Their role in such matters is less well established than is that of the neutrophils.

The discovery of unusually large numbers of circulating endothelial cells in patients with sickle cell disease brought a new perspective to the factors that might contribute to sickle cell pathology.[49] The circulating endothelial cells in sickle cell disease express "activation" proteins on their surface, indicating that they have been jarred into a new metabolic state.[50] At fault, most likely, is injury from hypoxia as well as from factors such as reactive oxygen species produced by damaged sickle erythrocytes. The number of circulating endothelial cells rise with sickle cell crisis. The issue of whether this change is a cause of the crisis or an effect an interesting and important area of investigation.

Inflammatory cytokines also appear to play a role in some of the complications of sickle cell disease. For instance, patients with the disorder have higher than normal levels of the neutrophil chemokine interleukin-8 that rise still further during sickle cell crisis.[51] The level of the substance P also rises with during vaso-occlusive sickle cell crisis.[52] This peptide promotes release of both TNF-α and Il-8. Cytokines form a complex web of regulatory and counterregulatory actions whose impact on the course of sickle cell disease likely exceeds current appreciation.

FELICITOUS FACTORS

Hemoglobin F

Coincident hematologic factors modulate the severity of sickle cell disease in some patients. Patients with homozygous hemoglobin S disease who have high levels of fetal hemoglobin often experience milder than average disease. This phenomenon is most dramatic in patients with hereditary persistence of fetal hemoglobin where a second mutation in the β-globin locus causes the γ-globin gene to continue producing fetal hemoglobin well into adulthood.

Two properties of fetal hemoglobin help moderate the severity of sickle cell disease. First, hemoglobin F molecules do not participate in the polymerization that occurs between molecules of deoxygenated hemoglobin S.[53] Second, higher concentrations of hemoglobin F in a cell infer lower concentrations of hemoglobin S. Polymer formation depends exponentially on the concentration of deoxygenated hemoglobin S. Each of these effects reduces the propensity toward polymer formation and sickling of the erythrocytes.

The Comprehensive Study of Sickle Cell Disease (CSSCD) examined predictive factors for life expectancy and risk factors for early death in nearly 4000 patients in the United States. A high level of fetal hemoglobin (>8.6%) augured improved survival.[54] Analysis of another subset of the data focused on leg ulcers in this cohort of patients. The data showed that fetal hemoglobin levels above 10% correlated with fewer chronic leg ulcers in children with sickle cell disease.[55]

Sickle cell disease is common in India and parts of the Middle East. Analysis of the genes shows a separate origin from the sickle cell disease seen in people of African heritage.[56] Many patients with this "Eastern" variety of sickle cell disease tend to run a milder disease course relative to that seen in people with the African variety of the disorder. Many of these patients have fetal hemoglobin levels that are quite high. Fetal hemoglobin levels averaged about 17% in one group of patients in Saudi Arabia.[57] This value exceeds by more than two-fold the level reported in the CSSCD. One investigation compared patients from Orissa State, India to Jamaican patients with sickle cell.[58] The Indian patients had a more benign course relative to the Jamaican cohort. The reported protective level of fetal hemoglobin in this study was on average 16.64%, with a range of 4.6–31.5%.

α-Thalassemia

Another factor that can lessen sickle cell disease severity is the coinheritance of α-thalassemia. α-thalassemia, like sickle cell disease, is a genetic variant that affects hemoglobin (see Chapter 14). In people of African descent, two-gene deletion α-thalassemia produces moderate microcytosis and a mild anemia. Two-gene deletion α-thalassemia in isolation is a clinically benign condition.

Investigations of sickle erythrocyte properties important to sickle cell disease, including irreversibly sickled cells, the fraction of red cells with a high hemoglobin concentration (dense cells), and red cells with reduced deformabilty, show a direct correlation with the number of α-globin genes.[59] A primary effect of α-thalassemia is reduction in the fraction of red cells that attained a high hemoglobin concentration. These "dense cells" result from potassium loss due to acquired membrane leaks. The overall deformability of dense sickle red cells is substantially lower than normal and they contribute substantially to vaso-occlusion.

Reduction in overall hemoglobin concentration due to absent α genes is not the only mechanism by which α-thalassemia reduces the formation of dense and irreversibly sickled cells. The red cell membrane redundancy produced by α-thalassemia (morphologically manifested as target cells) appears also to reduce red cell damage in sickle cell disease.[60] Membrane redundancy possibly protects against stretching and damage to the erythrocyte membrane when hemoglobin S polymerizes. The effect would be to minimize potassium leakage and cell dehydration.[61]

■ CLINICAL MANAGEMENT OF SICKLE CELL DISEASE

HYDROXYUREA

Hydroxyurea (Hydrea®) is the most important advancement in the care of people with sickle cell disease since the 1986 introduction of prophylactic penicillin. While hydroxyurea treatment requires care, the drug is neither an investigational nor esoteric intervention. Hydroxyurea is not aspirin. But neither is it warfain, which is easily the most dangerous drug in broad clinical use. Clinicians who do not shy from warfain administration can easily master a much safer drug such as hydroxyurea.

Hydroxyurea therapy is not appropriate for all people with sickle cell disease nor is it effective in everyone. The medication can dramatically alter the clinical course of many patients, however. No oracle exists to identify the patients who will respond to hydroxyurea. An important aspect of the care of patients with sickle cell disease is to assure that no one who might benefit from hydroxyurea is neglected. Although hydroxyurea is not essential to optimal management of sickle cell disease, the drug should be at least considered for patients with the disorder. The key data on the use of hydroxyurea in sickle cell disease comes from the Multicenter Study of Hydroxyurea in Sickle Cell Anemia.[62] The key facts are as follows.

1. Hydroxyurea reduces painful crises by half.
2. Hydroxyurea reduces hospital stays for painful crises by half.
3. Hydroxyurea reduces ACS by half.
4. Hydroxyurea reduces transfusion requirements.

Hydroxyurea appears also to lower mortality in adults with sickle cell disease.[63] Table 13-4 broadly summarizes the considerations surrounding the use

TABLE 13-4	HYDROXYUREA THERAPY IN SICKLE CELL DISEASE
Eligibility for Hydroxyurea	*Clinical Indications for Hydroxyurea*
• 18 years of age or older • Not pregnant	• Recurrent vaso-occlusive pain crises. Patients with three or more pain crises per year should be considered for hydroxyurea management. • Recurrent acute chest syndrome. • Frequent or chronic transfusion requirement.

of hydroxyurea. For patients not needing hydroxyurea, the issue should be reviewed yearly. For patients started on the drug, ongoing assessment of its efficacy is vital. The drug should be stopped in the absence of a clinical benefit.

Pediatric studies confirm hydroxyurea safety in children 5 years of age and older.[64] No definitive data show that hydroxyurea ameliorates clinical problems in children with sickle cell disease, however. Existing reports with limited numbers of patients are quite favorable in this respect, but cannot be the sole basis of such a momentous decision about treatment.[65] The role of hydroxyurea remains a major focus of research in the management of pediatric sickle cell disease. A multi-institutional study of hydroxyurea in infants and young children is in progress (Baby HUG).

PAIN MANAGEMENT

Chronic pain is a predominant problem for many patients with sickle cell disease. The etiology of chronic pain in the disorder is unclear. Organ injury and necrosis produced by years of intermittent ischemia from vaso-occlusion likely play a large role. The severity of the pain varies greatly and can change over time. No universally applicable formula exists for management of chronic pain. Physicians frequently face the greatest management challenges from patients with persistent severe pain controlled by chronically administered opioid analgesics.

Nonsteroidal Anti-inflammatory Drugs

Nonsteroidal anti-inflammatory drugs (NSAIDs) can control chronic pain in many patients with sickle cell disease. The agents can be used alone or in conjunction with opioid analgesics. Most commonly, NSAIDs are used intermittently to control flares of pain. The issue of renal dysfunction and associated complications makes most specialists chary of chronic NSAID use. Physicians who opt for NSAID-based pain management *must closely monitor renal function*. Equally important is awareness that the clinical chemical profile of renal function in sickle cell disease differs importantly from that of normal people. Interpretation of BUN and creatinine values must be made in that light.

Opiod Analgesics

Chronic administration of opioid analgesics produces drug tolerance. Consequently, the quantity of medication needed to control chronic severe pain exceeds that associated with a severe but self-limited painful episode, such as torn knee ligaments. In the absence of an objective measure of pain intensity, appropriate management of chronic pain with opioids requires an ongoing dialogue between the doctor and patient.

Whenever possible, patients should start taking analgesics at home before the pain crescendos. Maintaining pain at a tolerable level is easier than reducing it from an intense apogee. Patients manage many severe sickle pain episodes at home with analgesics, fluids, and rest. If the pain progresses despite the use of reasonable quantities of medication, emergency medical care is the next option.

Health care providers often view sickle cell disease pain as episodic bouts secondary to occlusion of the microcirculation. Frequently absent is the realization that severe chronic pain more loosely associated with vaso-occlusion also occurs. Chronic sickle cell pain is more common in adults than in children reflecting permanent damage to the microcirculation and tissues after years of recurrent sickle-related injury.

Opioid analgesic management of sickle cell disease pain requires constant reevaluation both of efficacy and necessity. The drugs can dull the sensorium and impair normal judgment and function of even the most scrupulously careful patient. A delicate and often difficult balance must be struck between relief of pain and functional impairment. With any medical condition that produces chronic pain, the issue of how best to use opioid analgesics taxes physician skill in the extreme.

TRANSFUSIONS

Sporadic

Patients with sickle cell disease are anemic, by definition. Baseline hemoglobin values vary between patients but are stable for each individual. Most patients are conditioned to tolerate their degree of anemia making routine transfusion unnecessary. Raising the hemoglobin value rarely provides clinical benefit, unless the baseline value has fallen to 5 g/dL or so (hematocrit of approximately 15%), at which point oxygen-carrying capacity is seriously compromised. Also, such low hemoglobin values leave little leeway for further decline. On the other hand, transfusing patients with sickle cell disease to hemoglobin values of 11 or 12 g/dL (hematocrits in the mid- to upper-30s) can be dangerous, since blood viscosity increases substantially at higher hemoglobin levels with secondary vaso-occlusion possibly resulting.

A key factor that can contribute to significantly low baseline hemoglobin values in patients with sickle cell disease is low-grade renal insufficiency. Erythropoietin supplementation can markedly improve the hemoglobin value and clinical well being of these patients. Another possible intervention is therapy with hydroxyurea. On occasion, relatively low doses of hydroxyurea (e.g., 25 mg/kg/day) dramatically raise hemoglobin values to the range of 9 or 10 g/dL. Most elevations are more modest if they occur. Nonetheless, a rise in hemoglobin from 5 to 7 g/dL can dramatically improve the clinical status and well being of some patients.

Chronic Transfusions

The role of chronic transfusion therapy is best documented for stroke victims.[66] Chronic transfusion therapy is less well established for other issues in sickle cell disease including recurrent severe episodes of sickle pain, ACS, priapism and prophylaxis of pregnancy complications. The utility of chronic transfusion therapy is limited by complications, most notably alloimmunization and iron overload.

With the virtual elimination of transfusion-related infections, iron overload currently is the most dread and deadly complication of chronic transfusion therapy. Hepatic injury including fibrosis and cirrhosis along with cardiomyopathy and congestive heart failure lead the parade of associated problems. The only proven treatment for transfusional iron overload is indefinite parenteral administration of the iron chelator, deferoxamine (Desferal®) 12 hours per day for 5 days each week. Patients hold opinions of deferoxamine treatment that range from dislike to abhorrence. Deferoxamine is a highly effective iron chelator. However, adherence to the prescribed regimen is low with a consequently poor clinical response. Oral iron chelators newly introduced to the market might improve this picture.

Alloimmunization

Alloimmunization against minor red cell antigens is a major problem for patients with sickle cell disease who receive frequent transfusions (see acute chest syndrome). Kell, E, and C are the most problematic minor antigens. The rate of alloimmunization approaches 40% in some reports.[67] Occasionally, patients develop such severe problems with alloantibodies that transfusion becomes nearly impossible.

Limited phenotype matching for these antigens markedly reduces the incidence of alloimmunization.[68] The procedure involves screening for minor red cell antigens known to be problematic for chronically transfused patients with sickle cell disease. Limited phenotype matching increases the cost of transfusion for patients with sickle cell disease. Avoidance of subsequent alloimmunization and the need for extensive screening entailed by this complication ultimately saves the transfusion service money both in manpower and materiel, however.[69] Most importantly, the approach abrogates the danger to patients created by transfusion time delays necessitated by extensive crossmatching for alloantibodies. Some people tragically have died during the search for appropriately matched blood.

HEMATOPOIETIC STEM CELL TRANSPLANTATION

Hematopoietic stem cell transplantation can cure sickle cell disease.[70] The procedure works best in children with HLA-matched siblings as stem cell donors. Bone marrow and cord blood both provide adequate quantities of hematopoietic stem cells for the procedure.[71] The 5-year disease-free survival in children is about 80%.

The variable nature of sickle cell disease creates an important dilemma with respect to transplantation, however. Some people with sickle cell disease lead full lives where the problems encountered are managed relatively easily by conventional approaches. In contrast, other patients have devastatingly severe disease and suffer early mortality. Hematopoietic stem cell transplantation is an appropriate intervention for people in the latter group. The procedure works best, however, before severe end organ damage and debility develop.

Early forecasts of which patients will fit the transplantation profile are difficult. Even a modifier of sickle cell disease severity as well-established as Hb F levels has shortcomings because the correlations are statistical values that apply to populations. The clinical triad in children noted earlier of severe anemia, dactylitis and persistent neutropenia is another possible guide. Nonetheless, predictions for an individual remain a dicey business. Until better forecasts are possible for individual patients, selection of transplant candidates will be a delicate affair (Tables 13-5 and 13-6).

TABLE 13-5 | **KEY DIAGNOSTIC ISSUES IN SICKLE CELL DISEASE**

Problem	Manifestation	Approach
Acute chest syndrome	• Falling oxygen saturation with P_{O_2} <80 mm Hg on room air • Chest x-ray infiltrates • Fever • Leukocytosis	• Simple transfusion • Exchange transfusion • Antibiotics • Ventilation support • Bronchodilators
Splenic sequestration crisis	• Enlarging spleen on examination • Left upper quadrant pain • Falling hemoglobin	• Simple transfusion
Stroke	• Acute hemiplegia/hemiparesis • Severe headache • Nausea, vomiting	• Exchange transfusion
Aplastic crisis	• Reticulocyte count low or zero • Falling hemoglobin • Fever, vaso-occlusive pain	• Simple transfusion
Septicemia	• Fever • Leukocytosis • Peripheral blood bands • Lethargy • Confusion	• Cultures • Broad-spectrum antibiotics
Acute bone marrow necrosis	• Severe pain • Leucocytosis • Nucleated red cells • Falling hemoglobin	• Simple transfusion • Exchange transfusion • Monitor for acute chest syndrome
Multiorgan failure	• Falling oxygen saturation with P_{O_2} <80 mm Hg on room air • Chest x-ray infiltrates • Fever • Leucocytosis • Confusion • Rising BUN/Creatinine	• Exchange transfusion • Antibiotics • Ventilator support

TABLE 13-6	KEY MANAGEMENT ISSUES IN SICKLE CELL DISEASE
Issue	*Comment*
Hydroxyurea	Hydroxyurea should be considered in patients where pain significantly restricts lifestyle.
Penicillin prophylaxis	Daily penicillin or equivalent in children from ages 6 months to 7 years.
Pneumococcal immunization	Children and adults. Repeat every 5–7 years.
Hepatitis B immunization	Children and adults.
Viral influenza immunization	Adults every year.
Limited phenotype-matched red cell transfusion	Children and adults. Reduces the risk of red cell alloimmunization.
Severe acute pain crisis	• Parenterally administered short-acting opioids for immediate pain control. • Patient controlled analgesia when possible. • Avoid meperidine for long-term pain management due to potential of triggering seizures.
Renal dysfunction	• Monitor BUN and creatinine regularly. • Assess glomerular filtration rate if the creatinine is persistently greater than 1.0. • Consider interventions to spare renal function including ACE inhibitors and protein restriction. • Avoid chronic NSAID use.
Retinopathy	• Yearly ophthalmology examination with indirect ophthalmoscopy. • Laser treatment of early proliferative lesions.
Avascular necrosis of bone	• Avoid chronic NSAID use to prevent renal disease. • Minimize weight bearing. • Intra-articular injection of cortisol. • Consider marrow decompression of femoral head. • Prosthesis as last resort.
Strokes	• Transcranial dopler beginning at 2–3 years of age, repeated every 6–12 months through age 12.

References

1. Herrick J. 1910. Peculiar elongated and sickle shaped red blood corpuscles in a case of severe anemia. Arch Intern Med 6:517–527.

2. Pauling L, Itano HA, Singer SJ, Wells IC. 1949. Sickle cell anemia a molecular disease. Science 110:543–548.

3. Ingram V. 1956. A specific chemical difference between globins of normal and sickle-cell anaemia haemoglobins. Nature 178:792–794.

4. Wang X, Seaman C, Paik M, Chen T, Bank A, Piomelli S. 1994. Experience with 500 prenatal diagnoses of sickle cell diseases: The effect of gestational age on affected pregnancy outcome. Prenat Diagn 14(9):851–857.

5. Panepinto JA, Magid D, Rewers MJ, Lane PA. 2000. Universal versus targeted screening of infants for sickle cell disease: A cost-effectiveness analysis. J Pediatr 136(2):201–208.

6. Watson J, Staldman A, Shields GS. 1948. The significance of the paucity of sickle cells in newborn Negro infants. Am J Med Sci 215:419–423.

7. Miller ST, Sleeper LA, Pegelow CH, et al. 2000. Prediction of adverse outcomes in children with sickle cell disease. N Engl J Med 342(2):83–99.

8. Gaston MH, Verter JI, Woods G, et al. 1986. Prophylaxis with oral penicillin in children with sickle cell anemia. A randomized trial. N Engl J Med 314(25):1593–1599.

9. Zimmerman R. 2001. Pneumococcal conjugate vaccine for young children. Am Fam Physician 63(10):1991–1998.

10. Kinney TR, Ware RE, Schultz WH, Filston HC. 1990. Long-term management of splenic sequestration in children with sickle cell disease. J Pediatr 117(2 Pt 1):194–199.

11. Smith-Whitley K, Zhao H, Hodinka RL, et al. 2004. Epidemiology of human parvovirus B19 in children with sickle cell disease. Blood 103(2):422–427.

12. Wang WC, Kovnar EH, Tonkin IL, et al. 1991. High risk of recurrent stroke after discontinuance of five to twelve years of transfusion therapy in patients with sickle cell disease. J Pediatr 118(3):377–382.

13. Kinney TR, Sleeper LA, Wang WC, et al. 1991. Silent cerebral infarcts in sickle cell anemia: A risk factor analysis. The cooperative study of sickle cell disease. Pediatrics 103:64–645.

14. Pegelow CH, Adams RJ, McKie V, et al. 1995. Risk of recurrent stroke in patients with sickle cell disease treated with erythrocyte transfusions. J Pediatr 126(6):896–899.

15. Seibert JJ, Glasier CM, Kirby RS, et al. 1998. Transcranial Doppler, MRA, and MRI as a screening examination for cerebrovascular disease in patients with sickle cell anemia: An 8-year study. Pediatr Radiol 28(3):138–142.

16. Adams RJ, Brambilla DJ, Granger S, et al. 2004. Stroke and conversion to high risk in children screened with transcranial Doppler ultrasound during the STOP study. Blood 103(10):3689–3694.

17. Platt OS, Thorington BD, Brambilla DJ, et al. 1991. Pain in sickle cell disease. Rates and risk factors. N Engl J Med 325(1):11–16.

18. Castro O, Brambilla DJ, Thorington B, et al. 1994. The acute chest syndrome in sickle cell disease: Incidence and risk factors. The cooperative study of sickle cell disease. Blood 84:643–649.

19. Vichinsky E, Neumayr L, Earles A, et al. 2000. Causes and outcomes of the acute chest syndrome in sickle cell disease. N Engl J Med 342:1855–1865.

20. Vichinsky EP, Haberkern CM, Neumayr L, et al. 1995. A comparison of conservative and aggressive transfusion regimens in the perioperative management of sickle cell disease. The

Preoperative Transfusion in Sickle Cell Disease Study Group. N Engl J Med 333(4):206–213.

[21] Emre U, Miller ST, Gutierez M, Steiner P, Rao SP, Rao M. 1995. Effect of transfusion in acute chest syndrome of sickle cell disease. J Pediatr 127(6):901–904.

[22] Milner PF, Squires JE, Larison PJ, Charles WT, Krauss JS. 1985. Posttransfusion crises in sickle cell anemia: Role of delayed hemolytic reactions to transfusion. South Med J 78(12):1462–1469.

[23] Rosse WF, Gallagher D, Kinney TR, et al. 1990. Transfusion and alloimmunization in sickle cell disease. The cooperative study of sickle cell disease. Blood 76(7):1431–1437.

[24] Mankad VN, Williams JP, Harpen MD, et al. 1990. Magnetic resonance imaging of bone marrow in sickle cell disease: Clinical, hematologic, and pathologic correlations. Blood 75(1):274–283.

[25] Vichinsky E, Williams R, Das M, et al. 1994. Pulmonary fat embolism: A distinct cause of severe acute chest syndrome in sickle cell anemia. Blood 83:3107–3112.

[26] Johnson K, Stastny JF, Rucknagel DL. 1994. Fat embolism syndrome associated with asthma and sickle cell-beta(+)-thalassemia. Am J Hematol 46(4):354–357.

[27] Hassell KL, Eckman JR, Lane PA. 1994. Acute multiorgan failure syndrome: A potentially catastrophic complication of severe sickle cell pain episodes. Am J Med 96(2):155–162.

[28] Powars D, Johnson C, 1996. Priapism. Hematol Oncol Clin North Am 10(6):1363–1372.

[29] Mantadakis E, Cavender JD, Rogers ZR, Ewalt DH, Buchanan GR. 1999. Prevalence of priapism in children and adolescents with sickle cell anemia. J Pediatr Hematol Oncol 21(6):518–522.

[30] Fuselier HA Jr, Ochsner MG, Ross RJ. 1980. Priapism: Review of simple surgical procedure. J Urol 123(5):778–781.

[31] Gbadoe AD, Atakouma Y, Kusiaku K, Assimadi JK. 2001. Management of sickle cell priapism with etilefrine. Arch Dis Child 85(1):52–53.

[32] Hernigou P, Bachir D, Galacteros F. 2003. The natural history of symptomatic osteonecrosis in adults with sickle-cell disease. J Bone Joint Surg Am 85-A(3):500–504.

[33] Powars DR, Elliott-Mills DD, Chan L, et al. 1991. Chronic renal failure in sickle cell disease: Risk factors, clinical course, and mortality. Ann Intern Med 115(8):614–620.

[34] Wigfall DR, Ware RE, Burchinal MR, Kinney TR, Foreman JW. 2000. Prevalence and clinical correlates of glomerulopathy in children with sickle cell disease. J Pediatr 136(6):749–753.

[35] Falk RJ, Scheinman J, Phillips G, Orringer E, Johnson A, Jennette JC. 1992. Prevalence and pathologic features of sickle cell nephropathy and response to inhibition of angiotensin-converting enzyme. N Engl J Med 326(14):910–915.

[36] Gonzalez-Carrillo M, Rudge CJ, Parsons V, Bewick M, White JM. 1982. Renal transplantation in sickle cell disease. Clin Nephrol 18(4):209–210.

[37] Collins F, Orringer E. 1982. Pulmonary hypertension and cor pulmonale in the sickle hemoglobinopathies. Am J Med 73(6):814–821.

[38] Clarkson J. 1992. The ocular manifestations of sickle-cell disease: A prevalence and natural history study. Trans Am Opthalmol Soc 90:481–504.

[39] Farber M, Jampol LM, Fox P, et al. 1991. A randomized clinical trial of scatter photocoagulation of proliferative sickle cell retinopathy. Arch Ophthalmol 109(3):363–367.

[40] Smith JA, Espeland M, Bellevue R, Bonds D, Brown AK, Koshy M. 1996. Pregnancy in sickle cell disease: Experience of the Cooperative Study of Sickle Cell Disease. Obstet Gynecol 87(2):199–204.

[41] Koshy M, Burd L. 1991. Management of pregnancy in sickle cell syndromes. Hematol Oncol Clin North Am 5(3):585–596.

[42] Rank BH, Carlsson J, Hebbel RP. 1985. Abnormal redox status of membrane-protein thiols in sickle erythrocytes. J Clin Invest 75(5):1531–1537.

[43] Repka T, Hebbel R. 1991. Hydroxyl radical formation by sickle erythrocyte membranes: Role of pathologic iron deposits and cytoplasmic reducing agents. Blood 78(10):2753–2758.

[44] Hebbel RP, Schwartz RS, Mohandas N. 1985. The adhesive sickle erythrocyte: Cause and consequence of abnormal interactions with endothelium, monocytes/macrophages and model membranes. Clin Haematol 14(1):141–161.

[45] Lard LR, Mul FP, de Haas M, Roos D, Duits AJ. 1999. Neutrophil activation in sickle cell disease. J Leukoc Biol 66(3):411–415.

[46] Fadlon E, Vordermeier S, Pearson TC, et al. 1998. Blood polymorphonuclear leukocytes from the majority of sickle cell patients in the crisis phase of the disease show enhanced adhesion to vascular endothelium and increased expression of CD62. Blood 91:266–274.

[47] Abboud M, Laver J, Blau CA. 1998. Granulocytosis causing sickle-cell crisis. Lancet 35:959.

[48] Saleh AW, Hillen HF, Duits AJ. 1999. Levels of endothelial, neutrophil and platelet-specific factors in sickle cell anemia patients during hydroxyurea therapy. Acta Haematol 102(1):31–37.

[49] Solovey A, Lin Y, Browne P, Choong S, Wayner E, Hebbel RP. 1997. Circulating activated endothelial cells in sickle cell anemia. N Engl J Med 337(22):1584–1590.

[50] Solovey AA, Solovey AN, Harkness J, Hebbel RP. 2001. Modulation of endothelial cell activation in sickle cell disease: A pilot study. Blood 97(7):1937–1941.

[51] Duits AJ, Schnog JB, Lard LR, Saleh AW, Rojer RA. 1998. Elevated IL-8 levels during sickle cell crisis. Eur J Haematol 61(5):303–305.

[52] Michaels LA, Ohene-Frempong K, Zhao H, Douglas SD. 1998. Serum levels of substance P are elevated in patients with sickle cell disease and increase further during vaso-occlusive crisis. Blood 92(9):3148–3151.

[53] Goldberg MA, Husson MA, Bunn HF. 1977. Participation of hemoglobins A and F in polymerization of sickle hemoglobin. J Biol Chem 252(10):3414–3421.

[54] Platt OS, Brambilla DJ, Rosse WF, et al. 1994. Mortality in sickle cell disease. Life expectancy and risk factors for early death. N Engl J Med 330(23):1639–1644.

[55] Koshy M, Entsuah R, Koranda A, et al. 1989. Leg ulcers in patients with sickle cell disease. Blood 74(4):1403–1408.

[56] Trabuchet G, Elion J, Baudot G, et al. 1991. Origin and spread of beta-globin gene mutations in India, Africa, and Mediterranea: Analysis of the 5′ flanking and intragenic sequences of β-S and β-C genes. Hum Biol 63(3):241–252.

[57] Miller BA, Olivieri N, Salameh M, et al. 1987. Molecular analysis of the high-hemoglobin-F phenotype in Saudi Arabian sickle cell anemia. N Engl J Med 316(5):244–250.

[58] Kar BC, Satapathy RK, Kulozik AE, et al. 1986. Sickle cell disease in Orissa State, India. Lancet 2(8517):1198–1201.

[59] Embury SH, Clark MR, Monroy G, Mohandas N. 1984. Concurrent sickle cell anemia and alpha-thalassemia. Effect on pathological properties of sickle erythrocytes. J Clin Invest 73(1):116–123.

[60] Steinberg M, Embury S. 1986. Alpha-thalassemia in blacks: Genetic and clinical aspects and interactions with the sickle hemoglobin gene. Blood 68(5):985–990.

[61] Embury SH, Backer K, Glader BE. 1985. Monovalent cation changes in sickle erythrocytes: A direct reflection of alpha-globin gene number. J Lab Clin Med 106(1):75–79.

[62] Charache S, Terrin M, Moore R, et al. 1995. Effect of hydroxyurea on the frequency of painful crises in sickle cell anemia. Investigators of the multicenter study of hydroxyurea in sickle cell anemia. N Engl J Med 332:1317–1322.

[63] Steinberg MH, Barton F, Castro O. 2003. Effect of hydroxyurea on mortality and morbidity in adult sickle cell anemia: Risks and benefits up to 9 years of treatment. JAMA 289(13):1645–1651.

[64] Kinney T, Helms R, O'Branski E, et al. 1999. Safety of hydroxyurea in children with sickle cell anemia: Results of the HUG-KIDS study, a phase I/II trial. Pediatric Hydroxyurea Group. Blood 94:1550–1554.

[65] Ferster A, Tahriri P, Vermylen C. 2001. Five years of experience with hydroxyurea in children and young adults with sickle cell disease. Blood 97(11):3628–3632.

[66] Scothorn D, Price C, Schwartz D, et al. 2002. Risk of recurrent stroke in children with sickle cell disease receiving blood transfusion therapy for at least five years after initial stroke. J Pediatr 140:348–354.

[67] Cox JV, Steane E, Cunningham G, Frenkel EP. 1988. Risk of alloimmunization and delayed hemolytic transfusion reactions in patients with sickle cell disease. Arch Intern Med 148(11):2485–2489.

[68] Vichinsky EP, Luban NL, Wright E. 2001. Stroke-prevention trial in sickle cell anemia. Transfusion 41(9):1086–1092.

[69] Tahhan H, Holbrook C, Braddy L, Brewer L, Christie J. 1994. Antigen-matched donor blood in the transfusion management of patients with sickle cell disease. Transfusion 34:562–569.

[70] Vermylen C. 2003. Hematopoietic stem cell transplantation in sickle cell disease. Blood Rev 17(3):163–166.

[71] Locatelli F, Rocha V, Reed W. 2003. Related umbilical cord blood transplant in patients with thalassemia and sickle cell disease. Blood 101(6):2137–2143.

THALASSEMIA

Dr. Thomas B. Cooley, a pediatrician from Detroit, gave the first description of thalassemia in 1925 at the annual meeting of the American Pediatric Society. He reported on five young children with severe anemia, splenomegaly, and unusual bone abnormalities. Prior to this, children with such findings were said to have "von Jaksch's anemia," an ill-defined syndrome that included leukemia, infections, and doubtless a potpourri of other conditions. Two years later, Cooley published his classic paper detailing this new clinical entity.[1] He referred to the condition as "erythroblastic anemia" because of the many nucleated red cells on the peripheral blood smear. "Mediterranean anemia" was another term used to describe the disorder, reflecting the Italian or Greek ethnicity of the affected children. Other clinicians and investigators widely adopted the eponym "Cooley's anemia" to describe the entity. Subsequent descriptions of children with similar conditions from Italy and Greece as well as the United States indicated that Cooley's anemia was more than an isolated curiosity. In 1932, Whipple and Bradford coined the term *thalassemia* from the Greek word *thalassa*, which means the sea (in this case, the Mediterranean).

Somewhat later, a mild microcytic anemia was described in family members of patients with Cooley's anemia. Affected individuals had no symptoms and lacked any of the clinical features seen within the family probands. Clinicians soon realized that this mild anemia represented heterozygous inheritance of abnormal genes. The homozygous state produced the severe disorder Cooley's anemia.

The thalassemias are a group of hereditary anemias that result from diminished synthesis of one of the two globin polypeptide chains, α and β, that combine to form adult hemoglobin A ($\alpha_2\beta_2$). In contrast to the hemoglobinopathies, the thalassemias usually produce no hemoglobin subunits other than normal α and β chains. These normal subunits can combine however in many proportions different from those seen with the normal hemoglobins. Normal hemoglobin A (Hb A) contains both α and β subunits, and the most important thalassemias are grouped as either α- or β-thalassemia.

■ GENETIC BASIS OF THE THALASSEMIAS

α-GLOBIN LOCUS

Each chromosome 16 has a ζ-globin gene and two α-globin genes aligned sequentially on the chromosome (Figure 14-1). For practical purposes, the two α-globin genes (termed $\alpha 1$ and $\alpha 2$) are identical. Since each cell has two chromosomes 16, a total of four α-globin genes exist in each cell. Each of the four genes produces about one-quarter of the α-globin chains needed for hemoglobin synthesis. The mechanism controlling this coordination is mysterious. Promoter elements reside 5' to each α-globin gene. In addition, a powerful enhancer region called the locus control region (LCR) is required for optimal gene expression. The LCR resides 5' upstream of the α-globin locus by many kilobases. The mechanism by which such distant DNA elements control globin gene expression is the source of intense investigation.

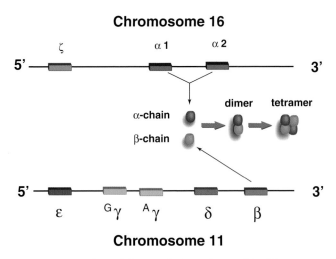

FIGURE 14–1 *Hemoglobin synthesis and assembly. Chromosome 16 is the location of the "α-like" globin gene cluster, while the "β-like" globin gene cluster exists on chromosome 11. The globin genes in each group have internal similarity while differing significantly from their counterparts in the other gene cluster. During development, the globin genes sequentially turn on and off beginning at the 5′ end of the gene cluster. The two α-globin genes on chromosome 16 (α1 and α2) produce the α-globin subunit in adult hemoglobin A. The β-globin gene on chromosome 11 produces the β-globin subunit. The quantity of globin subunit produced by the β-globin gene precisely matches the α-globin subunit production of the two α-globin genes. The individual globin subunits quickly associate to an αβ dimer. The two dimers associate to form an $\alpha_2\beta_2$ tetramer, which is the functional hemoglobin molecule.*

β-GLOBIN LOCUS

The genes in the β-globin locus are arranged sequentially from 5′ to 3′ beginning with the epsilon (ε) gene and ending with the adult β-globin gene. The sequence of the genes is ε, γ, δ, and β. Two copies of the γ gene exist on each chromosome 11 designated as $^G\gamma$ and $^A\gamma$. The other globin genes are present as single copies. Therefore, each cell has two adult β-globin genes, one on each of the two chromosomes 11. These two β-globin genes express their globin protein in a quantity that precisely matches that of the four α-globin genes. The mechanism that maintains this balanced gene expression remains elusive.

Solitary γ- and β-globin chains are extremely unstable. One α-globin chain and one β-globin chain combine to form a dimer (αβ) immediately following synthesis as shown in Figure 14-1. However, the globin dimer cannot bind oxygen. Two dimers combine to form a tetramer ($\alpha_2\beta_2$), which is the functionally complete hemoglobin molecule capable of reversible oxygen binding. Any process that interferes with the production of the $\alpha_2\beta_2$ hemoglobin tetramer creates a pathological condition. The thalassemias profoundly derange hemoglobin tetramer synthesis.

TABLE 14-1 | **HUMAN HEMOGLOBINS**

Embryonic Hemoglobins	*Fetal Hemoglobin*	*Adult Hemoglobins*
Gower 1—zeta$_2$epsilon$_2$ ($\zeta_2 \varepsilon_2$)	Hemoglobin F— alpha$_2$gamma$_2$ ($\alpha_2 \gamma_2$)	Hemoglobin A— alpha$_2$beta$_2$ ($\alpha_2 \beta_2$)
Gower 2—alpha$_2$epsilon$_2$ ($\alpha_2 \varepsilon_2$)		Hemoglobin A2— alpha$_2$delta$_2$ ($\alpha_2 \delta_2$)
Portland—zeta$_2$gamma$_2$ ($\zeta_2 \gamma_2$)		

ONTOGENY OF HEMOGLOBIN SYNTHESIS

The globin genes are activated in sequence during development, moving from $5'$ to $3'$ on the chromosome. The ζ gene of the α-globin gene cluster is expressed only during the first few weeks of embryogenesis (Table 14-1). Thereafter, the α-globin genes take over. For the β-globin gene cluster, ε-gene expression occurs first during embryogensis. The γ gene is expressed during fetal development. Just before birth, the production of γ globin begins to decline in concert with a rise in β-globin synthesis. A significant amount of fetal hemoglobin persists for 7 or 8 months after birth. However, most people have only trace amounts ($<2.0\%$) of fetal hemoglobin after the first year of life. The combination of two α subunits and two β subunits forms complete hemoglobin A.

The δ-globin gene, located between the γ- and β-globin genes on chromosome 11, produces a small amount of δ globin in children and adults. The product of the δ-globin gene is called hemoglobin A2 ($\alpha_2\delta_2$), and normally comprises less than 3.5% of hemoglobin in children and adults.

■ β-THALASSEMIA SYNDROMES

The β-thalassemia syndromes reflect abnormalities of the β-gene complex located on chromosome 11.[2] More than 150 different mutations have been described. Most of these are single nucleotide substitutions. Mutations that disrupt the function of the β-globin gene promoter reduce the rate of gene transcription. Deletions or mutations that produce abnormal cleavage or splicing of β-globin RNA can also produce thalassemia. The abnormal message often is unstable and is degraded prior to translation. In other cases, translation begins only to abort before the process is complete. Some mutations completely eliminate β-chain production and are designated as "β^0-thalassemias." Other mutations dampen but do not abrogate β-globin synthesis, producing the "β^+-thalassemias." The precise level of β-globin gene synthesis varies among the specific β^+-thalassemia mutations.

The variable degree of β-subunit expression produces a spectrum of clinical expression that at times is bewildering. The impact of nonhematological factors such as hypersplenism adds an additional layer of complexity. Nonetheless, a rough correlation exists between the genetic classification and the clinical presentation.

- Thalassemia trait (minor)—normal β^A gene/thalassemic gene (β^0 or β^+)
- Thalassemia intermedia—often two β^+ genes.
- Thalassemia major—two β^+ genes (where the plus is not substantial); β^+ gene/β^0 gene; β^0 gene/β^0 gene.

The relationship between genetics and clinical expression is approximate, at best. The presumed genotype of a person with thalassemia can only be confirmed by identification of the thalassemia genes using careful genetic analysis.

The β-thalassemia genes have a worldwide distribution, being particularly prevalent in southern Italy and Greece where gene frequencies of 2–5% or more exist. A high prevalence of β-thalassemia also occurs in the Middle East, the Indian subcontinent, southern China, and Southeast Asia. About 1400 children with β-thalassemia are born each year in Egypt, while in India the figure is close to 10,000. β-Thalassemia is rare in people of north European ancestry and is found in about 0.5% of African Americans. The high prevalence of thalassemia in tropical areas likely derives from a relative resistance to malaria in people who are heterozygous for the condition (balanced polymorphism) (see Chapter 6).

HETEROZYGOUS β-THALASSEMIA (THALASSEMIA MINOR, THALASSEMIA TRAIT)

Heterozygosity for a β-thalassemia gene lowers β-chain synthesis with a consequent reduction in hemoglobin A production and a mild anemia. Hemoglobin levels are 1.0–2.0 g/dL lower than in normal persons of the same age and gender. The anemia often worsens during pregnancy. This mild anemia usually produces no symptoms, and longevity is normal.

Microcytosis and red cell hypochromia characterize thalassemia trait. Target cells, ovalocytes, and basophilic stippling on the peripheral blood smear are usual findings (Figure 14-2). Mean corpuscular volume (MCV) and mean corpuscular hemoglobin (MCH) determined by electronic cell counters are both low. The MCV characteristically falls below 75 fL, with a mean MCV of 68 fL in typical β-thalassemia trait. The MCV is disproportionately low for the degree of anemia, reflecting a red cell count that is normal or elevated despite a low hemoglobin value. Iron studies (transferrin saturation and serum ferritin) are normal and administration of iron does not improve the anemia.

The RDW is normal in thalassemia trait. This observation can be an early clue that distinguishes β-thalassemia trait from iron deficiency anemia, where the RDW typically is high. The ratio of MCV/RBC (Mentzer index) is <11 in thalassemia trait but >12 in iron deficiency. A hemoglobin electrophoresis confirms the diagnosis of β-thalassemia trait in an individual with microcytic erythrocytes by quantifying the level

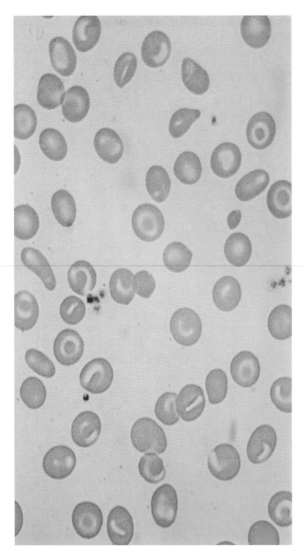

FIGURE 14–2 *Peripheral blood smear in thalassemia trait. The red cells are small and hypochromic. Target cells are prominent. (From Kamff CT, Jandl JH. 1991.* Blood: Atlas and Sourcebook of Hematology, *2nd edn. Boston: Little, Brown and Company. Figure 12-3, p. 29.)*

of the normal, minor hemoglobin component Hb A2 ($\alpha_2\delta_2$). The normal values for Hb A2 range between 1.5% and 3.4%. Erythrocyte microcytosis and elevated quantities of Hb A2 (>3.5%) confirm the diagnosis of what is called *classical* thalassemia trait, the most common form of β-thalassemia trait. Levels of Hb F ($\alpha_2\gamma_2$) are normal (<2.0%) in about half of the individuals with classical thalassemia trait and only moderately elevated (2.0–7%) in the remainder.

A less common form of β-thalassemia trait, β–δ thalassemia trait, results from a deletion of the δ-globin gene and most of or the entire β-globin gene. Familial microcytosis, normal levels of Hb A2, and high levels of Hb F (5–15%) are typical of the condition. Lepore hemoglobin trait, another variant of β-thalassemia, is characterized by the presence of 5–10% hemoglobin Lepore, a hemoglobin that migrates electrophoretically in the position of hemoglobin S. Lepore hemoglobin, a fusion product resulting from an unequal crossover between β and δ genes, is associated with decreased β-chain synthesis. Occasionally, a so-called *silent carrier* can be identified as having a β-thalassemia gene on the basis of being the parent of a child with severe thalassemia. The silent carrier has slight or no microcytosis and no elevation of Hb A2 or Hb F.

The rationale for establishing a diagnosis of β-thalassemia trait is to avoid unnecessary treatment with medicinal iron and to provide genetic counseling. A couple where the partners have β-thalassemia trait faces a 25% risk of having a child with homozygous β-thalassemia with each pregnancy. Populations with a high prevalence of thalassemia trait can be screened in order to provide genetic counseling. In Connecticut more than 10,000 people of Mediterranean ancestry were screened for thalassemia by measuring MCV, followed by Hb A2 determination when MCV values fell below 75 fL. In pregnancies at risk of producing a child with homozygous β-thalassemia, prenatal diagnosis can be performed by as early as 10–12 weeks of gestation using fetal DNA obtained by chorionic villus biopsy. This approach has greatly reduced the incidence of new cases of β-thalassemia major in Italy and Cyprus as well in many Greek American and Italian American communities in the United States.

HOMOZYGOUS β-THALASSEMIA (THALASSEMIA MAJOR, COOLEY'S ANEMIA)

Homozygosity or double heterozygosity for β-thalassemia genes usually produces severe anemia due to the marked reduction in synthesis of the β-globin chains of Hb A. The muted synthesis of Hb A does not however explain the marked hemolysis and ineffective erythropoiesis that feature prominently with these disorders. These problems are a consequence of *unbalanced* globin chain synthesis. In homozygous β-thalassemia, α-globin chains produced in normal amounts accumulate, denature, and precipitate in red cell precursors within the bone marrow and in circulating erythrocytes. These precipitated α-globin chains, so-called Fessas bodies, damage the membrane of the red cells leading to their destruction within the bone marrow (ineffective erythropoiesis). The injury also causes rapid destruction of the erythrocytes that reach the peripheral blood (hemolysis).

The fetus and the newborn infant with homozygous β-thalassemia are clinically and hematologically normal since Hb F ($\alpha_2\gamma_2$) predominates during fetal development. However, in vitro assays demonstrate reduced or absent β-chain synthesis. Increasingly, diagnosis of homozygous β-thalassemia in the United States comes with neonatal hemoglobinopathy screening, which is now conducted in 47 of the United States and the District of Columbia. Hemoglobin patterns of affected infants show only Hb F and no Hb A.

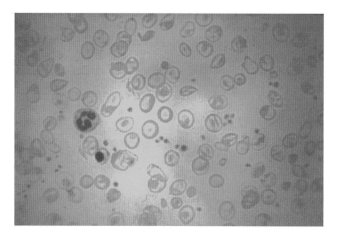

FIGURE 14–3 *Peripheral blood smear in thalassemia major. The red cell morphology is strikingly abnormal with marked hypochromia, many microcytes, bizarre poikilocytes, and target cells. Note the large, thin wrinkled, and folded erythrocytes containing irregular inclusions. Supravital stain shows these to be aggregates of precipitated α-globin chains. Nucleated red cells are invariably present.*

The clinical onset of β-thalassemia major occurs gradually over the first 6–12 months after birth when the normal postnatal switch from synthesis of γ-chains to β-chains causes a slow decline in hemoglobin F levels. By the age of 6–12 months, progressive pallor, irritability, growth retardation, jaundice, and hepatosplenomegaly due to extramedullary hematopoiesis characterize the clinical picture of most affected infants. By 2 years of age, 90% of infants are anemic and symptomatic to the point that transfusions are necessary. The hemoglobin level sometimes falls to values as low as 3.0–5.0 g/dL. Progressive changes in the facial and cranial bones reflect massive expansion of the erythroid marrow, producing characteristic and disfiguring cosmetic changes.

The red cell morphology is strikingly abnormal with marked hypochromia, many microcytes, bizarre poikilocytes, and target cells (Figure 14-3). A characteristic finding is that of large, thin wrinkled, and folded erythrocytes often containing irregular inclusions that supravital stain shows to be aggregates of precipitated α-globin chains. Nucleated red cells are invariably present. The reticulocyte count is moderately elevated at 5–8%. The white blood cell count, corrected for nucleated red cells, also is moderately elevated. The platelet count is normal or increased but can be low if the spleen is enlarged. Splenectomy produces thrombocytosis ($>750,000/mm^3$) and large numbers of nucleated red cells. High indirect bilirubin levels reflect rapid turnover of hemoglobin due to the ineffective erythropoiesis and hemolysis.

Hemoglobin F dominates the hemoglobin electrophoretic pattern. Hemoglobin A is absent when the thalassemia is due to homozygous β^0-thalassemia genes. Small amounts of Hb A occur when one or both genes are from the β^+-thalassemia subgroup.

Hemoglobin A2 values tend to parallel the levels of Hb A; they can be high or low and are of little diagnostic value.

The severe anemia necessitates regular red cell transfusions in more than 80% of children with homozygous β-thalassemia by 1–2 years of age. Life expectancy of untreated thalassemia major is less than 5 years. Prior to about 1970, children with severe, symptomatic anemia received transfusions only intermittently. Hemoglobin levels at the time of transfusion often were as low as 4.0–6.0 gm/dL. The clinical features of infrequently transfused thalassemia major patients reflected severe anemia: irritability, fatigability, listlessness, and anorexia were prominent symptoms. Cardiomegaly, flow murmurs, scleral icterus, and gallstones were common. Growth retardation was marked and puberty was rare.

The extreme ineffective erythropoiesis associated with poorly transfused thalassemia major evoked massive hypertrophy of the erythroid marrow, with expansion of the erythroid tissue by as much as 30-fold. Marrow expansion in the maxilla and facial bones produced severe cosmetic deformity including overgrowth and protrusion of the upper jaw with malocclusion and jumbling of the teeth. The malar eminences were prominent, giving the eyes a mongoloid slant (Cooley's facies) and producing a strikingly similar appearance among these children (Figure 14-4). Expansion of the marrow cavity of the cranial bones caused enlargement of the skull with frontal and parietal bossing. Radiographs showed widened dipole with perpendicular bone trabeculae giving a classic hair-on-end appearance. Expansion of the marrow cavities of the long bones produced marked cortical bone thinning with pathological fractures being a common sequela. Extramedullary hematopoiesis in the liver and spleen caused abdominal enlargement due to progressive hepatosplenomegaly. Paraspinal masses due to extramedullary hematopoiesis sometimes developed, with occasional spinal cord compression.

The average age at death was 15–20 years. Few patients survived into the late twenties. This shortened survival derived not only from the severe anemia, but also from a progressive increase in the body iron burden, largely a consequence of transfusions and increased dietary iron absorption. Each unit of transfused blood delivers about 250 mg of iron to the body iron stores with no physiological means for its removal. Large iron accumulations in the liver, pancreas, endocrine glands, and heart produced fibrosis and permanent tissue damage.

Failure of sexual development was frequent, reflecting early damage to the hypothalamic-pituitary-gonadal axis. Diabetes mellitus, hepatic fibrosis, and endocrinopathies including hypothyroidism and hypoparathyroidism were a consequence of iron deposition in these organs. Myocardial siderosis and fibrosis developed by the second decade of life, manifested by cardiac tachyarrhythmias and ultimately by refractory congestive heart failure, the most common cause of death.

Beginning in the 1970s, more vigorous transfusion programs, called "hypertransfusion," were instituted with the aim of maintaining a minimum hemoglobin level of 10.0 g/dL. The goal was to reduce the consequences of severe anemia and marrow hypertrophy. Hypertransfusion has significant advantages over a limited transfusion regimen and should be employed whenever possible. Activity, exercise tolerance, and sense of well-being are improved. The deforming cosmetic changes of the face

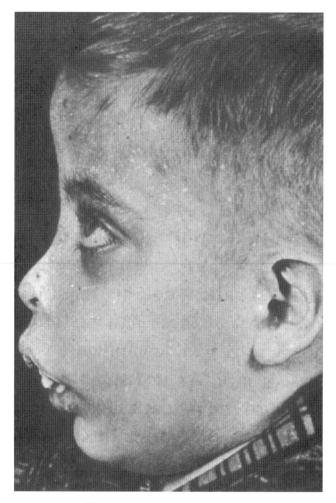

FIGURE 14–4 *Thalassemia facies.*

are averted. Osteoporosis of the long bones is lessened as are pathologic fractures. Splenomegaly is less prominent. Growth is enhanced. The iron accumulation of patients receiving hypertransfusion is not significantly greater than that produced by minimal transfusion programs. Hypertransfusion alone does not increase longevity in thalassemia major, but considerably improves the quality of life.

By the second decade of life, these patients have massive total body iron accumulation as indicated by substantially high levels of serum ferritin ($>2500\,\text{ng/mL}$) and by increased tissue iron deposition, as quantified by liver biopsy or SQUID (*S*uperconducting *qu*antum *i*nterference *d*evice) analysis. Minimally transfused patients developed massive splenomegaly, requiring splenectomy in early life. Massive splenomegaly is unusual in children on hypertransfusion regimens.

With age, patients often develop transfusion requirements that exceed 200 mL of red cells per kilogram body weight per year. In this circumstance, splenectomy often is performed to improve survival of transfused red cells. Because of the higher risk of bacterial septicemia following splenectomy, especially in children younger than 6 years, immunization with pneumococcal and *Haemophilus influenzae Type B* vaccines is recommended. Children younger than 6 years of age require prophylactic antibiotic therapy.

THALASSEMIA INTERMEDIA

Clinical phenotype defines thalassemia intermedia. Patients have an anemia that is more severe than occurs in thalassemia trait and less severe than is seen with thalassemia major. Most commonly, the question in such patients is whether the diagnosis is thalassemia intermedia or thalassemia major. Thalassemia intermedia is not defined by a precise hemoglobin value; rather the hemoglobin value and the patient's tolerance of the anemia determine whether thalassemia intermedia is the appropriate label.

Most thalassemia patients with hemoglobin values much below 7 or 8 g/dL require transfusions and therefore fall under the heading of thalassemia major. On the other hand, some patients can maintain a baseline hemoglobin value of about 9–10 g/dL. Here, exercise tolerance and energy levels are significantly better than is the case with lower values. The key issue then is whether the accelerated bone marrow activity needed to maintain this hemoglobin level causes unacceptable side effects such as bone abnormalities or splenic enlargement. This is a judgment decision. Most physicians with a patient at the critical borderline would advise transfusion to prevent the bone abnormalities in particular, even if they are modest. The patient then would be *clinically* classified as having thalassemia major. Other physicians after weighing risks and benefits might suggest avoiding the complications of chronic transfusion. The same patient then would be *clinically* classified as having thalassemia intermedia. The thalassemia is more severe than thalassemia trait, but the patient does not receive chronic transfusions, as occurs with thalassemia major.

A patient can change status. All patients with significant anemia due to thalassemia have some degree of splenomegaly. The spleen plays an important role in clearing damaged red cells from the blood stream. Since all red cells in patients with severe thalassemia are damaged to some degree, erythrocyte clearance by the spleen accelerates the rate of cell loss. Enhanced erythropoiesis compensates for this loss. In some instances, removal of the spleen reduces the rate of red cell destruction just enough so that patients can manage without transfusion and still not have unacceptable side effects. In this case, the patient converts *clinically* from thalassemia major to thalassemia intermedia.

The molecular basis of β-thalassemia intermedia is complex and puzzling. Most people with the syndrome are homozygotes or compound heterozygotes either with two mild β-thalassemia alleles or two severe alleles plus a modifier such as α-thalassemia. Uncommonly, two severe alleles with no known modifier unexpectedly manifest the milder intermedia state. Conversely, β-thalassemia intermedia with one defective β-globin gene usually reflects excessively severe imbalance in globin synthesis due to a very severe β-globin mutation or a condition that produces an excess number of α-globin chains.

The α-globin gene status is an important moderator of clinical expression in β-thalassemia. Patients with β-thalassemia can independently inherit two-gene deletion α-thalassemia due to a defect involving the α-globin genes on chromosome 16. The dampened production of α-globin subunits reduces the degree of α/β-subunit imbalance. (The β-thalassemia defect decreases β-subunit production while the α-thalassemia defect lowers α-subunit production.) Since α/β-subunit imbalance in erythroid cells is key to the anemia in thalassemia, the coinheritance of β-thalassemia and α-thalassemia can paradoxically lessen the severity of the anemia. Conversely, the coinheritance of β-thalassemia and either five or six α-globin genes exacerbates α/β-chain imbalance and worsens the degree of anemia.

Significant overlap in the distribution of α-thalassemia and β-thalassemia occurs in many regions of the world, including India and Southeast Asia. Coinheritance of α-thalassemia and β-thalassemia is therefore more common than would be expected at first blush. α-Thalassemia is less common in people of Mediterranean ancestry, but at times is a moderating factor in these patients as well.

HEMOGLOBIN E/β-THALASSEMIA

Although the presence of hemoglobin E is a hemoglobinopathy, discussion of the condition falls most appropriately under the thalassemia umbrella. Other hemoglobinopathies have clinically significant manifestations when paired with a thalassemia gene. For instance, the gene for sickle cell disease paired with a β-thalassemia gene produces a severe phenotype that resembles homozygous sickle cell disease, namely sickle β-thalassemia. Hemoglobin E is singular in that the aberrant hemoglobin, either in heterozygous combination with hemoglobin A or as a homozygous condition, has a relatively mild phenotype. This contrasts with the combination of hemoglobin E with a β-thalassemia gene where a severe condition results that in most cases clinically resembles either thalassemia intermedia or thalassemia major.

Hemoglobin E is one of the most common hemoglobin variants in the world, with its epicenter of expression in Southeast Asia. In some regions of Thailand, up to 15% of people carry the hemoglobin E gene. Therefore, hemoglobin E/β-thalassemia is one of the most important genetic causes of severe anemia in the world. The increase in worldwide population migration means that hemoglobin E is increasingly frequent in nations around the globe.

Hemoglobin E has a mutation at the 26th amino acid position of the hemoglobin β subunit that replaces the normal glutamic acid with a lysine residue. For complex biochemical and biophysical reasons, erythroid precursors produce hemoglobin E at a rate lower than that of hemoglobin A.[3] In people with heterozygous hemoglobin β^A/β^E, hemoglobin E comprises between 30% and 35% of the hemoglobin in the cell. The red cell characteristics of these heterozygotes superficially resemble those seen in thalassemia trait. The MCH is lower than normal. The MCV is also depressed, with a median value of about 73 fL. Together, the result is small red cells with a normal mean corpuscular hemoglobin concentration (MCHC), as is the case with thalassemia trait.[4] People with heterozygous hemoglobin β^A/β^E have no symptoms.

People with homozygous hemoglobin E are also asymptomatic. Hemoglobin levels are normal or only slightly depressed. Patients have a mean MCV 67 fL and a normal MCHC. Both reticulocyte count and red cell survival are within normal limits.[5] Target cells are prominent on the peripheral smear.

In contrast to benignity of hemoglobin E trait and the homozygous hemoglobin E state, hemoglobin E/β-thalassemia produces an anemia that is unexpectedly severe and surprisingly variable. Although some patients with hemoglobin E/β-thalassemia are asymptomatic or have mild disease, about half require chronic transfusions and resemble patients with thalassemia major.[6] Reports on the condition commonly note hemoglobin values that range between 3 and 13 g/dL with no clear explanation for this remarkable variation. The only agreed upon moderating factor is elevated hemoglobin F levels. Hemoglobin F, however, is not a major contributor to most cases of clinically mild or moderate hemoglobin E/β-thalassemia.[7]

■ α-THALASSEMIA

The α-thalassemia syndromes are prevalent in people of southeastern Asian ancestry and are due usually to deletion of one or more of the four α-globin genes on chromosomes 16. In general, the severity is proportional to the number of deleted α-globin genes. DNA analysis allows quantification of the number of α-globin genes.

SILENT CARRIER (α-2-THALASSEMIA TRAIT, -α/$\alpha\alpha$)

People with a single α-globin gene deletion are clinically and hematologically normal. The presence of a small amount (1–3%) of the fast migrating hemoglobin Barts (γ_4) on neonatal hemoglobin electrophoresis is sometimes a clue to the presence of single α-globin gene deletion. In later life, determination of the number of α-globin genes by DNA analysis is the sole laboratory means of making the diagnosis.

Family history is a powerful tool in the analysis of all types of thalassemia. A careful history sometimes provides strong support for the diagnosis of single-gene deletion α-thalassemia. For instance, a child with hemoglobin H disease sometimes has one parent with two-gene deletion α-thalassemia and one parent who appears to be normal. Since the third absent α-globin gene in the child could have come only from the "normal" parent, this parent by exclusion has single-gene deletion α-thalassemia.

α-1-THALASSEMIA TRAIT (-α/-α OR --/$\alpha\alpha$)

Mild microcytic anemia is the clinical manifestation with deletion of two of four α-globin genes. At birth, a relative microcytosis exists along with 5–8% hemoglobin

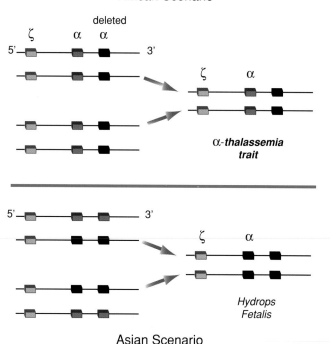

FIGURE 14–5 *Offspring of parents with two-gene deletion α-thalassemia. The upper panel shows the African orientation of two-gene deletion α-thalassemia (α-thalassemia trait). The most severe combination possible for the offspring produces α-thalassemia trait. The lower panel shows the Asian orientation of two-gene deletion α-thalassemia trait. The most severe combination possible for the offspring produces hydrops fetalis.*

Barts on hemoglobin electrophoresis. Hemoglobin Barts disappears by 3–6 months of age, and the hemoglobin electrophoresis thereafter is normal. After the newborn period, a definitive diagnosis by DNA Southern blot analysis often is impractical for this mild disorder. Exclusion of other causes of microcytic anemia such as β-thalassemia trait or iron deficiency leaves two-gene deletion α-thalassemia as a presumptive diagnosis. α-1-Thalassemia trait can arise in either of two ways: the two deleted α genes can exist on the same chromosome 16 (designated as cis deletions) or one gene can be deleted from each of the chromosomes 16 (designated as trans deletions; Figure 14-5).

  The cis orientation of α-gene deletion is usual in people of Southeast Asian heritage, while trans deletions are the norm in people of African ethnicity. The distinction carries important clinical implications. While α-thalassemia is common in African peoples, the trans configuration of the α-globin gene deletion means that a maximum of two genes can be deleted in any individual. Consequently, the more severe α-thalassemia syndromes are not seen in these populations.

HEMOGLOBIN H DISEASE (--/-α)

Deletion of three α-globin genes produces hemoglobin H disease with a marked imbalance between α- and β- globin chain synthesis. Excess free β chains accumulate and combine to form a tetramer of β chains (β_4) called hemoglobin H. Hemoglobin H is unstable and precipitates within red cells, particularly at the plasma membrane. This precipitated material produces membrane damage, including oxidant injury by reactive oxygen species. The reticuloendothelial system removes the damaged erythrocytes from the circulation producing a chronic microcytic, hemolytic anemia. Laboratory findings include a moderately severe microcytic anemia (hemoglobin values of 6.0–10.0 gm/dL) along with evidence of hemolysis.[8] Supravital staining of the red cells demonstrates clumps of precipitated hemoglobin H called Heinz bodies. Hemoglobin H has a fast mobility on hemoglobin electrophoresis and accounts for 10–15% of the total hemoglobin.

Many patients with hemoglobin H disease have a hemoglobin variant, Hb Constant Spring, on electrophoresis. In these instances the genotype is ($-/\alpha^{CS}\alpha$). Hb Constant Spring is an abnormally long α chain created by a mutation in the termination codon of the α-globin gene with consequent readthrough into the $3'$ untranslated region of the message. Hb Constant Spring mRNA is unstable and rapidly degraded, producing a lower than expected representation of α^{CS} in the hemoglobin mix.

Hb Constant Spring is the most prevalent nondeletional α-thalassemia condition, with a gene frequency of about 8% in Southeast Asia. However, the hemoglobin variant occurs in nearly 50% of people with Hb H disease in this region of the world. Ironically, anemia is more severe in patients with Hb Constant Spring than is the case for routine three-gene deletion Hb H disease.[9] The average hemoglobin in these patients is about 2 g/dL lower than that seen in three-gene deletion Hb H disease although the degree of microcytosis is less pronounced. Splenomegaly is more striking in these patients and they are more likely to require transfusions.

FETAL HYDROPS SYNDROME (--/--)

Deletion of all four α-globin genes produces the syndrome of hydrops fetalis with stillbirth or death in the immediate postnatal period. In the absence of α-chain synthesis, such fetuses cannot synthesize any of the normal human hemoglobins with the exception of embryonic hemoglobins gower 1 and Portland (see Table 14-1). At birth, hemoglobin electrophoresis shows predominantly Barts hemoglobin (γ_4) and small amounts of hemoglobin H (β_4) as well as embryonic hemoglobins.

The high oxygen affinity of Barts hemoglobin makes it ineffective in oxygen transport with consequent intrauterine manifestations of severe hypoxia out of proportion to the degree of anemia. A number of infants with this syndrome identified by prenatal diagnosis and treated with intrauterine and postnatal transfusions have survived. These patients require chronic transfusions to survive, but some have developed normally. As with thalassemia major, the only cure is bone marrow transplantation. At present, termination of the pregnancy is usually recommended because of a high frequency of severe maternal toxemia caused by carrying a hydropic fetus.

■ HEREDITARY PERSISTENCE OF FETAL HEMOGLOBIN

Thalassemia results from an imbalance in the α/β-globin chain ratio in erythroid cells. Any phenomenon that moderates or corrects that imbalance will improve or eliminate the thalassemia. As shown in Figure 14-1, both the α- and β-globin gene clusters contain genes encoding globin chains whose production is restricted to brief windows during life. Particularly intriguing in this regard are the γ-globin genes on chromosome 11 that encode the β-like subunits found in Hb F ($\alpha_2\gamma_2$). Hb F exists in large quantities only during fetal development. The hemoglobin has a higher oxygen affinity than Hb A, but its functional activity is in a range that allows physiologically acceptable oxygen delivery.

For the β-thalassemias, γ-globin could possibly act as a "stand in" for the missing β-globin, allowing affected persons to survive using Hb F in the stead of Hb A. The syndromes called hereditary persistence of fetal hemoglobin (HPFH) involve genetic alterations that foster abundant production of Hb F long after its normal shut off time. Coincident inheritance of HPFH and β-thalassemia permits ongoing production of γ-globin subunits after birth and compensates for the functionally defective β-globin genes. The persistent production of γ-globin partially or completely corrects the imbalance in α/β-globin chain ratio and moderates the severity of the thalassemia.

A myriad of genetic events can prompt persistent production of Hb F. As with all genes, promoter elements in the 5′ untranslated region adjacent to the each of the two γ-globin genes are vital to the expression of γ-globin subunits. Perturbations in DNA structure within these regions can override the normal shutoff of γ-globin gene expression late in fetal development. Most often these promoter modifications are point mutations. Other DNA sequences called enhancers exist 3′ to the β-globin gene and can also modulate globin gene expression. Deletions of critical regions within the β-globin gene complex can produce scenarios in which these enhancers foster γ-globin synthesis into the postnatal phase of life.

The deletional forms of HPFH generally involve removal of very large segments of DNA that stretch from just 3′ to the γ-globin genes into the 3′ segment well beyond the β-globin gene (Figure 14-6). The basis of the sustained production of Hb F is unclear, but the change could reflect the closer proximity of 3′ enhancer segments to the two γ-globin genes that results from the deletion. The deletions completely remove the δ-globin and β-globin genes, eliminating production of both Hb A and Hb A2 by the affected chromosome. The heterozygous state produces no anemia, and 20–30% of the hemoglobin in red cells is Hb F. Hb F is evenly distributed within the erythrocytes, a manifestation called pan-cellular Hb F. Homozygotes for deletional HPFH are healthy with red cells that are slightly microcytic and contain 100% Hb F.

The nondeletional forms of HPFH derive from point mutations in the promoter regions of the γ genes that override the signals that normally shut off γ-globin gene transcription. The mutations probably alter the interactions of the promoter with trans acting regulator proteins. Hb F levels vary between 3% and 30%, with a distribution that can be either pan-cellular or heterocellular.

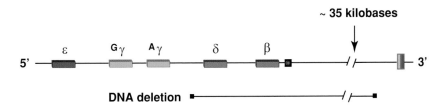

■ β-globin gene enhancer

▌ Enhancer-like element

FIGURE 14–6 *Deletional hereditary persistence of fetal hemoglobin. A region of DNA with enhancer-like activity exists on chromosome 11 at about 35 kilobases 3' of the β-globin gene. A deletion of a segment of DNA on the chromosome such as that shown in the figure eliminates the δ- and β-globin genes. The deletion also moves the previously distant enhancer-like DNA region into close proximity to the γ-globin genes. This juxtaposition activates γ-globin gene activity by mechanisms yet unclear. (Adapted from Forget B. 1998. Ann N Y Acad Sci 850:38–44).*

Either form of HPFH can moderate the severity of β-thalassemia by producing Hb F in quantities sufficient to compensate for the deficit in Hb A synthesis. In these instances, the degree of anemia correlates with the vigor of Hb F production associated with the particular HPFH syndrome. Sometimes, patients who would have thalassemia major on the basis of their β-gene mutations have instead only mild anemia, thanks to the effect of HPFH.

■ **SEQUELAE OF THALASSEMIA**

The sections on the severe thalassemia syndromes such as thalassemia major and hemoglobin E/β-thalassemia detail the complications that arise due to the anemia, including hepatosplenomegaly, osteoporosis, and high-output congestive heart failure. Chronic transfusion therapy for severe thalassemia eliminates most of these problems, but introduces a new set of concerns. Table 14-2 outlines some of the major problems in patients with thalassemia who regularly receive transfusions. Iron overload dominates the picture, with cardiac and hepatic complications occupying center stage.

Congestive cardiomyopathy is the most common cardiac defect produced by iron overload, but other problems have been described including pericarditis, restrictive cardiomyopathy, and angina without coronary artery disease. A strong correlation exists between the cumulative number of blood transfusions and functional cardiac derangements in patients with thalassemia.[10] Echocardiographic assessment of patients with β-thalassemia major who receive concurrent chelation therapy with deferoxamine shows no difference in fractional shortening relative to controls.[11] The clear message is that effective chelation therapy prevents major cardiac complications due to transfusional iron overload.

TABLE 14-2 | **SEQUELAE OF THALASSEMIA IN CHRONICALLY TRANSFUSED PATIENTS**

Trigger	*Effect*
Iron overload	Cardiac • Arrhythmias • Congestive heart failure Hepatic • Fibrosis, cirrhosis • Hepatocellular carcinoma Endocrine • Short stature (growth hormone deficiency) • Diabetes • Infertility
Infection	Hepatitis C HIV
Other	Thrombosis Pulmonary arterial hypertension Leg ulcers

The physical examination is surprisingly benign even in patients with heavy cardiac iron deposition. Once evidence of cardiac failure appears, however, heart function rapidly deteriorates, often without response to medical intervention. Biventricular failure produces pulmonary congestion, peripheral edema, and hepatic engorgement. An S3 cardiac gallop, bibasilar rales, and tender hepatosplenomegaly are prominent features on clinical examination. This potentially lethal cardiac complication has been reversed on occasion by vigorous iron extrication. Iron deposition in the bundle of His and the Purkinje system impairs signal conduction from the atrial pacemaker to the ventricles. Patients sometimes die suddenly, presumably due to arrhythmias.

Echocardiography in children and radionuclide ventriculography in adults are the noninvasive diagnostic techniques used most commonly to assess the cardiac impact of transfusional iron overload. Unfortunately, both approaches provided information of only limited utility. The correlation between echocardiographic abnormalities and the number of transfusions is rough at best. Exercise radionuclide ventriculograms is more sensitive in the detection of cardiac dysfunction in patients with iron overload, but has significant shortcomings nonetheless. Reports from investigational cardiac MRI show the technique to be more sensitive to cardiac iron deposition than either of the current clinical approaches.[12] However, significant refinement is needed to bring the approach into the clinical arena.

The other major transfusion-related problem for patients with severe thalassemia is viral infection due to blood contamination. The advent of screening for the most important viruses, hepatitis C and HIV, has greatly lessened but not eliminated the risk of infection. The number of thalassemia patients with hepatitis C has declined in the United States due to the screening procedures for both blood donors and the units of blood themselves. Significant issues with bloodborne infection remain in many countries where screening is more difficult and bloodborne viruses are more prevalent in the population. Hepatitis C is extraordinarily common in Egypt, for instance, where between 15% and 20% of people are infected with the virus.[13] The disease prevalence is even higher in some regions of the Nile delta.[14] The problem derives from efforts to eradicate schistosomiasis using parenteral drug administration in the 1970s before isolation of the hepatitis C virus (HCV).

The nature of the HCV was a mystery until the 1990s. A member of the Flaviviridae family of RNA viruses, the HCV, destroys hepatic parenchymal cells over times ranging from years to decades. Hepatic fibrosis and cirrhosis are the consequences of chronic infection. Without intervention 10% or more of people develop end-stage liver disease.[15]

Hepatitis C viral infection produces relatively little inflammation or immune response as it slowly destroys hepatic parenchymal cells. Consequently, progression of the disease often is quite insidious. Abnormalities in liver biochemical enzymes such as aspartate aminotransferase and alanine aminotransferase typically are remarkably mild. Progression to cirrhosis increases the risk of hepatocellular carcinoma.[16] Hepatic iron overload independently predisposes to hepatocellular carcinoma. The combination of the two is particularly minatory.

Pulmonary arterial hypertension is increasingly recognized as an insidious and sometimes deadly problem in patients with transfusion-dependent thalassemia. The problem possibly stems from a predisposition to venous thrombosis with chronic showering of the pulmonary arterial bed with microthrombi. Over time these small episodes lead to fixed damage to the vascular bed and high pulmonary arterial resistance.

The emergence of pulmonary arterial hypertension as a problem in these patients is due both to longer survival and better control of problems such as iron overload that long dominated the clinical picture. Right-sided heart failure develops producing arterial and ventricular filling and ejection abnormalities. Dependent edema is a common sequela. Passive hepatic congestion can produce painful enlargement of the organ that sometimes is superimposed on hepatomegaly related to the thalassemia. Hepatic fibrosis and cirrhosis are serious concerns particularly in a setting that also includes substantial hepatic iron overload.

■ IRON CHELATION

Because no physiological mechanism for iron excretion exists, iron-chelating compounds that bind the element and promote its excretion in urine and bile are essential to the treatment of transfusional iron overload in patients with thalassemia. The only approved iron chelator in the United States is deferoxamine (Desferal, DF), which is a siderophore produced by *Streptomyces pilosus*. Deferoxamine is an effective and nearly specific iron-chelating agent with low toxicity. For maximal effectiveness the chelator must be given either subcutaneously or intravenously over an extended period of time. The drug is usually infused subcutaneously over 8–10 hours during sleep using a battery-driven infusion pump. The usual dose is 40–50 mg/kg, five nights each week. Regular use of DF prevents endocrine, cardiac, and hepatic abnormalities related to iron overload and significantly extends life expectancy.

Iron overload promotes the production of a number of reactive oxygen species of which the hydroxyl radical is the most damaging ($^\bullet$OH).[17,18] The molecule is both extremely short-lived and extremely active in its interaction with biological molecules. Lipid peroxides, protein disulfide bridges, and DNA cross-linking are some of the problems that occur with iron-mediated generation of reactive oxygen species.[19]

Much of the clinical benefit of deferoxamine derives from its positive impact on the heart. Cardiac cells are particularly sensitive to oxidant-mediated injury since they must perform a number of complex functions that include contraction and transmission of electrical impulses. Iron loaded in the cells exists primarily as hemosiderin, which is innocuous.[20] This iron is in equilibrium, however, with a very small pool of so-called "free iron" in the cell. This pool of iron is so small that its size has never been satisfactorily determined. Better termed, "loosely-bound" iron, this material catalyzes the formation of reactive oxygen species through Fenton chemistry. These reactive oxygen species are the agents of cell injury.

With iron loading, cardiac cells in culture begin to fail, loosing their characteristic rhythmic beating pattern. Deferoxamine prevents generation of reactive oxygen species by the Fenton reaction and can restore normal cellular activity.[21] This ability to intercept loosely bound iron occurs in heart cells in vivo. The clinical outcome is restoration of cardiac function.

The degree to which aggressive chelation therapy can reverse cardiac dysfunction has been a subject of vigorous debate. A number of short-term reports suggest that chelation can restore function in patients with significant cardiac compromise.[22] One group of investigators examined a cohort of patients with β-thalassemia major who were transfused while receiving chelation therapy.[23] Analysis of the data showed that only repeated plasma ferritin values of greater than 2500 ng/mL were associated with cardiac-related death.

Other investigators reviewed the outcome of aggressive treatment of patients with transfusional iron overload and marked cardiac dysfunction.[24] Some of the 19 patients suffered from severe congestive heart failure, others had cardiac arrhythmias, and a few had both problems. The patients received intravenously administered deferoxamine on a 24-hour per day regimen with dramatic effect. The mean ejection fraction of the patients with congestive heart failure improved from 30% to 50%. Arrhythmias were controlled and no patient suffered sudden death. The plasma ferritin values exceeded 10,000 ng/mL in many of the patients at the onset of treatment. These values declined, but never approached normal values.

The fact that deferoxamine improved cardiac function despite clear evidence of continued massive iron overload points to a key pharmacological characteristic of the drug. The chelator binds the minute quantity of bioactive "free" iron in cells, thereby eliminating iron-mediated cell damage. The cells and tissue still contain large iron deposits in the form of ferritin and hemosiderin. However, iron does not damage cells as long as the chelator is present in the body. A 6-day chelation regimen provides protection superior to a 4-day regimen not because of the trivial difference between the two in the degree of iron mobilization, but the enhanced protection reflects the fact that the chelator shields the patient 85% of the time with a 6-day regimen and only 57% of the time with a 4-day regimen.

Deferoxamine's ability to abrogate the injurious properties of intracellular bioactive iron is the key to its beneficial effect. Deferoxamine is best thought of as an *iron neutralizing compound*. Although the drug facilitates excretion of storage iron, the clinical benefit of the chelator derives from its capacity to neutralize toxic "free" iron.

These data point to the fact that cardiomyopathy and arrhythmias in patients with transfusional iron overload are not fixed lesions. Unlike the situation with ischemic cardiomyopathy, the cardiac myocytes are not necessarily destroyed by the pathologic events producing the dysfunction. Iron overload injures myocytes by production of free radicals that interfere with their function. Until fixed lesions occur (these cells will eventually die), the injury can be halted and reversed by chelators that block production of free radicals. Aggressive intervention with cardiac support and chelation therapy can be lifesaving for patients with iron-induced cardiac dysfunction.

Despite its excellent pharmacological profile with respect to the treatment of iron overload, deferoxamine has drawbacks. Side effects include frequent hard, painful swellings at the injection sites that in many patients necessitate use of permanent venous access devices such as the Portocath®. Less common problems include visual and auditory neurotoxicity as well as osteoporosis. The most severe drawback to deferoxamine therapy, however, is patient nonadherence with the complex, very expensive, and often uncomfortable regimen.

For patients who adhere to the cumbersome transfusion and chelation regimens, longevity to age 35 years and well beyond can be expected. In contrast, those who are noncompliant with the chelation regimen usually die during their teens or in their early 20s from iron-mediated end-organ failure, with cardiac toxicity as the preeminent problem.

Poor patient compliance with deferoxamine therapy prompted a search for other chelating agents, with a particular focus on drugs that are active with oral administration. The oral iron chelator, deferiprone (L1), showed efficacy in short-term clinical trials, but produces reversible agranulocytosis in a significant number of patients. In addition, long-term deferiprone therapy fails to control adequately the body iron accumulation and possibly worsens hepatic fibrosis. Although the drug is marketed in India and several other countries, deferiprone is not approved for use in the United States or Canada. Other oral chelating agents are under scrutiny. One of the most promising, Exjade®, has recently been approved for use in the US by the FDA and has become an additional tool in the fight against transfusional iron overload. Oral iron chelators enhance iron excretion but have not been shown to prevent long-term organ injury, which is the true test of their efficacy.

■ DEFINITIVE TREATMENT OF THALASSEMIA

Chronic red cell transfusion is a stopgap measure in the management of thalassemia. For β-thalassemia, HPFH is a natural experiment that shows the benefit of sustained high levels of Hb F production. A technique that artificially mimics HPFH is the Holy Grail of thalassemia therapeutics. Despite improved understanding of gene regulation, the means to flip the switch that activates γ-globin gene activity remains elusive.

Investigators have examined a number of drugs in this context and all have come up wanting. Candidate agents have included small molecules such as hydroxyurea, γ-aminobutyrate, and 5-azacytadine. Clinically trivial enhancement of γ-globin production, inconsistent drug activity, as well as unacceptable toxicity has plagued these efforts. The ongoing exploration of globin gene switching has been an exercise akin to opening a Russian matryoshka doll. Each layer has a more intricate figure underneath.

Currently, allogeneic hematopoietic stem cell transplantation is the sole definitive treatment for thalassemia.[25] The intervention is effective for both α- and β-thalassemia. Hematopoietic stem cell transplantation should be considered for any patient with a histocompatible marrow donor, which usually is a sibling. Complications with transplants involving marrow from matched, unrelated donors make this

TABLE 14-3	**KEY DIAGNOSTIC ISSUES IN THALASSEMIA**	
Issue	*Manifestation*	*Approach*
β-thalassemia trait versus iron deficiency anemia	• Mild anemia • Microcytosis • Target cells	• Normal RDW in thalassemia; elevated RDW in iron deficiency • Elevated Hb A2 in thalassemia
Two-gene deletion α-thalassemia	• Anemia • Microcytosis • Target cells	• Iron, transferrin saturation to rule out iron deficiency • Hb electrophoresis to rule out β-thalassemia trait • Family history of hemoglobin H disease or hydrops fetalis • DNA Southern blot of α-globin genes
Cardiac injury from iron overload	• Congestive heart failure • Arrhythmias • Sudden death	• Echocardiogram; sensitivity is low • Radionucleotide ventriculogram; sensitivity is low • Cardiac MRI • Early implementation of a vigorous iron chelation regimen

approach unacceptable at present. More than 500 transplants have been carried out worldwide, with most taking place in Italy. For well-chelated children without evidence of liver disease, event-free survival 3 years after transplantation exceeds 80%.[26] Results in patients with hepatic disease and in most adults fall significantly short of this mark, however. Even with children who are good transplant candidates, the relatively high immediate mortality associated with the procedure stands in contrast to the many years of reasonably normal life that can be obtained with appropriate transfusion and chelation therapies. This tradeoff makes decisions regarding transplantation difficult for many families.

The advent of modern transfusion and chelation therapy has substantially changed the profile of thalassemia major in the United States by greatly extending the lives

TABLE 14-4	KEY MANAGEMENT ISSUES IN THALASSEMIA
Issue	*Comment*
Transfusion management in thalassemia major	Patients should be transfused sufficiently often to maintain an Hb ≥ 10 g/dL immediately prior to transfusion. This hypertransfusion approach greatly reduces the incidence and severity of problems related to erythroid hyperplasia. Iron loading is not substantially greater than that occurs with casual transfusion programs.
Thalassemia intermedia	Thalassemia intermedia is a clinical diagnosis. Patients have anemia more severe than that in thalassemia trait. The anemia is both less severe than in thalassemia major *and* does not produce unacceptable side effects from erythroid hyperplasia in the absence of transfusions. A patient with thalassemia intermedia whose clinical state later demands chronic transfusion is reclassified as thalassemia major at that time.
Transfusional iron overload	Regular, vigorous chelation therapy is the only effective treatment for this problem. Deferoxamine administration for a minimum of 5 days per week is essential to obtain benefit. Some oral chelators exist and others are in development. Evidence that these agents protect organs from long-term iron damage does not currently exist.
Hepatitis C	Hepatitis C infection is a significant problem for patients with transfusion-dependent thalassemia. This infection combined with iron overload produces substantial liver injury and a high risk of hepatocellular carcinoma. Interferon and ribavirin therapy is the current treatment of choice.

of these patients.[27] A former childhood disorder is increasingly a disease of adults. Widespread screening of individuals from populations where β-thalassemia trait is prevalent has enabled prenatal diagnosis of affected fetuses. In Greek American and Italian American communities, the number of affected infants has sharply decreased.

The number of children with thalassemia in the United States is rising however as a result of the increase in the number of Americans of Southeast Asian ancestry. These more recent arrivals to the country have not yet achieved the cohesive approach to thalassemia that proved so successful in other American communities. Until this goal is reached, thalassemia will remain an important issue in American medicine (Tables 14-3 and 14-4).

References

1. Cooley TB, Witwer ER, Lee P. 1927. Anemia in children with splenomegaly and peculiar changes in bones: Report of cases. Am J Dis Child 34:347–355.
2. Olivieri NF. 1999. The beta-thalassemias. N Engl J Med 341:99–109.
3. Wasi P, Winichagoon P, Baramee T, Fucharoean S. 1982. Globin chain synthesis in heterozygous and homozygous hemoglobin E. Hemoglobin 6:75–78.
4. Fairbanks VF, Gilchrist GS, Brimhall B, Jereb JA, Goldston EC. 1979. Hemoglobin E trait revisited: A cause of microcytosis and erythrocytosis. Blood 53:109–115.
5. Fairbanks VF, Oliveros R, Brandabur JH, Willis RR, Fiester RF. 1980. Homozygous hemoglobin E mimics b-thalassemia minor without anemia or hemolysis: Hematologic, functional and biosynthetic studies of first North American cases. Am J Hematol 8:109–121.
6. Rees DC, Styles L, Vichinsky EP, Clegg JB, Weatherall DJ. 1998. The hemoglobin E syndromes. Ann N Y Acad Sci 850:334–343.
7. Fucharoen S, Ketvichit P, Pootrakul P, Siritanaratkul N, Piankijagum A, Wasi P. 2000. Clinical manifestation of beta thalassemia/hemoglobin E disease. J Pediatr Hematol Oncol 22:552–557.
8. Chui DH, Fucharoen S, Chan V. 2003. Hemoglobin H disease: Not necessarily a benign disorder. Blood 101:791–800.
9. Chen FE, Ooi C, Ha SY, et al. 2000. Genetic and clinical features of hemoglobin H disease in Chinese patients. N Engl J Med 343:544–550.
10. Scopinaro F, Banci M, Vania A, et al. 1993. Radioisotope assessment of heart damage in hypertransfused thalassaemic patients. Eur J Nucl Med 20:603–608.
11. Lattanzi F, Bellotti P, Picano E, et al. 1993. Quantitative ultrasonic analysis of myocardium in patients with thalassemia major and iron overload. Circulation 87:748–754.
12. Prennell DJ, Bland JM. 2003. Deferiprone versus desferrioxamine in thalassemia, and T2* validation and utility. Lancet 361:182–184.
13. Strickland GT, Elhefni H, Salman T, et al. 2002. Role of hepatitis C infection in chronic liver disease in Egypt. Am J Trop Med Hyg 67(4):436–442.
14. Darwish MA, Faris R, Darwish N, et al. 2001. Hepatitis C and cirrhotic liver disease in the Nile delta of Egypt: A community-based study. Am J Trop Med Hyg 64:147–153.
15. Seeff LB, Hoofnagle JH. 2003. Appendix: The National Institutes of Health Consensus Development Conference Management of Hepatitis C 2002. Clin Liver Dis 7:261–287.

[16] Gupta S, Bent S, Kohlwes J. 2003. Test characteristics of alpha-fetoprotein for detecting hepatocellular carcinoma in patients with hepatitis C. A systematic review and critical analysis. Ann Intern Med 139:46–50.

[17] McCord JM. 1993. Human disease, free radicals, and the oxidant/antioxidant balance. Clin Biochem 26:351–353.

[18] Farber JL. 1994. Mechanisms of cell injury by activated oxygen species. Environ Health Perspect 102:17–24.

[19] Enright HU, Miller WJ, Hebbel RP. 1992. Nucleosomal histone protein protects DNA from iron-mediated damage. Nucleic Acids Res 20:3341–3346.

[20] Bonkovsky, HL. 1991. Iron and the liver. Am J Med 301:32–43.

[21] Link G, Konijn AM, Hershko C. 1999. Cardioprotective effect of alpha-tocopherol, ascorbate, deferoxamine, and deferiprone: Mitochondrial function in cultured, iron-loaded heart cells. J Lab Clin Med 133:179–188.

[22] Aldouri MA, Wonke B, Hoffbrand AV, et al. 1990. High incidence of cardiomyopathy in beta-thalassaemia patients receiving regular transfusion and iron chelation: Reversal by intensified chelation. Acta Haematol 84:113–117.

[23] Olivieri NF, Nathan DG, MacMillan JH, et al. 1994. Survival in medically treated patients with homozygous beta-thalassemia. N Engl J Med 331:574–578.

[24] Davis B, J. Porter. 2000. Long-term outcome of continuous 24-hour deferoxamine infusion via indwelling intravenous catheters in high-risk beta-thalassemia. Blood 95(4):1229–1236.

[25] Lucarelli G, Galimberti M, Polchi P, et al. 1993. Marrow transplantation in patients with thalassemia responsive to iron chelation therapy. N Engl J Med 329:840–844.

[26] Lucarelli G, Galimberti M, Giardini C, et al. 1998. Bone marrow transplantation in thalassemia. The experience of Pesaro. Ann N Y Acad Sci 850:270–275.

[27] Pearson HA, Giardina P, Cohen A. 1996. The changing profile of thalassemia major. Pediatrics 97:352–356.

Enzymopathies

G6PD DEFICIENCY

Glucose-6-phosphate dehydrogenase (G6PD) deficiency is the most common erythrocyte enzyme defect, affecting over 400 million people. The initial descriptions of the disorder arose in the wake of peculiar outbreaks of hemolytic anemia in military personnel in the Pacific theater during World War II following prophylactic treatment with the antimalarial drug Primaquine.[1] A number of unusual attributes characterized the hemolytic episodes and whetted interest in the relationship between Primaquine and hemolysis. Although the problem involved a significant number of people, only a minority of the group who used the drug were affected. The episodes of hemolysis were self-limiting, with a sometimes explosive early phase followed by spontaneous recovery. After the initial hemolytic episode, susceptible people could continue Primaquine treatment without further problem. A break of several months in Primaquine exposure saw a recrudescence in hemolytic sensitivity.

     The demographics of the problem also were unusual. The hemolytic episodes occurred almost exclusively in people of African heritage, pointing to an ethnic component of the susceptibility. The familial pattern of drug sensitivity reinforced belief

TABLE 15-1 | **CLINICAL CLASSIFICATION OF G6PD SYNDROMES**

Class	Residual G6PD Activity (% normal)	Clinical Characteristics
I	<20	Chronic nonspherocytic hemolytic anemia (CNSHA). Neonatal jaundice.
II	<10	Severe episodic hemolysis often related to drugs or other oxidant exposure. Fava bean mediated hemolysis. Neonatal jaundice.
III	10–60	Episodic hemolysis often related to drug exposure. Hemolysis with infections. Neonatal jaundice in premature infants.
IV	90–100	No clinical symptoms.
V	>100	No clinical symptoms.

in the genetic nature of the disorder. Furthermore, men were the almost sole victims of Primaquine-induced hemolysis, indicating an X-linked pattern of inheritance. In retrospect the episodes of hemolysis were a result of a form of G6PD deficiency that originated in sub-Saharan Africa and spread to the New World as part of the African diaspora driven by the slave trade.

Further investigation uncovered the existence of many other types of G6PD deficiencies with varying manifestations and severity. Over time, more than 400 descriptions of mutations in the gene encoding G6PD appeared in the literature.[2] While some of the mutations, such as those affecting African Americans, are common, most are extremely rare. Also, the clinical characteristics of the G6PD deficiency varied significantly. The WHO devised a classification that divided G6PD deficiency into five groups, depending on the clinical manifestations (Table 15-1). The strikingly different presentations, clinical characteristics, and manifestations seen within these subgroups reflect the degree to which the G6PD enzyme levels fall below the normal range.

■ CLASSIFICATION OF G6PD DEFICIENCY SYNDROMES

Table 15-1 outlines the five clinical classes of G6PD variant syndromes as categorized by the WHO. The Class I G6PD deficiency phenotype derives from a marked erythrocyte enzyme deficiency. The extreme sensitivity of these cells to oxidant stress produces ongoing hemolysis with a moderately severe chronic nonspherocytic hemolytic anemia (CNSHA), with an associated marked reticulocytosis as the most common manifestation. Class II syndromes exhibit extreme enzyme deficiency in which G6PD values average less than 10% of the normal value. Affected patients are healthy at baseline but are susceptible to fulminant and sometimes life-threatening episodes of hemolysis when exposed to certain oxidizing agents. The Class III syndromes have mild to moderate enzyme deficit. This group was the primary subject of the Primaquine studies. The Class IV G6PD deficiency syndromes show at most only mildly depressed enzyme levels and no clinical symptoms. Class V, a phenotype also without clinical manifestations, rounds out the categorization of the condition with G6PD enzymes whose activity exceeds the normal value.

The G6PD deficiency syndromes show patterns of geographic and ethnic clustering. The Class III variety is the most prevalent form in people of African ethnic heritage, as noted earlier. Class II G6PD deficiency occurs commonly, but not exclusively, in people of Mediterranean background.[3] Both Class II and Class III G6PD deficiency variants are common in China and Southeast Asia.[4] Knowledge of a patient's ethnic background greatly aids in the evaluation and treatment of hemolytic episodes where G6PD deficiency is the possible culprit.

CLASS I G6PD DEFICIENCY

Patients who fall under this rubric typically have chronic hemolytic anemia that often is moderate in severity, thanks to a robust compensatory reticulocyte response. Class I G6PD deficiency manifests most commonly as congenital nonspherocytic hemolytic anemia. The very low G6PD levels in the erythrocytes render these cells incapable of withstanding the normal levels of oxidant stress visited upon all erythrocytes. The compensating reticulocytosis commonly ranges between 10% and 40%. Interestingly, splenomegaly is not a major manifestation of the condition. Occasional patients with congenital nonspherocytic hemolytic anemia due to G6PD deficiency develop recurrent infections. This problem apparently reflects dampening of neutrophil-generated reactive oxygen species that are essential to the bacteriocidal capability of these phagocytes.[5,6]

The marked elevation of bilirubin levels that sometimes occurs in the neonatal period raises the risk of kernicterus. Although hemolysis contributes to the high bilirubin levels, an additional factor is a neonatal deficiency of the hepatic glucuronyl transferase enzyme with consequent impairment of bilirubin metabolism. Neonatal hyperbilirubinemia often arises in association with Gilbert's syndrome.[7–9] Supportive treatment including phototherapy or even exchange transfusions may be necessary to control hyperbilirubinemia.

Most patients with CNSHA hemolytic anemia due to G6PD deficiency maintain hemoglobin levels in the range of 8–10 g/dL and compensate for anemia reasonably well. Epistatic factors may influence the degree of the anemia associated with the condition, since siblings sometimes have very disparate courses. Rarely, an anemia arises whose severity necessitates chronic transfusion to maintain a reasonable level of activity and comfort. The lack of splenic enlargement associated with congenital nonspherocytic hemolytic anemia due to Class I G6PD deficiency parallels the failure of splenectomy to benefit most such patients.

TABLE 15-2 | REPRESENTATIVE AGENTS CAUSING HEMOLYSIS IN G6PD DEFICIENCY[*]

Class	Agents
Antibiotics	Sulphonamides, Co-trimoxazole (Bactrim, Septrin), Dapsone, Chloramphenicol, Nitrofurantoin, Nalidixic acid
Antimalarials	Chloroquine, Hydroxychloroquine, Primaquine, Quinine, Mepacrine
Other drugs	Aspirin, Phenacitin, Sulphasalazine, Methyldopa, pharmacological doses of vitamin C, Hydralazine, Procainamide, Phenothiazine, vitamin K, penicillamine
Anthelmintics	β-Naphthol, Stibophen, Niridazole
Chemicals	Mothballs (naphthalene), Methylene blue
Foods	Raw fava beans (broad beans)
Infections	Bacterial infection; viral infection, hepatitis

[*]The drugs and agents listed are representative examples only. Susceptibility to hemolytic episodes varies depending on the subtype of G6PD deficiency. Definitive information comes from the WHO Glucose-6-phosphate Working Group, Bull WHO 1989, 67:610.

The maintenance of a hemoglobin value that is both stable and substantive depends on the brisk and ongoing production of new red cells. Any phenomenon or process that heightens hemolysis can precipitate life-threatening anemia. Even small quantities of oxidant drugs such as those listed in Table 15-2 can trigger massive hemolysis and a dramatic fall in hematocrit. Equally dangerous are events that dampen production of new erythrocytes. Parvovirus B19 infection, for instance, shuts off erythropoiesis for several days, creating an anemia of life-threatening severity.

CLASS II G6PD DEFICIENCY

Favism is a striking phenomenon that occurs in many people with Class II G6PD deficiency where spectacular and occasionally life-threatening hemolysis follows consumption of raw, uncooked fava beans (*Vicia fava*). These innocent legumes of the broad bean family are common throughout the world and are nutritional staples for millions of people. The form of G6PD deficiency common in the Mediterranean renders red cells particularly susceptible to hemolysis after consumption of raw fava beans. The syndrome has been known for centuries without, of course, an understanding of its basis. In some Mediterranean countries, hospitals geared up each year during planting or harvesting of the beans for the expected influxes of people stricken with favism. In some regions, such as Sardinia, the economic and social burden of favism was enormous.

The particulars of the syndrome are puzzling and suggest that factors other than exposure to the bean contribute to or modify the degree of hemolysis. Perhaps the most curious aspect of favism is that not every exposure to the beans produces hemolysis in people with the Mediterranean variety of G6PD deficiency. Some people consume fava beans for years without difficulty and then are felled by a hemolytic episode. Others are so sensitive to the active agent in fava beans that hemolysis can develop after mere exposure to pollen from the plant. Interestingly, hemolysis is more common in children than in adults, with as many as three-quarters of episodes occurring in children between the ages of 2 and 10 years.

As many as 48 unremarkable hours commonly pass following ingestion of the beans. The child then develops lethargy, sometimes in conjunction with confusion and a mild fever. Nausea, abdominal pain, and diarrhea are other nonspecific manifestations. A more telling feature (in retrospect) is back pain, which commonly accompanies acute hemolytic episodes of any cause. The alarming and illuminating aspect of the illness that usually brings the child to medical attention is the passage of dark red or brown urine. Physical examination at this point reveals frank jaundice, pallor, and tachycardia. Moderately severe anemia quickly follows, often with the hemoglobin falling to range of 4–7 g/dL. Although extremely severe cases that threaten circulatory collapse sometimes demand transfusion therapy,[10] most children recover without this intervention. The hemoglobin level usually returns to normal in 4–6 weeks.

The precise basis of hemolysis induced by fava beans in people with the Mediterranean variety of G6PD deficiency is unclear. The likely mediators are vicine and convicine, constituents in the beans that are metabolized to compounds capable of generating reactive oxygen species. The extreme deficiency of G6PD leaves the red cells compromised and very susceptible to oxidant damage and consequent hemolysis. The delay in the onset of manifestations following consumption of fava beans probably represents the time required to convert the latent compounds to their active metabolites. Favism is only one clinical manifestation of Class II G6PD deficiency. People with the condition are also susceptible to oxidizing compounds and drugs such as those listed in Table 15-2. Neonatal jaundice with possible kernicterus is another issue in Class II G6PD deficiency. The problem of hyperbilirubinemia in the newborn reflects both decreased hepatic Conjugation of bilirubin as well as hemolysis.

An interesting neonatal syndrome sometimes designated "Greek Baby Jaundice" is common in newborns from Greece and the islands of the Aegean Sea, characterized by extreme hyperbilirubin and a risk of kernicterus. Affected babies can be shown to have Type II G6PD deficiency; however, unknown environmental factors must also be operative, because the syndrome is not seen with any frequency in children of Greek families who have emigrated to North America or Australia.

CLASS III G6PD DEFICIENCY

Class III G6PD deficiency is associated with only a modest depression of the erythrocyte enzyme level (Table 15-1). The most commonly encountered variety of condition in the United States is that seen in African Americans, which is designated as the A⁻ subtype of G6PD deficiency. People with the condition ordinarily have a normal hematological profile and most are unaware of any issue with respect to their red cells. Problems arise only with stressful conditions such as exposure to drugs (Table 15-2) that can produce significant red cell oxidant damage.

Most drugs and chemicals that produce problems do so after an initial conversion to metabolites that then generate oxidant species. The result is a delay of 1–2 days between drug exposure and the manifestations of hemolysis. An investigation of hemolysis possibly related to G6PD deficiency must include potential exposures occurring in the days preceding the attack. The severity of hemolytic reactions varies substantially between patients. Furthermore, separate episodes of hemolysis experienced by a single patient can vary in course and severity. Other as yet poorly understood modifying factors likely contribute to the inconsistent hemolytic reactions in patients with G6PD deficiency of the A⁻ variety.

On the first day of the hemolytic reaction, patients commonly experience jaundice and dark urine. Some develop back pain and a few experience low-grade fever. A general malaise afflicts the patient often without specific localizing features. Pallor is a prominent aspect of the clinical complex, but detection often requires more than a glancing observation in patients with dark skin. Pale conjunctivae, mucous membranes, and nail beds are the features most easily assessed. The low hemoglobin value often produces prominent retinal pallor in which the eye grounds take on a salmon color.

The hemoglobin often falls to levels that are 3–4 g/dL below baseline. Palpitations and dyspnea are common complaints and tachycardia accompanies these symptoms. The precipitous decline in the hemoglobin value produces lightheadedness and dizziness in many patients. Older people can experience serious secondary side effects including angina and peripheral edema. Nausea and sometimes vomiting are less frequent clinical features.

The focus on drugs as agents of hemolysis in G6PD deficiency is an understandable result of the key role played by drug exposure in bringing the disorder to the medical spotlight. Worldwide, however, infection likely is the most common cause of hemolysis due to deficiency of the enzyme. Bacterial processes, such as *Streptococcus pneumoniae* infections, are quite prominent in this regard. Viral hepatitis often is at the root of episodes of hemolysis in people with G6PD deficiency. The variability in the association between infection and hemolysis exceeds that seen with the drug insult. The precise mechanism by which infection produces hemolysis in people with G6PD deficiency is unknown. Many factors undoubtedly contribute in small ways to the final effect. One speculation on mechanism posits that reactive oxygen species generated by phagocytes in the battle with bacteria somehow set off a chain reaction with inadvertent oxidant injury to susceptible erythrocytes.[11]

Hemolytic episodes in people with Class III G6PD deficiency rarely produce the life-threatening scenarios that can arise with Class I or Class II deficiency. The proportion of cells in the circulation that are susceptible to oxidant-mediated hemolysis is much lower than in the latter two conditions. Recovery from the acute hemolytic reaction proceeds due to replenishment of the circulation with young erythrocytes containing sufficient G6PD to resist further oxidant assault. A recovery phase occurs within about 10 days of the initial insult even with continued administration of the offending drug. By 3–4 weeks of chronic exposure to the oxidant drug, a new steady state ensues wherein a higher reticulocyte count (usually about twofold greater than baseline) maintains a normal hemoglobin value. Interestingly, the K_m of the G6PD A$^-$ variant for G6P is normal. The problem for the red cell is poor enzyme stability that leads to depletion in older erythrocytes (see below). The fresh reticulocytes have abundant and active G6PD with which to resist oxidant assault. Neonatal jaundice associate with Class III G6PD may occur in babies whose mothers ingested mothballs prior to delivery; and hyperbilirubinemia may occur in premature African American babies, even without known drug exposures.

CLASS IV AND V G6PD VARIANTS

Class IV and V G6PD variants are rare anomalies that do not produce clinical problems. People with Class IV variants have G6PD activity that is either normal or only slightly below normal. The very unusual Class V variants have G6PD activity that exceeds the normal value. The lack of clinical symptoms associated with these variants means that serendipity commonly underlies their discovery.

■ LABORATORY MANIFESTATIONS OF G6PD DEFICIENCY

Hemolysis due to G6PD deficiency invariably lowers the hemoglobin level. The degree of decline depends on the class of the deficiency state and the magnitude of the oxidant insult. Mild episodes might register a fall in hemoglobin of only 1 or 2 g/dL to values of 9 or 10 g/dL. In contrast, the hemoglobin might plunge to values as low as 3 or 4 g/dL in people with severe G6PD deficiency.

The intravascular red cell destruction produces prominent hemoglobinemia and hemoglobinuria. Massive release of hemoglobin into the circulation reduces haptoglobin levels to zero. Methemalbumin is prominent when looked for. Urinary hemosiderin appears within several days of the hemolytic episode and can persist for weeks following the insult. While assay for hemopexin is usually a research tool, the protein is invariably absent in the aftermath of hemolysis due to G6PD deficiency.

Hemolysis due to G6PD deficiency dramatically alters erythrocyte morphology. Some deformed red cells appear to have bites taken out of them, producing the characteristic "bite cells" that mark this type of hemolysis (Figure 15-1). Occasional spherocytes and other nonspecifically deformed red cells also appear in the peripheral blood. Prominent polychromasia reflects the large number of reticulocytes that pour out in the wake of the hemolytic episode.

Clumps of denatured hemoglobin, called Heinz bodies, form within the raddled red cells. Visualization of Heinz bodies by ordinary microscopy is difficult due to the subtle nature of these inclusions. Wright-Geimsa staining shows dark, irregular bulges or blisters at the edges of some cells presumably due to clusters of Heinz bodies in

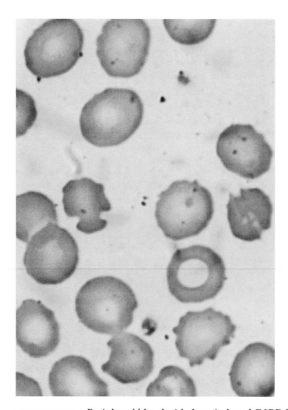

FIGURE 15–1   *Peripheral blood with drug-induced G6PD hemolysis. The smear is 3 days into the acute hemolytic episode. Several bite cells appear on the smear along with other nonspecific shape anomalies. Small bulges exist along the edge of some of the cells. (From Kapff CT and Jandl JH. 1991. Blood: Atlas and Sourcebook of Hematology, 2nd edn. Boston: Little, Brown and Company. Figure 23-1, p. 53. Reproduced with permission of the publisher.)*

the region. Although phase contrast microscopes easily show these anomalous bodies within erythrocytes, most clinical laboratories lack these relatively sophisticated instruments. A more readily available means of visualizing Heinz bodies involves staining the red cells with crystal violet or methyl violet in supravital preparations (Figure 15-2). However, Heinz bodies are not evident after 24–48 hours.

Heinz bodies cause a number of problems for red cells. Methemoglobin accumulates due to the dearth of NADPH to support methemoglobin reductase activity. Hemoglobin denatures and the oxidized heme slips out of its usual site in the heme-binding pocket. The resulting amalgam forms hemichromes that can themselves facilitate further formation of reactive oxygen species. This downward spiral due to oxidant injury dooms the G6PD-deficient erythrocytes.

Heinz bodies also adhere to the red cell membrane where they disrupt architecture, promote oxidation and cross-linking of lipids and proteins, and impair function of membrane-associated enzymes including ion channels. Cross-links of membrane structures produce rigid red cells with impaired ability to pass through capillaries.

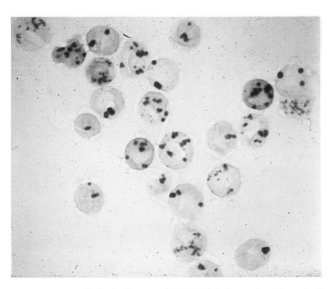

FIGURE 15-2 *Heinz body prep of G6PD deficient cells. The red cells are ghostly outlines with the Heinz bodies appearing as dark inclusions.*

The spleen briskly clears the circulation of these decrepit red cells. Disturbed ion channel activity produces erythrocyte swelling and rupture. Some cells show bizarre distributions of hemoglobin with protein confined to one portion of the cell and a ghostly appearance to the remainder.

Reticuloendothelial cells rapidly remove these spavined erythrocytes from the circulation. Sometimes an erythrocyte rips free of the reticuloendothelial cell, leaving a large rent in its membrane. The cells appear to have bites taken out of them, giving rise to the common moniker "bite cells." Many such cells are scalloped and some have thin peduncles reflecting narrow escapes from reticuloendothelial cell assault. The spleen eventually clears the circulation of these aberrant erythrocytes.

Levels of unconjugated bilirubin rise during the hemolytic acute attack, mirroring the jaundice on physical examination. Small rises in the level of conjugated bilirubin occur occasionally, particularly with massive hemolysis. Transient, small elevations in BUN occur most often in the wake of marked hemolysis.

The high RDW in the condition reflects the tremendous size variation of red cells that include reticulocytes, cell fragments, and distorted cells. The augmented marrow activity that produces the reticulocytosis also raises production of neutrophils. This at times confuses the distinction between hemolysis due to infection and that due to oxidant agents. The platelet count typically varies little from baseline.

■ G6PD AND RED CELL METABOLISM

The monomer subunit of G6PD is a 59-kDa polypeptide. Two subunits join to create a protein dimer that includes a tightly bound NADP molecule. The enzymatically

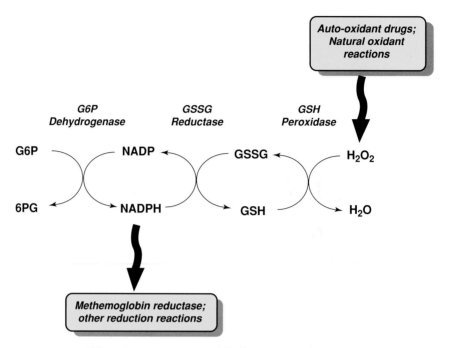

FIGURE 15–3 *Schematic representation of the hexose monophospate (HMP) shunt. G6PD dehydrogenase converts glucose-6-phosphate (G6PD), the initial product of glycolysis, into 6-phosphogluconate (6PG) with the coupled conversion of NADP to NADPH. This reaction is the sole source of NADPH in the red cell, which is needed for a number of important metabolic functions including the rescue of hemoglobin from constant oxidation to methemoglobin. A host of normal metabolic processes generate hydrogen peroxide (H_2O_2) as a usual byproduct. This compound, along with other pernicious reactive oxygen species that it produces, has the potential of wrecking widespread cell injury including the cross-linking of lipids and proteins. In the last step of the HMP shunt, glutathione peroxidase converts this destructive chemical to water.*

inactive dimer is in equilibrium with the fully functional tetramer form of the molecule. Structural studies show that the NADP lodges near the dimer contact point and is essential to molecular stability.[12]

G6PD provides red cells with crucial protection against oxidant damage. Glucose-6-phosphate is the first metabolite produced in glycolysis. The Embden-Meyerhof pathway is the primary metabolic route for the compound, producing ATP along the way and generating lactate in the final step. A portion of the glucose-6-phosphate takes an alternate route involving the hexose monophosphate (HMP) shunt. The metabolic steps of the HMP eventually swing back to merge with the Embden-Meyerhoff pathway leading to lactate. Along the way, however, the HMP shunt produces several compounds important to the health of the cell.

Figure 15-3 is a simplified representation of the HMP shunt. G6PD catalyzes the first step that converts glucose-6-phosphate to 6-phosphogluconate. The NADPH generated from NADP in the process provides the cell with a metabolite that is central to many reductive biochemical reactions. Hydrogen peroxide (H_2O_2) produced by natural processes in the cell oxidizes heme iron from the Fe(II) valance state to Fe(III), thereby daily converting as much as 3% of hemoglobin to functionally inactive methemoglobin. The NADPH-dependent enzyme, methemoglobin reductase, regenerates hemoglobin from methemoglobin allowing continued normal oxygen delivery.

H_2O_2 transforms into other reactive oxygen species including the highly volatile hydroxyl radical ($^{\bullet}OH$). These destructive molecules attack carbon–carbon double bonds of unsaturated fatty acids, producing fatty acid hydroperoxides that promote further cleavage and cross-linking of carbon–carbon bonds in membrane lipids. The damaged regions of membrane loose their fluidity and accumulate aggregates of proteins that normally are integral to or closely associated with the membrane. These changes alter both the biophysical and biochemical properties of red cell membranes and promote hemolysis. As Figure 15-2 shows, glutathione peroxidase defuses H_2O_2 before it can wreck havoc on the cell, a job shared with catalase. Glutathione peroxidase performs the additional valuable function of decomposing fatty acid peroxides.

G6PD deficiency blunts the efficiency of this entire cascade of events. The degree of enzyme deficiency markedly influences the clinical character of the condition. Syndromes in which the G6PD deficit is only mild or moderate, such as occurs with Class III deficiency, show hemolysis only with major insults that rain vast quantities of H_2O_2 on the cell. People with Class I G6PD deficiency in contrast are in such delicate balance with the forces producing oxidant cell stress that a relatively minor upswing in cellular oxidant activity can mean disaster.

Red cell G6PD levels normally decline slowly with age, due to among other things protein inactivation by oxidant damage. Reticulocyte levels of G6PD in fact exceed by nearly fivefold those of the oldest erythrocytes. Figure 15-4 schematically shows that the normal decay of G6PD maintains sufficient levels of the enzyme to protect erythrocytes from exorbitant oxidant damage out to the end of the cell life span. The enzyme produced by the *G6PD A*$^-$ gene is unstable and decays much more rapidly than normal. Consequently, older cells fall below the protective threshold and are vulnerable to the type of oxidant stress produced by Primaquine, for instance. After the initial bout of hemolysis following exposure to an oxidant drug, the compensatory reticulocytosis produces young cells containing sufficient enzyme to defend the cell integrity. A new steady state maintains the hemoglobin in the normal range even with continued exposure to the oxidant drug.

The G6PD Mediterranean deficiency, in contrast, results from an extremely unstable enzyme whose half-life in the cell is exceedingly short. As indicated in Figure 15-3, most of the cells fall into the oxidant danger zone soon after their production. The massive hemolysis seen with this form of G6PD deficiency reflects the large number of vulnerable erythrocytes in the circulation. Maximally augmented erythropoiesis often fails to keep pace with the rate of hemolysis creating a potentially life-threatening situation.

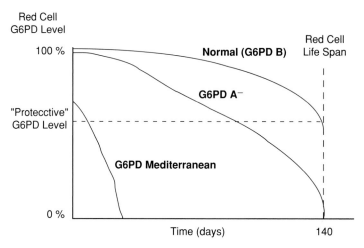

FIGURE 15–4 *Schematic representation of the time-dependent decay of red cell G6PD. Normal G6PD (G6PD B) decays naturally over the life of the red cell but maintains a level sufficient to protect against oxidant assault such as that produced by Primaquine. In contrast to G6PD B, G6PD A⁻ begins in the normal range but decays more rapidly due to a structural mutation. A cohort of older cells comprising up to 30% of those in circulation are susceptible to hemolysis when bombarded with excessive quantities of oxidants. The more severe G6PD Mediterranean is very unstable and falls quickly to low levels that leave a large fraction of circulating red cells susceptible to destruction by oxidant assault.*

■ THE MOLECULAR BIOLOGY OF G6PD DEFICIENCY

The gene encoding G6PD located on the X-chromosome, X(q28), is over 20 Kb in length and contains 13 exons.[13] Most of the hundreds of known mutations are point mutations that produce some degree of reduced enzymatic activity. A few mutants have normal or even enhanced enzymatic activity. The absence of a mutant that produces complete enzyme loss suggests that complete G6PD deficiency is incompatible with life.

Table 15-3 provides information on some common and representative examples of G6PD deficiency. The designation "G6PD B" attached to the normal enzyme derives from its mobility on gel electrophoresis relative to the more rapidly migrating band seen commonly in African Americans, which is designated "G6PD A⁺." The altered mobility of G6PD A⁺ derives from a nucleotide and amino acid difference relative to G6PD B, but the protein has full enzymatic activity. A mutation on the G6PD A⁺ background that lowers G6PD enzymatic activity is the basis of the G6PD A⁻ deficiency seen in African Americans.[14]

The mutations that produce the Class II G6PD variants tend to cluster in the region of the NADP binding site or the interface between the two dimers. Protein structural alterations in these regions appear to be particularly detrimental to enzymatic activity. NADP binds tightly to the G6PD dimer behaving more as a structural component than

TABLE 15-3	REPRESENTATIVE G6PD VARIANTS		
Common Distribution	*WHO Clinical Classification*	*Common Designation*	*Amino Acid Substitution*
Worldwide	IV	Normal; G6PD B	None
African ethnicity	IV	G6PD A$^+$	68 Val → Met
Sporadic	I	G6PD Marion	213 Val → Leu
Mediterranean	II	G6PD Mediterranean	188 Ser → Phe
Southeast Asia	II	G6PD Canton	463 Arg → Leu
African Ethnicity	III	G6PD A$^-$	68 Val → Met 126 Asn → Asp

as a simple enzyme substrate. Mutations that interrupt NADP binding severely dampen enzyme activity. The fact that G6PD activity is confined to the tetramer means that mutants disrupting the interface between dimers are particularly deleterious.

■ DIAGNOSIS OF G6PD DEFICIENCY

A number of enzyme assays exist that assess G6PD activity. Such tests have limitations in certain clinical settings, but are very useful and reliable within the parameters set by those limitations. The most discriminating assay detects the conversion of NADP to NADPH wherein a resonating structure forms in one of the molecule's rings and produces a characteristic UV absorption band. The assay is precise and provides a quantitative readout of G6PD activity, but is relatively complex. A simplified variant of that is particularly suitable for population screening is the fluorescent spot test. The test takes advantage of the change in UV absorption profile by an approach that requires a simple UV lamp rather than a sophisticated spectrophotometer.

A number of other simple screening tests for G6PD rely on biochemical changes produced by the active enzyme, including dye decolorization and reduction of methemoglobin. These semiquantitative tests are best at providing a "positive" or "negative" answer, which requires setting proper cutoffs for the reading. Used correctly, these tests are very useful in the detection of G6PD deficiency. A number of caveats exist, however.

The key drawback to all these approaches when applied to patients suspected of having hemolysis due to G6PD deficiency is that an acute hemolytic episode destroys the cohort of cells that are deficient in G6PD (Figure 15-3). Patients with the G6PD A$^-$ deficiency, for instance, often show normal testing readouts for more than 3 weeks after drug exposure. Patients with the more severe Class II defects are less of a problem since even very young red cells have substantial enzyme deficits. Physicians who order testing for G6PD deficiency must be aware of the laboratory procedure employed and alert to the possibility that it will elide a Class III G6PD deficiency in particular.

The ascorbate-cyanide test provides a broad screen for red cells that are sensitive to oxidant stress. The test involves inactivating catalase with cyanide followed by treatment with sodium ascorbate. The ascorbate produces reactive oxygen intermediates that convert hemoglobin to methemoglobin, seen as a brown pigment that is readily visible to the unaided eye. The ascorbate-cyanide test is a sensitive but not specific screen with respect to G6PD deficiency. Positive results occur in a variety of settings with red cells that are sensitive to oxidant stress, including pyruvate kinase deficiency. The test can be very useful in screening for Class III G6PD deficiency in the immediate aftermath of a hemolytic episode, however. The extreme oxidant stress of the ascorbate-cyanide test overwhelms red cells with low levels of G6PD that managed to survive the in vivo hemolysis. The positive test supports the existence of a red cell metabolic defect whose nature later can be definitely documented.

Depending on the urgency of obtaining a diagnosis of G6PD deficiency, one possible solution to the dilemma of testing in the aftermath of hemolysis is to wait for a few weeks and perform the assay after the patient has returned to steady state. When time is an issue, another approach is to test the patient's mother who is an obligate heterozygote for this X-linked disorder. However, heterozygotes sometimes have normal enzyme levels due to selective lyonization of the affected X-chromosome. Testing of the patient's brothers, who have a 50% chance of also having G6PD deficiency, can also provide indirect support for the diagnosis. The size and availability of the family dictates the usefulness of this approach to the issue.

TABLE 15-4	KEY DIAGNOSTIC POINTS WITH G6PD DEFICIENCY	
Issue	*Manifestation*	*Approach*
Congenital hemolysis	Anemia, reticulocytosis, elevated bilirubin	• Assess G6PD level. • Heinz body prep. • Osmotic fragility test.
Acute hemolysis following drug exposure	Falling hematocrit, reticulocytosis, elevated bilirubin, hematuria	• Obtain history of drug exposure over preceding several days. • Urine hemosiderin if hemolytic episode occurred several weeks before evaluation. • G6PD level. Low in Class I and II. Speciously normal in Class III.

TABLE 15-5	KEY MANAGEMENT POINTS WITH G6PD DEFICIENCY
Issue	*Comments*
Infection and hemolysis	Infection can produce severe hemolysis in Class III G6PD deficiency. Control of the infection and supportive care for anemia and hemolysis are indicated. Infection induces hemolysis inconsistently, even for a single patient.
Drug-induced hemolysis	Removing the offending drug is extremely important with Class I and II G6PD deficiency due to their very low enzyme levels. Continued use of the drug is possible with Class III G6PD deficiency. The moderate enzyme deficiency allows attainment of a new steady state with a mild increase over baseline of the reticulocyte count.
Diagnosis of G6PD deficiency following acute hemolysis	The severe enzyme deficiency of Class I and II G6PD deficiency shows up as a low enzyme levels even after acute hemolysis. Class III G6PD deficiency can show normal values in G6PD testing immediately after hemolysis due to the higher enzyme levels in the surviving cells. The test becomes abnormal only after 6–8 weeks when aged cells with low G6PD content again exist in the circulation.

Analysis of genomic DNA obtained from the circulating lymphocytes allows direct assay of the gene encoding G6PD and provides powerful insight into the patient's status. Most often, the procedure involves polymerase chain reaction that amplifies the gene encoding the mutant enzyme allowing its subsequent analysis by a number of sophisticated techniques. Despite its power and precision, DNA analysis has limitations. More than 400 mutants involving the *G6PD* gene are known, including many that are essentially genetic polymorphisms. This shortcoming is balanced by the fact that a few subtypes of true G6PD deficiency dominate in specific populations or ethnic groups, allowing a directed search for the most likely candidates. In the real world, the search for G6PD deficiency will be determined by factors such as the prevalence of the disorder and the availability of the various testing methods. Genetic testing is not an option in many regions of the world where G6PD deficiency is common and medical resources are scarce. As long as the physician remains aware of the probable culprit, the likelihood is good that an accurate determination will result irrespective of the final analytical approach (Tables 15-4 and 15-5).

References

[1] Beutler E. 1994. G6PD deficiency. Blood 84:3613–3636.
[2] Beutler E. 1992. The molecular biology of G6PD variants and other red cell enzyme defects. Annu Rev Med 43:47–59.

3   Cappellini MD, Martinez di Montemuros F, De Bellis G, Debernardi S, Dotti C, Fiorelli G. 1996. Multiple G6PD mutations are associated with a clinical and biochemical phenotype similar to that of G6PD Mediterranean. Blood 87:3953–3958.

4   Chiu DT, Zuo L, Chao L, et al. 1993. Molecular characterization of glucose-6-phosphate dehydrogenase (G6PD) deficiency in patients of Chinese descent and identification of new base substitutions in the human G6PD gene. Blood 81:2150–2154.

5   van Bruggen R, Bautista JM, Petropoulou T, et al. 2002 Deletion of leucine 61 in glucose-6-phosphate dehydrogenase leads to chronic nonspherocytic anemia, granulocyte dysfunction, and increased susceptibility to infections. Blood 100:1026–1030.

6   Iancovici-Kidon M, Sthoeger D, Abrahamov A, et al. 2000 A new exon 9 glucose-6-phosphate dehydrogenase mutation (G6PD "Rehovot") in a Jewish Ethiopian family with variable phenotypes. Blood Cells Mol Dis 26:567–571.

7   Kaplan M, Renbaum P, Levy-Lahad E, Hammerman C, Lahad A, Beutler E. 1997. Gilbert syndrome and glucose-6-phosphate dehydrogenase deficiency: A dose-dependent genetic interaction crucial to neonatal hyperbilirubinemia. Proc Natl Acad Sci USA 94:12128–12132.

8   Kaplan M, Hammerman C. 2002. Glucose-6-phosphate dehydrogenase deficiency: A potential source of severe neonatal hyperbilirubinaemia and kernicterus. Semin Neonatol 7:121–128.

9   Huang CS, Chang PF, Huang MJ, Chen ES, Chen WC. 2002. Glucose-6-phosphate dehydrogenase deficiency, the UDP-glucuronosyl transferase 1A1 gene, and neonatal hyperbilirubinemia. Gastroenterology 123:127–133.

10 Shibuya A, Hirono A, Ishii S, Fujii H, Miwa S. 1999. Hemolytic crisis after excessive ingestion of fava beans in a male infant with G6PD Canton. Int J Hematol 70:233–235.

11 Baehner RL, Nathan DG, Castle WB. 1971. Oxidant injury of caucasian glucose-6-phosphate dehydrogenase-deficient red blood cells by phagocytosing leukocytes during infection. J Clin Invest 50:2466–2473.

12 Au SW, Gover S, Lam VM, Adams MJ. 2000. Human glucose-6-phosphate dehydrogenase: The crystal structure reveals a structural NADP(+) molecule and provides insights into enzyme deficiency. Structure Fold Des 8:293–303.

13 Takizawa T, Huang IY, Ikuta T, Yoshida A. 1986. Human glucose-6-phosphate dehydrogenase: Primary structure and cDNA cloning. Proc Natl Acad Sci USA 83:4157–4161.

14 Vulliamy TJ, Othman A, Town M, et al. 1991. Polymorphic sites in the African population detected by sequence analysis of the glucose-6-phosphate dehydrogenase gene outline the evolution of the variants A and A⁻. Proc Natl Acad Sci USA 88:8568–8571.

PYRUVATE KINASE DEFICIENCY

In 1953, John Dacie and colleagues provided the first cogent description of patients with a congenital hemolytic anemia who were distinct from those with the previously recognized disorder hereditary spherocytosis.[1] This heterogeneous collection of patients had a number of important common features including the absence of spherocytosis, no detectable abnormal hemoglobin, and no antibody directed against the red cell. The osmotic fragility of freshly isolated cells was normal. Spleen size was normal or only modestly enlarged and splenectomy provided no clinical benefit. Later, investigators identified pyruvate kinase (PK) deficiency as the basis of this constellation of findings.[2]

PK deficiency is the second most common human erythrocyte enzyme deficiency, following glucose-6-phosphate dehydrogenase (G6PD) deficiency. These two conditions account for most cases of congenital nonspherocytic hemolytic anemia (CN-SHA). While the number of people with G6PD deficiency ranges in the millions, however, only several hundred cases of PK deficiency exist in the literature. Most reported cases involve people of Northern European background with an estimated incidence of 50 cases per million, but sporadic reports involving people throughout the world suggest a wider distribution to the condition than has generally been appreciated in the past.[3]

■ CLINICAL MANIFESTATIONS

PK deficiency has a wide expression spectrum, ranging from severe neonatal hemolysis and jaundice to mild conditions that evade discovery until adulthood. Typically, anemia, jaundice, or both appear in childhood. A few cases of very severe PK deficiency have appeared in utero and some have produced recurrent episodes of hydrops fetalis.[4,5] Most often, however, the fetuses survive the period of pregnancy with relatively little difficulty.[6] Early recognition that a fetus has PK deficiency, often the result of a good family history, allows appropriate application of the tools available to high-risk obstetrics teams. Occasionally, mild hemolysis characterizes CNSHA, for which the reticulocyte response compensates fully, leaving jaundice as the only clinical manifestation. Anemia when present is lifelong and varies little over time.

Hyperbilirubinemia occurs commonly in newborns with PK deficiency and can necessitate exchange transfusion. Some children with severe manifestations subsequently require transfusions to maintain an acceptable hemoglobin level. Splenectomy, usually after 5 years of age, typically reduces or eliminates the transfusion requirement for most such children. A paradoxical rise in the reticulocyte count commonly follows splenectomy, with values sometimes reaching 70% or more. The hyperactive erythroid production partially compensates for the anemia. Marrow expansion in the maxilla and facial bones can produce severe cosmetic deformity in children with extreme marrow erythroid hyperplasia. Prominent malar eminences give the eyes a mongoloid slant reminiscent of that seen with thalassemia. Expansion of the marrow cavity of the cranial bones caused enlargement of the skull with frontal and parietal bossing. In contrast to thalassemia, PK deficiency does not stunt general growth and maturation. Cholelithiasis is a common sequela of long-standing hemolysis and hyperbilirubinemia.

Iron overload is a concern in PK deficiency, but generally the serum iron and ferritin levels are normal or only mildly elevated.[7,8] The picture differs strikingly from that seen with thalassemia where iron absorption exceeds normal and commonly produces severe overload in the absence of transfusion. The difference likely represents the fact that PK deficiency is a hemolytic disorder with little ineffective erythropoiesis. The destruction of erythroid precursors in the marrow, which is the core of ineffective erythropoiesis, appears to be the key signal for augmented gastrointestinal iron uptake. Recurrent transfusion in severely affected patients can of course produce iron overload to a degree requiring chelation therapy.

Events that disturb the balance between erythropoiesis and hemolysis can be profoundly deleterious to patients with PK deficiency. A well-recognized threat is infection with human parvovirus B19. This adeno-associated virus causes "Fifth Disease," a normally benign childhood disorder associated with fever, malaise, and a mild rash. The virus has a tropism for erythroid progenitor cells and impairs cell division for a few days during the infection. Reticulocyte counts often fall literally to zero. Normal people experience, at most, a slight drop in hematocrit since the half-life of erythrocytes in the circulation is 40–60 days. The viral infection resolves in a few days with no long-lasting problem. Anemia of life-threatening severity occurs in children with PK deficiency whose survival depends on brisk reticulocyte production.[9] Early recognition of the problem along with transfusion support allows the child to weather the storm. Fortunately, the virus induces a profound immune response that prevents further episodes of infection. Nonetheless, other viral (and sometimes bacterial) infections that only modestly suppress erythropoiesis can pose a significant danger.

With proper management, most patients with PK deficiency reach adulthood. Women with PK deficiency can become pregnant and carry their fetuses to term, but the course is variable and depends greatly on the severity of the particular case of PK deficiency. The dangers to pregnancy posed in the past by PK deficiency have subsided with improved skill at obstetrical management.[10] Women with mild disease often tolerate pregnancy without intervention. Even some women with relatively severe PK deficiency can stay the course without the need for transfusion.[11] In severe cases, prophylactic blood transfusions aim at maintaining the hemoglobin concentration above an arbitrary threshold of 7–8 g/dL. Puerperal jaundice is an occasional feature in otherwise unremarkable pregnancies.[12]

PK deficiency occasionally arises in people with acquired defects in hematopoiesis including myelodysplasia and myelogenous leukemia.[13,14] The changes likely reflect the profound alterations in the basic metabolism of erythroid precursors, which occurs with these disorders. Acquired enzyme deficiencies of many types as well as thalassemic disturbances in globin production occur in some patients. These are rare events. However, myelodysplasia is far more common than hereditary PK deficiency, making acquired PK deficiency relatively prominent in the overall picture of the enzymopathy.

■ LABORATORY FEATURES OF PK DEFICIENCY

The anemia associated with PK deficiency commonly produces a hemoglobin value in the range of 5–11 g/dL. Some patients require transfusions while others are asymptomatic. Splenectomy usually raises the hemoglobin value in patients with severe disease. The robust rise in the reticulocyte number following splenectomy sometimes makes these cells the primary conveyors of oxygen in the body.

The erythrocyte morphology often is surprisingly bland in cases of PK deficiency. Macrocytosis and polychromophilia are invariant. Red cells with spicules or irregular contractions occur with more severe disease, and rare cases can display acanthocytes. More prominent morphological alterations occur following splenectomy. Howell-Jolly bodies and nucleated red cells make an appearance following the procedure. The astonishing rise in reticulocyte count that often follows splenectomy sometimes gives the smear a complete polychromatophilic cast. Occasional target cells, spherocytes, as well as cells with Pappenheimer bodies can also appear on the stage following removal of the spleen (Figure 16-1).

Neutrophil and platelet morphology are normal with PK deficiency. Splenectomy produces a visible increase in platelets on the smear that includes some giant platelets

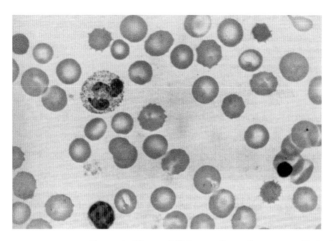

FIGURE 16–1   *Pyruvate kinase deficiency after splenectomy. Reticulocytes are prominent on the smear and crenated cells are numerous. The bristled edges seen in many of the cells are characteristic of the condition. (From Jandl JH. 1987. Blood: Textbook of Hematology. Boston: Little, Brown and Company. Figure 12-2, p. 353.)*

and occasional megakaryocyte fragments. The WBC often is slightly higher than normal.

Hyperbilirubinemia is invariant with PK deficiency, with most in the unconjugated state. Values in the range of 4–6 mg/dL are common, but some patients with severe disease have values as high as 20 mg/dL. As noted earlier, the bilirubin level commonly rises with pregnancy.

■ BIOLOGY OF PK DEFICIENCY

As shown in Figure 16-2, PK generates two equivalents of ATP during the conversion of phosphoenol-pyruvate to pyruvate in the penultimate step of the Embden-Meyerhof pathway. The block produced by PK deficiency not only deprives the cell of needed ATP but also disrupts the NAD cycle. Mitochondria in developing erythroid cells provide an alternate energy source, but are lost as the red cells mature. The severity of the PK deficiency determines the length of survival of the erythrocytes. The lifespan of severely defective cells is only a few days while those with more modest metabolic disturbances can survive for weeks.

Glycolytic intermediates produced prior to the PK block, such as 2,3-DPG, accumulate in the erythrocytes while the decline in NAD levels impairs important steps in intermediary metabolism. The factors that doom the cells are failed maintenance activities due to the energy deficit. ATP-dependent cation pumps fail, leading to potassium loss and cell shrinkage. Pathological levels of calcium accumulate in the cells and activate the Gardos channel with consequent further loss of cell potassium. The shrunken, crenated cells become rigid and are quickly cleared from the circulation by reticuloendothelial cells.

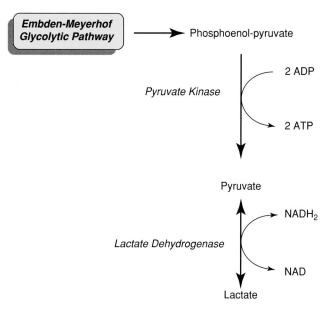

FIGURE 16–2 *Pyruvate kinase action. Pyruvate kinase catalyzes the conversion of phosphoenol-pyruvate to pyruvate in the penultimate step of the Embden-Meyerhof pathway. PK deficiency blocks this essential metabolic pathway whose importance in erythrocytes is magnified by the lack of mitochondria in these cells. The failure to produce ATP starves the cells of energy with deleterious effects on red cell metabolism, structural integrity, and survival. The blockade of the NAD cycle places further metabolic stress on the fey erythrocytes.*

PK is a homotetramer whose subunit content varies between tissues. Clinical PK deficiency affects the red cell form of the gene that is located on chromosome 1, while the enzyme types expressed in other tissues are normal. This fact explains the focal nature of the metabolic lesion. A variety of different point mutations in the gene underlie most cases of PK deficiency producing molecules with aberrant stability, enzyme kinetics, and membrane adhesion.[15] Most people with PK deficiency are compound heterozygotes for two aberrant genes. The clinical expression depends on the nature of the interaction between the abnormal subunits. In groups where consanguinity is high, PK deficiency involving homozygous variants can arise. This appears to underlie the severe PK deficiency that exists in the Amish deme in Pennsylvania.[16] Frameshift gene modifications, RNA splicing variants, and promoter mutations can also produce PK deficiency, but are unusual.[17–19]

■ DIAGNOSIS OF PK DEFICIENCY

The first steps in the diagnosis of PK deficiency involve elimination of other more common causes of chronic nonspherocytic hemolytic anemia, with G6PD deficiency being the most important consideration. The absence of spherocytes and a normal osmotic fragility test mitigate against hereditary spherocytosis. The absence of sickle cells or target cells along with a normal hemoglobin electrophoresis rules out sickle cell disease or thalassemia as the basis for the hemolysis. PK deficiency sometimes becomes apparent only later in life, meaning that acquired disorders should be eliminated, including immune-mediated hemolysis.

The ascorbate-cyanide test provides a broad screen for red cells that are sensitive to oxidant stress. The test involves inactivating catalase with cyanide followed by treatment with sodium ascorbate. The ascorbate produces reactive oxygen intermediates that convert hemoglobin to methemoglobin, seen as a brown pigment that is readily visible to the unaided eye. The ascorbate-cyanide test is a sensitive but not specific screen with respect to PK deficiency. Positive results occur with a variety of conditions with red cells that are sensitive to oxidant stress, including G6PD deficiency. A negative result with this inexpensive and readily available screening tool rules PK deficiency out of consideration, however.

The demonstration of a low erythrocyte PK level makes the diagnosis.[20] The process requires exquisite attention to detail to avoid error. For instance, reticulocytes and white cells must be removed from the preparation since the high levels of PK in these cells can swamp the low signal from the erythrocytes. Even with these careful steps, dissociation often exists between the in vitro assessment of PK levels and the degree of hemolysis.[21] Multiple mutants of the enzyme that commonly exist in compound heterozygous states contribute further to the difficulties in diagnosis. Nonetheless, a careful workup that includes a good family history usually resolves the issue.

TABLE 16-1 | KEY DIAGNOSTIC POINTS IN PYRUVATE KINASE DEFICIENCY

Issue	Manifestation	Approach
Suspected inherited PK deficiency	Hemolysis, jaundice, splenomegaly	• Rule out common causes of hemolysis including G6PD deficiency. • Ascorbate-cyanide test to demonstrate red cell susceptibility to oxidants. • Specific test for PK deficiency.
Suspected acquired PK deficiency	Hemolysis, anemia	• Rule out common causes of acquired hemolysis including immune-mediated hemolysis. • Ascorbate-cyanide test to demonstrate red cell susceptibility to oxidants. • Specific test for PK deficiency.

TABLE 16-2	KEY MANAGEMENT POINTS IN PYRUVATE KINASE DEFICIENCY
Issue	*Comment*
Splenectomy	Splenectomy often improves the anemia in PK deficiency, but variably so. The reticulocyte count often *rises* following removal of the spleen.
Pregnancy	Patients with PK deficiency can do well during pregnancy with good obstetrical management. Transfusion is sometimes needed to maintain a hemoglobin value in the range of 8 g/dL.
Acute illness	Hemoglobin levels fall with acute illness. Transfusions to stabilize the anemia allow patients to weather the crisis.

■ TREATMENT OF PK DEFICIENCY

No specific treatment exists for PK deficiency. Most patients maintain an acceptable hemoglobin value without intervention. Splenectomy can improve the hemoglobin level in patients with severe disease, but the outcome is unpredictable. Some patients require chronic or intermittent transfusion therapy to maintain acceptable hemoglobin levels. Often transfusions are needed to weather a particularly trying event such as a severe infection or pregnancy, after which the patient returns to the baseline state. Reports exist of successful bone marrow transplantation in patients with severe PK deficiency, but this intervention remains unconventional[22] (Tables 16-1 and 16-2).

References

1. Dacie JV, Mollison PL, Richardson N, Selwyn JG, Shapiro L. 1953. Atypical congenital hemolytic anemia. Q J Med 22:79–91.
2. Tanaka KR, Valentine WN, Miwa S. 1962. Pyruvate kinase (PK) deficiency hereditary non-spherocytic hemolytic anemia. Blood 19:267–277.
3. Beutler E, Gelbart T. 2000. Estimating the prevalence of pyruvate kinase deficiency from the gene frequency in the general white population. Blood 95:3585–3588.
4. Ferreira P, Morais L, Costa R, et al. 2000. Hydrops fetalis associated with erythrocyte pyruvate kinase deficiency. Eur J Pediatr 159:481–482.
5. Gilsanz F, Vega MA, Gomez-Castillo E, Ruiz-Balda JA, Omenaca F. 1993. Fetal anaemia due to pyruvate kinase deficiency. Arch Dis Child 69(5 Spec No):523–524.
6. Ghidini A, Sirtori M, Romero R, Yarkoni S, Solomon L, Hobbins JC. 1991. Hepatosplenomegaly as the only prenatal finding in a fetus with pyruvate kinase deficiency anemia. Am J Perinatol 8:44–46.
7. Andersen FD, d'Amore F, Nielsen FC, van Solinge W, Jensen F, Jensen PD. 2004. Unexpectedly high but still asymptomatic iron overload in a patient with pyruvate kinase deficiency. Hematol J 5:543–545.

8   Zanella A, Bianchi P, Iurlo A, et al. 2001. Iron status and HFE genotype in erythrocyte pyruvate kinase deficiency: Study of Italian cases. Blood Cells Mol Dis 27:653–661.

9   Duncan JR, Potter CB, Cappellini MD, Kurtz JB, Anderson MJ, Weatherall DJ. 1983. Aplastic crisis due to parvovirus infection in pyruvate kinase deficiency. Lancet 2(8340):14–16.

10 Amankwah KS, Dick BW, Dodge S. 1980. Hemolytic anemia and pyruvate kinase deficiency in pregnancy. Obstet Gynecol 55(3 Suppl):42S–44S.

11 Ghidini A, Korker VL. 1998. Severe pyruvate kinase deficiency anemia. A case report. J Reprod Med 43:713–715.

12 Esen UI, Olajide F. 1998. Pyruvate kinase deficiency: An unusual cause of puerperal jaundice. Int J Clin Pract 52:349–350.

13 Boivin P, Galand C, Hakim J, Kahn A. 1975. Acquired red cell pyruvate kinase deficiency in leukemias and related disorders. Enzyme 19:294–299.

14 Kornberg A, Goldfarb A. 1986. Preleukemia manifested by hemolytic anemia with pyruvate-kinase deficiency. Arch Intern Med 146:785–786.

15 Wang C, Chiarelli LR, Bianchi P, et al. 2001. Human erythrocyte pyruvate kinase: Characterization of the recombinant enzyme and a mutant form (R510Q) causing nonspherocytic hemolytic anemia. Blood 98:3113–3120.

16 Kanno H, Ballas SK, Miwa S, Fujii H, Bowman HS. 1994. Molecular abnormality of erythrocyte pyruvate kinase deficiency in the Amish. Blood 83:231123–231126.

17 Manco L, Ribeiro ML, Maximo V, et al. 2000. A new PKLR gene mutation in the R-type promoter region affects the gene transcription causing pyruvate kinase deficiency. Br J Haematol 110:993–997.

18 Kugler W, Laspe P, Stahl M, Schroter W, Lakomek M. 1999. Identification of a novel promoter mutation in the human pyruvate kinase (PK) LR gene of a patient with severe haemolytic anaemia. Br J Haematol 105:596–598.

19 Kanno H, Fujii H, Wei DC, et al. 1997. Frame shift mutation, exon skipping, and a two-codon deletion caused by splice site mutations account for pyruvate kinase deficiency. Blood 89:4213–4218.

20 Hirono A, Forman L, Beutler E. 1988. Enzymatic diagnosis in non-spherocytic hemolytic anemia. Medicine (Baltimore) 67:110–117.

21 Valentini G, Chiarelli LR, Fortin R, et al. 2002. Structure and function of human erythrocyte pyruvate kinase. Molecular basis of nonspherocytic hemolytic anemia. J Biol Chem 277:23807–23814.

22 Tanphaichitr VS, Suvatte V, Issaragrisil S, et al. 2000. Successful bone marrow transplantation in a child with red blood cell pyruvate kinase deficiency. Bone Marrow Transplant 26:689–690.

Membrane Disorders

CHAPTER 17

ANEMIAS ASSOCIATED WITH ERYTHROCYTE MEMBRANE ABNORMALITIES

The plasma membrane is the crucial demarcation between the interior of the cell and the rest of the world. The membrane is a restraint against escape of components vital to cell health and growth. At the same time, the plasma membrane is the barrier that protects the cell against the unwanted intrusion of external factors, both animate and inanimate. The shape of cells and their mechanical properties owe much to the characteristics of the plasma membrane.

Erythrocytes are the simplest cells in the body. They lack both nuclei and mitochondria and have an interior composition dominated by hemoglobin. In contrast to the simplicity of the cell interior, the red cell membrane is a complex structure composed of a host of specific proteins as well as a variety of lipids. The outer layer consists of a lipid bilayer containing phospholipids and cholesterol that are in dynamic equilibrium with plasma lipids. Floating in the lipid sea are a number of intrinsic membrane proteins and glycoproteins, including blood group glycoproteins and a variety of ion channels that maintain cellular ionic and osmotic balance by pumping ions either into or out of the cell.

Beneath the lipid membrane is a complex cytoskeleton of membrane proteins that includes α and β spectrin, actin, protein 4.2, and band 3. These proteins are prominent components of an intricate lattice that undergirds the plasma membrane itself. The protein ankyrin physically bridges the cytoskeleton and the membrane, connecting β spectrin to band 3, an intrinsic membrane glycoprotein (Figure 17-1). Defects involving the cytoskeletal proteins produce a number of red cell disorders.[1]

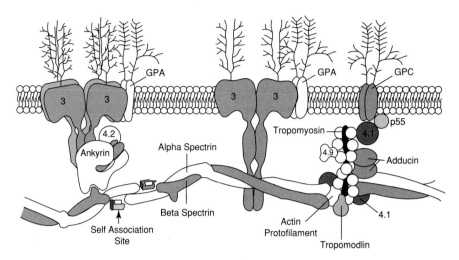

FIGURE 17–1 *Schematic diagram of the red cell membrane cytoskeleton. A complex lattice-work of proteins whose dominant members are α and β spectrin exists immediately below the red cell lipid bilayer. Ankyrin links the cytoskeleton to the membrane by forming a bridge between β spectrin and the intrinsic membrane protein, band 3. Actin and protein 4.2 are also prominent members of the red cell cytoskeleton. (From Lux SE, Palek J. 1995. Disorders of the red cell membrane. In: Handin RJ, Lux SE, Stossel TP, eds. Blood: Principles and Practice of Hematology. Philadelphia, Lippincott-Raven. Figure 54-20, pp. 1701–1818.)*

■ HEREDITARY SPHEROCYTOSIS

Hereditary spherocytosis (HS) is the most common cause of familial hemolytic anemia in peoples of north European background with an estimated frequency in the United States of about 1/5000. The disorder occurs in other ethnic groups, but with lower prevalence. An inherited deficiency of the cytoskeleton proteins, α and β spectrin sometimes accompanied by decreased quantities of ankyrin, underlies most cases of HS. Less frequently, the culprit is an inherited deficiency of band 3 or protein 4.2. These membrane abnormalities greatly increase permeability to ionic sodium with a consequent decrease in red cell survival due to eythrocyte "conditioning" during repeated sojourns through the spleen.

The sluggish percolation of erythrocytes through the splenic circulation produces major red cell stress. The increased cation permeability creates a need for energy production that cannot be met in the relatively acidic and hypoglycemic splenic environment. Inability to maintain the lipid bilayer, an energy-dependent process, ultimately results in loss of erythrocyte membrane. Reduction in surface area without loss of cell volume imparts a spherical shape to the red cells (Figure 17-2). Spherocytic red cells are rigid and progressively loose the ability to filter through the splenic circulation. Splenic reticuloendothelial cells selectively remove these damaged cells producing the hemolytic process characteristic of the disorder. Thus, HS is primarily a red cell abnormality that requires the spleen to produce hemolysis.

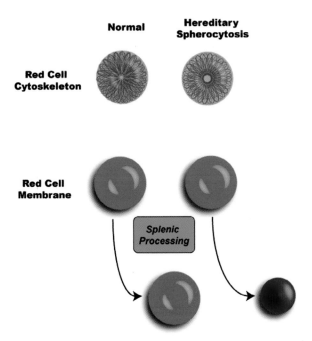

FIGURE 17–2 *Schematic diagram of the cytoskeleton in normal and HS red cells. The upper row of the diagram highlights the cytoskeleton in the cells, showing the reduction associated with HS. The middle row shows that both normal and HS red cells initially exist as biconcave discs. The relatively acidic and hypoglycemic splenic environment stresses both cells. The cytoskeleton deficit of the HS cells results in membrane loss and the formation of spherocytic red cells, as shown in the bottom row.*

CLINICAL MANIFESTATIONS

Hemolytic anemia of variable severity, unconjugated hyperbilirubinemia and acholuric jaundice, reticulocytosis, and clinical splenomegaly along with a family history of anemia, jaundice, splenectomy, and gallstones are frequent features of patients with HS. In many patients, enhanced red cell production compensates for the decreased erythrocyte survival and anemia is absent or mild. While HS produces a tremendously broad spectrum of anemia, within a single family the severity of the anemia tends to run true.

HS commonly presents in the neonatal period with anemia and hyperbilirubinemia that can necessitate exchange transfusion or phototherapy to prevent kernicterus. During the first year or so of life, some children require periodic red cell transfusions. Many children with these early problems improve over time and maintain reasonable levels of hemoglobin that support normal growth and physical activity. Severe HS can profoundly expand the erythroid marrow in some children with consequent unsightly cosmetic changes to the face.

Pigmented gallstones often develop as early as 3–4 years of age, meaning that children with HS should be monitored by abdominal ultrasound examinations.[2] The risk of cholelithiasis is even greater in patients with coexisting Gilbert's syndrome.[3] As in other chronic hemolytic conditions, children with HS are susceptible to transient "aplastic crises" characterized by severe anemia and reticulocytopenia in association with parvovirus B19 infections. Extreme degrees of anemia can also occur during other intercurrent viral infection such as infectious mononucleosis presumably because of increased splenomegaly. Adults with HS usually have moderate anemia (8–10 gm/dL), reticulocytosis, acholuric jaundice, and splenomegaly. Interestingly, some people with mild to moderate HS come to clinical attention only in the wake of a transient aplastic crisis due to infection with parvovirus B19.[4,5]

LABORATORY DIAGNOSIS

Prevenient laboratory findings pointing to HS include a peripheral blood smear with variable numbers of small, dense red cells that lack biconcavity (microspherocytes) (Figure 17-3). Some patients with severe disease show an almost exclusive picture of spherocytes on the blood smear. In contrast, spherocytes are sometimes elusive in patients with mild HS. Polychromasia reflecting reticulocytosis often is prominent. The MCHC is high (>36%) as is the RDW. These findings usually indicate a diagnosis of HS, but with many spherocytes on the blood smear, autoimmune hemolytic anemia, or in a newborn, ABO immune hemolysis merit consideration.

Osmotic fragility testing will confirm the diagnosis of HS. Red cells are mixed with a series of hypotonic saline solutions ranging from isotonic saline to distilled water. After a brief incubation, the solutions are centrifuged to sediment intact red

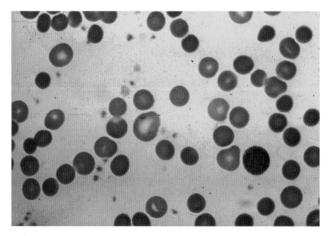

FIGURE 17-3 *Peripheral blood in HS. The smear shows numerous dense spherocytes in addition to other relatively normal appearing red cells. The large bluish cells are reticulocytes.*

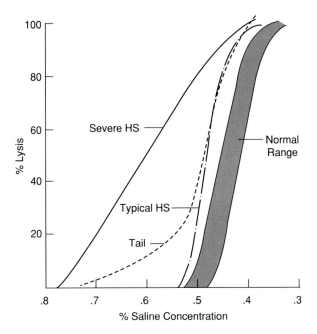

FIGURE 17–4 *Osmotic fragility curves. The shaded region in the figure shows the range over which normal cells lyse with lower ionic strength solutions. The dashed curve shows the pattern with HS where more hemolysis occurs than normal at every saline concentration. (From Nathan and Oski. 1998. In: Nathan DG, Orkin SH, eds. Hematology of Infancy and Childhood, 5th edn. Philadelphia, PA: Saunders. Figure 16-20.)*

cells and the hemoglobin content of the supernate is measured to quantify the degree of hemolysis at each saline concentration. Hemolysis in HS characteristically occurs at higher saline concentrations relative to normal controls (increased osmotic fragility) as shown in Figure 17-4. Sterile preincubation of the blood at 37°C for 24 hours increases the sensitivity of the test.

GENETICS

The inheritance pattern of HS most often is that of an autosomal dominant condition. However, in about 20% of cases, even careful examinations show both parents to be normal. Such "sporadic" cases of HS are believed to reflect new mutations that can be passed on to the next generation as an autosomal dominant feature. Rarely, cases of very severe HS appear to have a recessive transmission associated with a profound deficiency of spectrin. The various abnormal genes associated with HS have been identified and are located on chromosome 1, q22–23 (α spectrin), chromosome 8, p11.2 (ankyrin) chromosome 14, q23–24 (β spectrin), and chromosome 15, q15–21 (protein 4.2).

TREATMENT

Surgical removal of the spleen is the usual treatment for HS.[6] The timing of splenectomy is variable and at times somewhat controversial. In infants with severe anemia that requires frequent red cell transfusions to maintain normal growth and activity, early splenectomy is a consideration, although concern exists about the risk of

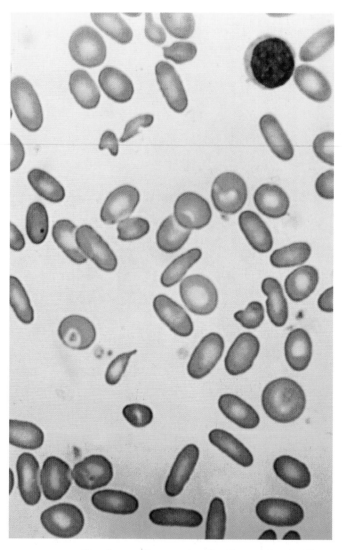

FIGURE 17-5 *Hereditary elliptocytosis. The elongated red cells are typical of hereditary elliptocytosis. (From Kapff CT, Jandl JH. 1991. Blood: Atlas and Sourcebook of Hematology, 2nd edn. Boston: Little, Brown and Company. Figure 19-1, p. 45. Reproduced with permission of the publisher.)*

overwhelming postsplenectomy sepsis.[7] The availability of protein-conjugated vaccines against *Streptococcus pneumoniae* and *Haemophilus influenzae* that are effective in infancy makes early splenectomy less risky, but prophylactic antibiotics are still recommended for the first 5–6 years of life. When possible, splenectomy should be deferred until the child is at least 5–6 years of age.

Whether splenectomy is necessary for all patients is debatable. Patients with fully compensated hemolysis are asymptomatic, but splenectomy can be indicated because of progressive splenomegaly. Cosmetic deformities due to marrow expansion can also prompt splenectomy in these children. Following splenectomy, anemia and hemolysis subside and the reticulocyte count declines into the normal range. However, the number of spherocytes on the peripheral blood smear increases markedly. Splenectomy eliminates the hemolytic process, eliminates the anemia, obviates the need for transfusions, and reduces the risks of aplastic crises and gallstones. Partial splenectomy has been advocated which may temporarily reduce the rate of hemolysis. However, the residual splenic tissue usually hypertrophies and the hemolysis resumes.[8,9]

■ HEREDITARY ELLIPTOCYTOSIS

Hereditary elliptocytosis (HE) or ovalocytosis is a heterogenous group of blood conditions characterized by elliptical red cells. The common, asymptomatic variety produces uniformly elliptical red cells but without hemolysis or increased erythrocyte production (Figure 17-5). The condition is transmitted as an autosomal dominant trait, meaning that a parent will also have elliptical red cells. Significant hemolysis afflicts a small subset of patients with elliptical erythrocytes who are designated as having "hereditary hemolytic elliptocytosis." During the neonatal period these patients can develop significant anemia and hyperbilirubinemia. Their blood smears show extreme poikilocytosis and spherocytosis whose magnitude exceeds the elliptocytosis. One of the parents usually has elliptical red cells. These patients tend to improve with passing time, but their blood smears show spherocytes as well as elliptical cells. HE is

TABLE 17-1 | DIAGNOSTIC ISSUES IN HEREDITARY SPHEROCYTOSIS

Issue	*Manifestation*	*Approach*
Neonatal presentation	Anemia, hyperbilirubinemia	● Review smear for spherocytes. ● Check red cell osmotic fragility. ● Rule out ABO isoimmune hemolysis of the newborn.
Gallstones	Often asymptomatic. Can produce abdominal pain, chills, fever, and severe jaundice.	● Ultrasound monitoring for gallstones. ● Cholecystectomy for large or symptomatic stones.

TABLE 17-2 | **MANAGEMENT ISSUES IN HEREDITARY SPHEROCYTOSIS**

Issue	*Comment*
Neonatal hyperbilirubinemia	Neonatal hyperbilirubinemia with the associated threat of kernicterus is a common presentation with HS. Some infants require phototherapy with or without exchange transfusion. The severity of the hemolysis often improves over time.
Splenectomy	Splenectomy relieves the hemolysis and anemia of HS. If possible, the procedure should be deferred until the child reaches 5 or 6 years of age to lessen the risk of systemic infection. Immunization against *Streptococcus pneumoniae* and *Haemophilus influenzae* is crucial. Prophylactic antibodies should be given until the age of 5 or 6 years.

caused by inherited deficiencies of the erythrocyte cytoskeleton, particularly α spectrin. If significant hemolytic anemia persists, splenectomy is a consideration since the procedure eliminates anemia in most patients (Tables 17-1 and 17-2).

References

[1] Gallagher PG, Lux S. 2003. Disorders of the erythrocyte membrane. In: Nathan DG, Orkin SH, Ginsburg D. Look AT, eds. Hematology of Infancy and Childhood. Philadelphia, PA: Saunders. Chapter 15, 560–684.

[2] Tamary H, Aviner S, Freud E, et al. 2003. High incidence of early cholelithiasis detected by ultrasonography in children and young adults with hereditary spherocytosis. J Pediatr Hematol Oncol 25:952–954.

[3] del Giudice EM, Perrotta S, Nobili B, Specchia C, d'Urzo G, Iolascon A. 1999. Coinheritance of Gilbert syndrome increases the risk for developing gallstones in patients with hereditary spherocytosis. Blood 94:2259–2262.

[4] Ng JP, Cumming RL, Horn EH, Hogg RB. 1987. Hereditary spherocytosis revealed by human parvovirus infection. Br J Haematol 65:379–380.

[5] Lefrere JJ, Courouce AM, Girot R, Bertrand Y, Soulier JP. 1986. Six cases of hereditary spherocytosis revealed by human parvovirus infection. Br J Haematol 62:653–658.

[6] Bader-Meunier B, Gauthier F. 2001. Long term evaluation of the beneficial effect of splenectomy for management of hereditary spherocytosis. Blood 97:2001

[7] Schilling RF. 1995. Estimating the risk for sepsis after splenectomy in hereditary spherocytosis. Ann Intern Med 122:187–188.

[8] De Buys Roessingh AS, Lagausie P, Rohrlich P, Berrebi D, Aigrain Y. 2002. Follow up of partial splenectomy in children with hereditary spherocytoisis. J Pediatr Surg 37:1459–1463.

[9] Sandoval C, Srtringel G, Weisberger J, Jayabose S. 1997. Failure of partial splenectomy to ameliorate the anemia of pyruvate kinase deficiency. J Pediatr Surg 32:641–642.

Immune Dysfunction

CHAPTER 18

ERYTHROBLASTOSIS FETALIS (IMMUNE HEMOLYTIC DISEASE OF THE NEWBORN)

In 1932, Dr. Louis K. Diamond and associates suggested that a single pathological process produced three supposedly distinct hematological syndromes of the newborn infant: universal edema (*hydrops fetalis*); anemia of the newborn; and *icterus gravis neonatorum.*[1] The new designation, *erythroblastosis fetalis,* emphasized the abundant presence of nucleated red cells in the blood and extramedullary organs of affected fetuses and infants. The decades following this description saw the discovery of the cause of erythroblastosis fetalis and the introduction of a series of diagnostic and therapeutic interventions that reduced the morbidity and mortality associated with the condition. Most importantly, the introduction of preventive measures has virtually eradicated the condition in much of the world. The story of the identification, treatment, and prevention of erythroblastosis fetalis, or immune hemolytic disease of the newborn (IHDN), is one of the great medical triumphs of the twentieth century.

■ ETIOLOGY OF IHDN

IHDN is a subset of the disorders discussed in the chapter on immune-mediated hemolysis (Chapter 19), which include autoimmune hemolytic anemia and transfusion-induced hemolysis. The former condition is a frankly pathologic state most commonly involving an immune regulatory system gone amok. The latter is an iatrogenic problem related to the introduction of foreign material (transfused red cells) into the blood stream.

IHDN is a blend of the two whose origin lies in the special relationship that exists between the mother and fetus. A partial state of immune tolerance allows the temporary coexistence of two genetically and antigenically distinct individuals. The tolerance is precarious with its integrity depending on the powerful physical barrier created by the placenta. The placenta is the gatekeeper that employs specific transport mechanisms to supply building blocks to the fetus while removing potentially toxic substances from the fetal environment.

The maternal and fetal circulations come into close juxtaposition in the placenta but do not commingle. The placenta has specific transport machinery to supply maternal antibodies of the IgG class to the fetus. These provide important protection to the immunologically immature newborn against pathogens that after birth descend like flies. The happy state functions flawlessly millions of times each year. However, on occasion problems do arise.

■ THE Rh ANTIGEN CULPRIT IN IHDN

The Rh antigen (Rhesus, referring to the important role this primate played in the early antigen characterization) is one of the many glycoprotein families expressed on the red cell membrane. Glycoproteins are quite immunogenic and most provoke some degree of antibody production when introduced into a foreign environment. Most of the red cell membrane glycoproteins have no assigned function, although they all presumably have some physiological role. The Rh proteins are part of an ancient and ubiquitous gene superfamily whose original members had a role in the regulation of cellular ammonium transport.[2] The current Rh gene family seen on red cells diverged from the primordial gene millions of years ago. Although the Rh proteins might have a residual role in ammonium homeostasis, the point remains open.[3]

The Rh blood group is widely expressed on red cells. The family has many members that differ by small structural variations. In the context of IHDN, the Rh D group is the key component. In routine clinical usage, the term "Rh positive" refers to red cells that express the Rh D antigen, ignoring all other Rh antigens. Red cells that lack Rh D are designated as "Rh negative." The importance of the Rh D antigen lies in what appears to be a historical genetic anomaly.

Most likely, in the anthropologically distant past all human red cells expressed the Rh D antigen. At some point in Europe, a mutation caused the loss of *RHD gene* expression.[4] Over time, the proportion of the Rh D-negative gene rose in the population to the point that currently about 15% of Caucasians are Rh D-negative. This remarkably high figure must reflect some past selective advantage since this is the sole means by which a variant can attain such a high gene frequency. The Rh D-negative phenotype is much less common in other ethnic groups. The 7–8% incidence of the Rh D-negative phenotype seen in African Americans likely reflects genetic admixture with Europeans. The Rh D-negative phenotype is fleetingly rare in East Asian peoples.[5,6]

■ Rh SENSITIZATION

Rh sensitization requires a specific clinical scenario in which the mother is Rh D-negative and the fetus is Rh D-positive.[7] The gene for Rh D expression in the fetus comes from the father, of course. However, several other factors must convene to trigger the production of antibodies to Rh D by the mother.

Most obviously, fetal blood must break the placental barrier and enter the maternal circulation. The likelihood of an antibody response rises with the volume of the leak. During the course of pregnancy, fetal red cells intermittently gain access to the maternal circulation in quantities ranging from 0.1 to 1.0 mL. These repeated small trespasses appear to provoke the antibodies against the Rh D antigen in the Rh D-negative mother.[8] Greater immunization occurs with the larger transplacental hemorrhages that accompany processes that severely disrupt the integrity of the placental barrier, such as toxemia. The largest risk of fetal to maternal blood transfer occurs at delivery. Rare causes of Rh D antigen sensitization include midtrimester spontaneous abortion and blood transfusion.

The Kleihauher-Betke stain allows simple detection of fetal red cells in the maternal circulation.[9] The test takes advantage of the relative resistance of fetal hemoglobin to alkaline denaturation. Maternal cells appear as washed-out ghosts while fetal cells stand out following the staining. Imprecise and subjective readouts often counterbalance the simplicity of this test. Fluorescence-activated cell sorter analysis using antibodies specific to human fetal hemoglobin or to Rh D detects minute numbers of fetal cells in the maternal circulation. Florescence microscopy is an alternate way to use this newer technology.[10]

Without preventive intervention, about 15% of Rh D-negative mothers will develop antibodies to Rh D during their first pregnancy where the fetus is Rh D-positive. Successive such pregnancies increase both the incidence of antibody production and its titer. For this reason, the severity of erythroblastosis fetalis increases with successive pregnancies in women so unfortunate as to suffer repetitions of the problem.

Other factors influence the rate and risk of Rh D immunization. Fetal red cells with a high density of Rh D antigen on the membrane are more likely to provoke an antibody response than are cells with a low antigen density.[11] Phenotypic characteristics of the father influence red cell density Rh D antigen. Interestingly, ABO incompatibility between mother and fetus lowers the risk of Rh immunization. The key fact in this setting is that the antibodies directed against ABO blood group antigens primarily are of the IgM class. IgM antibodies do not cross the placental barrier, thereby minimizing any hemolysis in utero. Furthermore, IgM antibodies directly and quickly lyse fetal red cells that cross into the maternal circulation. Few fetal cells reach the macrophage/lymphocyte system to prompt production of IgG antibodies against the Rh D antigen.

■ CLINICAL ASPECTS OF IHDN

The disease has a wide spectrum of severity that correlates with the level of maternal antibodies. First pregnancies are rarely affected. All pregnant women should have red cell grouping and typing in early pregnancy. Rh D-negative women should have their serum examined for the presence of anti-D antibodies by midtrimester. Should the mother have anti-D antibody, antibody titer determinations are in order. When the anti-D titer is high, the degree of fetal involvement is assessed.

In the most severely afflicted fetuses, the hemolytic process is so extreme that a progressively more severe anemia occurs in the midtrimester. In some fetuses, the anemia is extreme to the point of provoking congestive heart failure, resulting in universal edema and often in fetal death. At times, neutropenia and thrombocytopenia occur in association with the extreme anemia. Infants at high risk for intrauterine death can be salvaged by intrauterine transfusions and exchange transfusions permitting them to remain in utero until they attain a level of maturity consistent with safe delivery.[12]

Somewhat less severely affected infants are born alive, although they usually have substantial anemia with associated marked hepatosplenomegaly due to extramedullary hematopoiesis. Hyperbilirubinemia at the time of delivery is typical. The hemoglobin value at birth usually is less than 13.0 g/dL. The direct antiglobulin (Coombs') test is positive, reflecting antibody directed against the Rh D antigen. A plethora of nucleated red cells exist on the peripheral smear, true to the term erythroblastosis fetalis (Figure 18-1). The high level of unconjugated bilirubin at birth

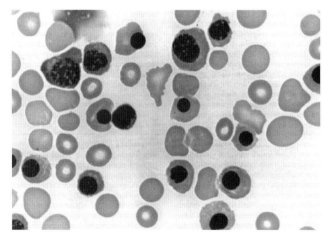

FIGURE 18–1 *Blood smear from a neonate with erythroblastosis fetalis. Erythroblasts of nearly all stages of normal development are present, accompanied by numerous polychromatophilic cells, scattered poikilocytes, and small numbers of spherocytes. (From Jandl JH. 1987. Blood: Textbook of Hematology. Boston: Little, Brown and Company. Figure 9-2, p. 293. With permission from the publisher.)*

rises following delivery since the placental connection is severed and the option of shunting the metabolite to the maternal circulation for disposal is lost.

Severe hyperbilirubinemia is the primary basis of morbidity and mortality in infants born with erythroblastosis fetalis. The high bilirubin level in these infants reflects both red cell destruction and the limited capacity of the liver to metabolize the compound.[13] Hyperbilirubinemia can cause severe neurological disease (kernicterus) and even death. Frequent sequelae of kernicterus include mental retardation, cerebral palsy, and deafness. The immature blood–brain barrier of the newborn cannot prevent free bilirubin in the plasma from entering the brain and damaging neurons. Albumin has a carrying capacity for bilirubin that approximates 20 mg/dL. Beyond this level the toxic metabolite is free in the plasma and able to cross into the neonate's brain.

Successful efforts that control bilirubin and maintain values below 20 mg/dL prevent most cases of kernicterus and its severe neurological consequences. Exchange transfusion through the umbilical vein is an effective means to this end.[14] The procedure involves the intermittent aspiration of 10–20 mL of fetal blood from the umbilical vein and its replacement with whole blood that is Rh negative and compatible with the mother's serum. An exchange volume of approximately twice the blood volume replaces 90% of the infant's red cells. A concentrated albumin solution is sometimes infused prior to the exchange absorbs additional bilirubin that is subsequently removed with the exchange procedure.

Bilirubin levels of mildly affected babies with less extreme hemolytic anemia can be near normal at birth but increase by 1–2 mg/dL daily to dangerously high postnatal levels. Such neonates usually require exchange transfusions but often they can be controlled by phototherapy. These infants are however at risk of developing very severe anemia in the first month of life because of the short survival of antibody-coated red cells. Close monitoring of these infants for the first 6–8 weeks of life is essential. Some require a simple transfusion with Rh D-negative red cells to stave off problems.

In the 1960s, prevention of Rh D isoimmunization and clinical erythroblastosis became possible.[15,16] Two groups, one in New York and the other in England, demonstrated that intravenous administration of anti-Rh immunoglobulin (Rhogam) to nonimmunized Rh D-negative mothers immediately postpartum could prevent primary immunization. The precise mechanism is not fully established, but a major reason could be that the antibody destroys fetal Rh D-positive red cells that have entered the maternal circulation in the peripartum period before they can evoke an immunological response in the mother.

This procedure has produced dramatic results. The incidence of erythroblastosis fetalis due to Rh D sensitization has decreased so greatly that it now is a rare disease in the United States and Europe. The gratifying outcome is that many physicians trained in recent decades have never seen the disorder.

Far less commonly, erythroblastosis fetalis results from maternal sensitization to other red cell antigens of the Rh system including C, c, and e. Antigens outside the Rh family such as Kell, Duffy, Kidd, and S/s on occasion produce similar problems if the mother lacks these antigens while carrying a fetus who expresses them. In the event of exchange transfusion to control hyperbilirubinemia, the transfused RBC should lack the offending blood group.

■ ABO HEMOLYTIC DISEASE OF THE NEWBORN

About 60% of persons lack A or B antigens on their RBC and are designated as having blood group O. Group O individuals have naturally occurring anti-A and anti-B antibodies in their serum (hemagglutinins). These antibodies are usually of the IgM class and so do not cross the placenta. However, some pregnant women occasionally develop IgG anti-A or anti-B antibodies that cross the placenta and induce hemolysis of either A-positive or B-positive fetal red cells. Most commonly, ABO hemolytic disease of the newborn involves an infant with blood group A and a mother with blood group O.

ABO erythroblastosis does not cause severe anemia in the fetus, so hydrops fetalis does not occur. Reticulocytosis exists at birth but the affected newborn usually lacks significant anemia. The blood smear shows polychromasia, a few nucleated RBCs, and intense spherocytosis. The direct Coombs' test (DAT) is usually positive, but can be weakly so. Jaundice often occurs in the first 24 hours of life, and monitoring of the serum bilirubin level is important. Extreme hyperbilirubinemia can require exchange transfusion or phototherapy to prevent kernicterus and its complications. In interesting contrast to IHDN due to Rh D incompatibility, hemolysis in the newborn due to ABO incompatibility occurs significantly more frequently in African American

TABLE 18-1 | KEY DIAGNOSTIC POINTS IN IHDN

Issue	*Manifestaion*	*Approach*
Maternal immunization to Rh D	• Rising antibody titers to Rh D	• Monitor antibody titers during pregnancy. • RhoGam immunization at delivery.
Hemolysis of fetal red cells	• Fetal hemolytic anemia	• Intrauterine transfusion or exchange transfusion through an umbilical or placental vein for severe anemia, to permit the extension of gestation.
Postpartum hyperbilirubinemia	• Rising neonatal bilirubin levels (20 mg/dL is *extremely* severe)	• Exchange transfusion and/or phototherapy.
Anemia in early infancy	Declining infant hemoglobin level	• Simple transfusion with Rh D-negative red cells.

infants than in Caucasians.[17] No child should be discharged from medical care before indicated. Extra vigilance is needed, however, for African American children when ABO incompatibility exists (Table 18-1).

References

[1] Diamond LK, Blackfan KD, Baty JM. 1932. Erythroblastosis fetalis and its association with universal edema of the fetus, icterus gravis neonatorum and anemia of the newborn. J Pediatr 1:269–309.

[2] Kitano T, Saitou N. 2000. Evolutionary history of the Rh blood group-related genes in vertebrates. Immunogenetics 51:856–862.

[3] Huang CH, Liu PZ. 2001. New insights into the Rh superfamily of genes and proteins in erythroid cells and nonerythroid tissues. Blood Cells Mol Dis 27:90–101.

[4] Colin Y, Cherif-Zahar B, Le Yan Kim C, Raynal V, Yan Huffel V, Cartron JP. 1991. Genetic basis of the RhD-positive and RhD-negative blood group polymorphism as determined by Southern analysis. Blood 78:2747–2752.

[5] Salmon D, Godelier M, Halle L, et al. 1988. Blood groups in Papua New Guinea Eastern Highlands. Gene Geogr 2(2–3):89–98.

[6] Lee CK, Ma ES, Tang M, Lam CC, Lin CK, Chan LC. 2003. Prevalence and specificity of clinically significant red cell alloantibodies in Chinese women during pregnancy—a review of cases from 1997 to 2001. Transfus Med 13:227–231.

[7] Hadley AG, Kumpel BM. 1993. The role of Rh antibodies in haemolytic disease of the newborn. Baillieres Clin Haematol 6:423–444.

[8] Jakobowicz R, Williams L, Silberman F. 1972. Immunization of Rh negative volunteers by repeated injections of very small amounts of Rh positive blood. Vox Sang 23:349–360.

[9] Holcomb WL, Gunderson E, Petrie RH. 1990. Clinical use of the Kleihauer-Betke test. J Perinat Med 18:331–337.

[10] Ochsenbein-Imhof N, Ochsenbein AF, Seifert B, Huch A, Huch R, Zimmermann R. 2002. Quantification of fetomaternal hemorrhage by fluorescence microscopy is equivalent to flow cytometry. Transfusion 42:947–953.

[11] Murry S. 1957. The effect of Rh genotypes on severity of haemolytic disease of the newborn. Br J Haematol 3:143–151.

[12] Diamond LK, Allen FH, Thomas WO, Jr. 1951. Erythroblastosis fetalis VII. Treatment with exchange tranfusion. N Engl J Med 244:621–631.

[13] Thaler MM. 1972. Perinatal bilirubin metabolism. Adv Pediatr 19:215–227.

[14] Pearson HA. 2003. The rise and fall of exchange transfusion. NeoReviews 7:171–174.

[15] Freda VJ, Gorman JG, Pollock W, Robertson JG, Jennings JR, Sullivan JF. 1967. Prevention of Rh isoimmunization. Progress report of the clinical trial in mothers. JAMA 199:390–394.

[16] Clark CA. 1967. Prevention of Rh haemolytic disease. Br Med J 4P:7–12.

[17] Kirkman HN, Jr. 1977. Further evidence for a racial difference in frequency of ABO hemolytic disease. J Pediatr 90(5):717–721.

The immune system is a vital defense mechanism against invasion by a variety of external pathogens ranging from bacteria and viruses to helminthes and parasites. The two divisions of the system, humeral immunity that involves the production of antibodies and cellular immunity that is conducted through the auspices of lymphocytes, work in concert toward this important end. Blood is the primary purveyor of the defense mechanisms, transporting both antibodies and lymphocytes to sites of need. As with any biological system, problems and breakdown can lead to injury and disease. These self-directed immune responses (autoimmune disorders) can strike any organ system due to poorly understood failures in immune tolerance. The resulting disorders range widely in scope and manifestations, including conditions such as systemic lupus erythematosus, type I diabetes mellitus, and vitiligo. Poor control of autoimmune processes can produce severe morbidity and, all-too-frequently, mortality.

As an organ, the erythron likewise is susceptible to immune-mediated injury. Immune-mediated hemolysis was one of the first medical conditions whose fundamental details were worked out. The need to better understand the problems and potential of blood transfusion spurred these efforts. The field took on a life and complexity of its own that led to the outgrowth of blood banking as a discipline separate from basic hematology. The need to understand the principles involved in immune reactions knows no disciplinary boundaries, however.

Antibodies are the principle weapons in immune-mediated destruction of red cells, triggering events that allow other components of the immune panoply including the macrophages of the reticuloendothelial system to complete the demolition. Figure 19-1 schematically represents the ways in which antibodies can trigger hemolysis. A key distinction is the hemolysis of endogenous versus transfused red cells. The former are normal body constituents while the latter are invaders from the point of view of the immune system. As an autoimmune process, issues involving hemolysis of endogenous red cells fall under the purview of hematology while those involving transfused red cells are generally considered to be blood-banking issues. A complete clinical understanding of the problem requires an overarching view of the process, however.

The antibodies in Figure 19-1 labeled as (1) are produced by the body's own immune system and attack endogenous red cells. This autoimmune hemolysis is a pathological process that involves dysfunctional immune regulation. Antibody (2) in Figure 19-1 attacks foreign antigens on transfused red cells. In their attack on transfused red cells, these antibodies, called isoantibodies or alloantibodies, perform the defensive job for which they are designed. The fact that the introduction of foreign erythrocytes is a medically indicated effort to stem a problem related to anemia is immaterial from the point of view of the immune defense system.

Antibody (3) in Figure 19-1 enters the system by way of serum from the transfused blood and potentially contains donor antibodies directed against the recipient (endogenous) red cells. The quantity of introduced antibody usually is small and produces only minor problems. The problem is most pronounced with the transfusion of whole blood. The current standard use of packed, washed red cells for transfusion virtually eliminates this transfusion complication.

The antibodies labeled (4) in Figure 19-1 are a special problem related to pregnancy. During fetal development, the mother can develop antibodies against fetal red cell antigens inherited from the father. These antibodies can cross the maternal–placental barrier and lyse fetal blood cells. This problem produces a dangerous and potentially lethal condition called isoimmune hemolysis of the newborn or erythroblastosis fetalis. Chapter 18 discusses this important and specialized problem.

A rare and more recently recognized condition evolves when the weapons of the immune system, either antibodies or effector lymphocytes, focus on erythroid precursors. Antibodies occasionally develop against erythropoietin or the erythropoietin receptor on developing erythroid precursor cells. Cellular immunity can damage or destroy these cells as well. The result is a singular process with very limited production of red cells by an erythron that generates all other blood components without difficulty. The severe and selective anemia is part of a process called pure red cell aplasia that falls best under the rubric of aplastic anemia.

■ COOMBS' TEST OR DIRECT ANTIGLOBULIN TEST

The Coombs' test or direct antiglobulin test (DAT) is so vital to the understanding and evaluation of immune-mediated hemolysis that a brief explanation of this tool is in

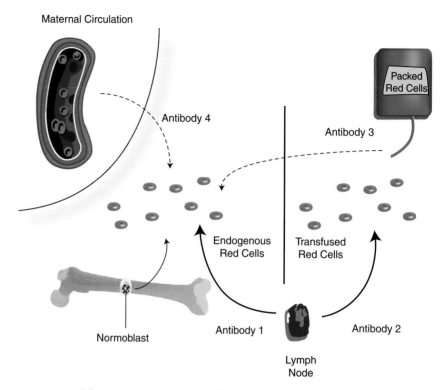

FIGURE 19–1 *Schematic representation of the components of immune-mediated hemolysis. Blood in the circulation is primarily produced in and released from the bone marrow as shown in the lower left of the figure. Transfusion shown in the upper right is the other way that red cells enter the circulation. The key distinction is that the endogenously produced cells are "self" and therefore elicit no immune response. Transfused cells are foreign elements and therefore are subject to normal immune defense operations. The natural antibodies to red cell ABO antigens are the most powerful barriers to transfusion. Natural antibodies also exist for the Rh antigens, but these are generally less potent. Antibody (2) in the figure represents these natural antibodies, which have the interchangeable names of "isoantibody" or "alloantibody." Correct typing and crossmatching in the blood bank allows the introduction of red cells that do not have the target antigens for antibody (2). Antibody (3) can be introduced into the circulation if plasma accompanies the transfused blood cells. The antibody (an alloantibody) reacts against the endogenous cells and can produce hemolysis. Whole blood transfusions face this problem, but the issue is moot with washed packed red cell transfusions that now are the treatment norm. Antibody (1) in the figure reacts against endogenous red cells and therefore is an autoantibody. The severity of the problem produced by autoantibodies depends on many factors that are discussed in detail in the text. Antibody (4) is a special case associated with pregnancy. Isoantibodies from the maternal circulation cross the placental barrier where reactions with fetal red cells produce hemolysis and other problems. The chapter on isoimmune disease of the newborn tackles this important issue.*

order. Immune hemolysis involves either IgM or IgG molecules that attach to red cell membrane antigens triggering a cascade of events that terminate in hemolysis. IgM, due to its large structure as five bridged immunoglobulin molecules in an outward facing ring, can activate complement directly, thereby mediating hemolysis without help from cellular components of the defense system. The solitary IgG molecule is unable to perform this feat, except with rare exception. IgG coats the circulating immune-marked red cells prior to their demise. The DAT is a simple means of assessing this fact.

The DAT reagent is a preparation of antibodies whose specificity is to human serum, specific pure preparations of human immuoglobulins, immunoglobulin Fc fragments, or complement components (usually C3). The process begins with a thorough washing of the cells to be tested in order to remove any adventitial plasma proteins that might adhere to the cell membrane. The only human plasma component left to react with the DAT reagent is IgG and C3 that remain attached to the red cell membrane by the strong interaction created as part of the immune coupling mechanism. IgM has the paradoxical property of dissociating from the membrane before the procedure is complete, meaning that the DAT does not detect IgM as a source of immune hemolysis.

Figure 19-2 shows two red cells each with an IgG molecule attached to the surface membrane. The DAT antibody directed against the IgG links the red cells. The process takes place many times in multiple orientations producing red cell agglutination that is visible to the naked eye. The readout is given as arbitrary values of 0–4+ depending on the degree of agglutination. Subjectivity in such instances is obvious. However, skilled technicians who read these tests become very proficient at providing reproducible answers in the DAT assay. Low power microscopy gives a better view of agglutination. However, the magnification often produces more confusion than clarification with respect to the readout so that visible assessment most often remains the standard.

Following the initial screen with the general DAT reagent, more specific information comes with the use of antibodies prepared solely against IgG, IgG subclasses, C3, or C4. The existence solely of complement in the DAT indicates that an antibody that binds and fixes complement has acted in vivo but dissociated from the membrane during the 37°C washings of the procedure. The offending antibody is termed a *cold-reactive* autoantibody and is either an IgM antibody or the singular Donath-Landsteiner IgG autoantibody that produces paroxysmal cold hemoglobinuria.

At times, the DAT is negative despite overwhelming clinical and other laboratory evidence for autoimmune hemolysis. This apparent paradox sometimes reflects a quantity of IgG on the red cell membrane that is insufficient to produce visible red cell agglutination. Other more sophisticated tests, such as an enzyme-linked immunosorbent assay (ELISA), often help to solve the dilemma. Rarely, an immunoglobulin such as IgA not detected by the DAT is the root of the problem. Expert intervention is needed to solve these problems.

■ AUTOIMMUNE HEMOLYSIS

Table 19-1 provides a classification of the immune-mediated hemolytic disorders. Primary autoimmune hemolysis has two major subgroups, each with its own

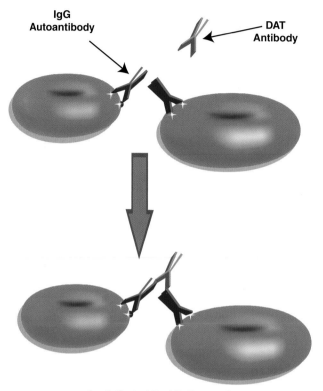

FIGURE 19–2   *Schematic representation of the DAT. The thoroughly washed red cells in the figure have only IgG autoantibody attached to the membrane surface. The strong bond created by binding between the antibody and antigen leaves the IgG in place while the washing removes loosely attached plasma proteins. The DAT antibody has recognition specificity for the IgG molecule. The DAT antibody binds to each of the IgG autoantibodies with one of its two arms, creating a bridge between the red cells. This process repeats many times in many directions and orientations. The result is agglutination of red cells to a degree that clusters of cells visible to the naked eye appear on the slide. Visible reading assigns values of 0–4+ to the degree of clustering.*

characteristics and causes. Warm-reactive autoantibodies of the IgG class are the usual culprits in this disorder. Antibodies of the IgM class most commonly cause cold-agglutinin disease. The singular Donath-Landsteiner antibody of paroxysmal cold hemoglobinuria has unique thermal properties that impart interesting and important characteristics to the disorder.

WARM-REACTIVE AUTOIMMUNE ANTIBODY HEMOLYSIS

Clinical Presentation

The onset of autoimmune hemolytic anemia (AIHA) can be fulminant, but often is insidious. Occasionally patients come to attention during an apparently routine

TABLE 19-1	**CLASSIFICATION OF IMMUNE HEMOLYTIC REACTIONS**
Autoimmune hemolytic reactions	Primary disease • Warm-reactive autoantibodies • Cold agglutinin disease • Paroxysmal cold hemoglobinuria
	Secondary disease • Autoimmune disorders • Malignancy • Infection • Drugs • Immune deficiency
Isoimmune hemolytic reactions	Hemolytic transfusion reactions
	Isoimmune hemolysis of the newborn

This classification is one approach of several that can order the participants in immune-mediated hemolysis. Some conditions could be assigned to more than one category but remain in one place for the sake of clarity. Cold agglutinin disease, for instance, can occur secondary to infection. The unique clinical character of the condition makes it best explained as a primary entity.

typing and screening due to intractable problems with agglutination produced by the autoantibody at various steps in the process. Jaundice can be the initial complaint when the pace and progress of the disorder are slow. The course of AIHA is quite variable, however. Sometimes the hemolysis stabilizes or even slows, producing a lull in disease progression. Other patients experience a fulminant course in which the hemoglobin drops two or more grams per deciliter over each 24-hour period with an attendant need for urgent and often intensive care.

In patients with explosive disease, symptoms related to anemia most often prompt medical attention. These include weakness, fatigue, and dyspnea. Palpitations and dizziness are common causes for complaint. Patients with angina at presentation demand attention commensurate with the gravity of this complaint. Pallor on physical examination is marked and often compounds jaundice, producing a sickly, sallow complexion. Many patients have prominent scleral icterus. Pale conjunctivae, nail beds, and mucous membranes are common findings on examination. A pale, salmon-colored retina is frequent. A midsystolic cardiac flow murmur is typical. Dependent edema is a sign of circulatory decompensation in the face of severe anemia.

The spleen size often is normal early in the course of the disorder, but enlarges over the course of a few weeks or even less. The spleen is soft and not tender. The organ is best appreciated with the patient lying in the left lateral position with the legs slightly bent to soften the abdominal muscles. Splenic palpation is much more difficult in these patients than in those with myelodysplastic disorders where the organ is "rock hard." A much less common finding is hepatomegaly, which often reflects right-sided congestive heart failure. Severe anemia can also prompt left-sided congestive heart failure with pulmonary edema. Lymphadenopathy suggests that the autoimmune process is secondary to a lymphoproliferative process such as lymphoma.

Less brisk autoimmune hemolysis provides a very different clinical picture. An unexplained anemia with hemoglobin values in the 10–11 g/dL range occurs in many such patients. The condition often occurs in older patients in whom the differential diagnosis of mild anemia can be extensive. The immediate clinical pressure on the provider is less, but the need to solve the mystery remains.

Anemia dominates the laboratory examination. With brisk autoimmune hemolysis, the hemoglobin level can fall to values in the range of 5 g/dL in the first 2–3 weeks of onset. The reticulocyte count rises in response to the anemia, with a steady state commonly achieved with reticulocyte values ranging between 20% and 40%. In contrast, patients with milder autoimmune hemolysis might maintain a hemoglobin value of 10 g/dL with a reticulocyte value of 5%. A feature on the peripheral smear that is virtually diagnostic of autoimmune hemolysis is that of small, intensely staining spherocytes, the so-called *microspherocytes* (Figure 19-3). These cells result from the loss of membrane segments to phagocytes attempting to clear the circulation of erythrocytes coated with antibody. Microspherocytes occasionally have a telltale small membrane projection as a remnant of the close encounter. Although microspherocytes resemble the cells that are seen with hereditary spherocytosis, their small size and intense staining distinguish them from the inherited membrane disorder.

Microspherocytes contrast with the large, pale polychromatic cells that also frequent the peripheral smear. Supravital staining with new methylene blue shows these cells to be reticulocytes. The combination of microspherocytes and reticulocytosis on the smear strongly supports the diagnosis of autoimmune hemolysis. A few nucleated red cells make an appearance in cases of very brisk hemolysis and reticulocytosis. Howell-Jolly bodies are common and of course increase in frequency following splenectomy.

An important morphological feature of a peripheral smear involving immune hemolytic anemia of any type is the relatively normal shape of the erythrocytes with the exception of microspherocytes. Most importantly, the cells lack features of mechanical membrane damage including spicules, spurs, rents, tears, or pedicles. The absence of these and other schistocyte features helps differentiate immune hemolysis from disseminated intravascular coagulation (DIC). Thrombocytopenia, anemia, and reticulocytosis dominate the latter disorder. However, the thrombocytopenia can be moderate with consequent clinical confusion with autoimmune hemolysis. The underlying cause of DIC and the required interventions differ drastically from those of autoimmune hemolysis. Proper distinction between the two conditions can be lifesaving.

The MCV is invariably high with autoimmune hemolysis reflecting the presence of large number of reticulocytes in the peripheral blood whose size typically exceeds that of erythrocytes by 10 fL or more. The WBC and platelet count are normal unless the disturbance stems from an underlying disorder that specifically affects these blood components. The high RDW typical of the condition reflects the variable red cell sizes, which range from microspherocytes to enormous reticulocytes. The serum

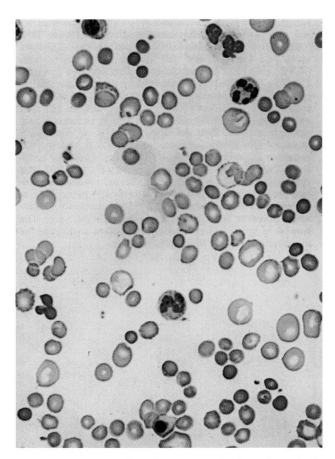

FIGURE 19-3 *Immune hemolytic anemia. The dimorphic red cell population with both micro-spherocytes and large, polychromatophilic cells is characteristic of severe immune hemolytic anemia. The former are antibody-coated erythrocytes that have lost membrane after being processed by reticuloendothelial cells. The latter are reticulocytes. In addition, the field contains a number of normoblasts that have been prematurely released into the circulation. (From Kapff CT, Jandl JH. 1991. Blood: Atlas and Sourcebook of Hematology. 2nd edn. Boston: Little, Brown and Company. Figure 17-1, p. 41. Reproduced with permission of the publisher.)*

haptoglobin level is typically low or zero. Some patients develop hemoglobinemia with brisk hemolysis, but this feature is unusual. The profile of the coagulation proteins is normal, which is an important distinction from the picture seen with DIC.

A high serum bilirubin value is a consistent feature of AIHA with values typically in the range of 5–6 mg/dL. Unconjugated bilirubin derived from erythrocyte destruction is the typical basis for the elevation in this laboratory value. A high serum LDH value reflects red cell hemolysis and release of this enzyme into the circulation. Liver enzymes such as ALT, AST, and alkaline phosphatase are normal.

TABLE 19-2 | **CAUSES OF AUTOIMMUNE HEMOLYTIC ANEMIAS**

Cause	*Examples*
Idiopathic	None
Lymphoproliferative disorders	• Chronic lymphocytic leukemia • Lymphoma • Multiple myeloma • Waldenstrom's macroglobulinemia
Autoimmune disorders	• Systemic lupus erythematosus • Rheumatoid arthritis • Ulcerative colitis
Infections	• Hepatitis C • HIV
Drugs	• α-Methyldopa • Cephalosporins

Etiology of Autoimmune Warm-Reactive Antibody Hemolysis

Table 19-2 lists some of the causes of AIHA. The idiopathic category tops the list. Common secondary causes of the disorder are the lymphoproliferative disorders and the autoimmune disorders.[1–4] Chronic lymphocytic leukemia (CLL) can be very subtle. In some patients the onset of AIHA is the first indication of the disorder. The CLL lymphocytes often have a normal morphology and the number of peripheral blood lymphocytes can be higher than normal by only a small amount. FACS analysis for lymphocyte surface antigens associated with CLL can be the only indication of the condition.

The autoimmune disorders are more common in the population as a whole, meaning that many cases of AIHA stem from these diseases. Anemia due to chronic inflammation is common with conditions such as rheumatoid arthritis and systemic lupus erythematosus. AIHA can produce an unexplained worsening of the baseline anemia in these patients. Screening for autoimmune hemolysis should always be a part of the workup for anemia exacerbations in these patients.

Infections, including HIV and hepatitis C, can also trigger autoimmune hemolysis.[5–7] Underlying immune dysfunction that is the primary component of the former infection and a prominent factor with the latter which no doubt contributes to the association. Sometimes apparently routine infections with viruses not noted for effects on the immune system can trigger AIHA.

Drugs are always the possible causes of AIHA.[8,9] α-Methyldopa is a less commonly used antihypertensive agent today but is a singular example of drug-induced

	TREATMENT OF AUTOIMMUNE-MEDIATED HEMOLYSIS
TABLE 19-3	
Intervention	*Example*
Remove offending agent	• Cephalosporin • α-Methyldopa
Treat underlying disorder	• Systemic lupus erythematosus • HIV
Immunomodulator drugs	• Corticosteroids • Rituximab • Cyclosporin A
Autoantibodies/sensitized red cells	Plasmapheresis/exchange transfusion
Block RE destruction of antibody-coated red cells	Intravenous immunoglobulin
Cytotoxic agents	• Cyclophosphamide • Azathioprine
Spleen	Splenectomy

hemolysis or red cell sensitization.[10] The drug induces red cell autoantibodies in 10–20% of patients after 4 or more months of use. These red cell antibodies are true autoantibodies directed against red blood cell membrane antigens rather than the drug or a drug-altered antigen. The target membrane antigen is usually within the Rh system, although often the antibody specificity is elusive. A warm-reacting IgG autoantibody is typical. Even with continued use of α-methyldopa, few patients who acquire these autoantibodies develop hemolytic anemia despite high titers of antibodies on their red cells. The basis of autoantibody formation remains a mystery.

Management of Autoimmune Warm-Reactive-Antibody-Mediated Hemolysis

Table 19-3 outlines the management strategy for autoimmune warm-reactive-antibody-mediated hemolysis. The approach depends on the nature of the problem, with the most important issue being the identification of any possible cryptic cause. With drugs, the obvious intervention is to remove the offending agent. Few drug treatment approaches have no alternative that effectively controls the primary medical condition without provoking a similar autoimmune hemolytic response. Likewise, control of an underlying disorder such as system lupus erythematosus can profoundly reduce or eliminate an associated autoimmune hemolytic condition. Exceptions exist in which control of the primary disorder has no effect on the hemolysis, but the logic and approach are sound.

The most taxing management issues surround idiopathic AIHA. Disordered immune regulation almost certainly is at the heart of most cases of idiopathic AIHA. In the absence of any guiding insights, the approach is completely empirical with results that too often are not optimal. The proximate cause of the problem is the autoantibodies in the circulation. An obvious and reasonable approach would be to remove these noxious agents, a feat that now is technically possible using plasmapheresis or exchange transfusion. The difficulties lie in the details, however. IgM is a large molecule that remains in the intravascular space, which allows effective removal by plasmapheresis. The confounding problem is that the rate of IgM production often matches or exceeds the rate at which the immunoglobulin can be effectively removed. Periods of relief from hemolysis often are brief. Cases do exist, however, in which patients fully recover after repeated treatments with plasmapheresis. Whether this is the cause or coincidence is unclear. The technical challenges with IgG autoantibodies are staggering since these molecules are smaller in size and spread throughout the extravascular space. The degree of effective reduction in IgG levels with plasmapheresis usually is small with disappointing results.

Another approach that aims at incapacitating the autoantibody is the infusion of large quantities of immunoglobulin. Some of the immunoglobulin molecules attach to the Fc receptors of the macrophages of the reticuloendothelial system, providing a temporary diversion from the antibody-coated red cells that would otherwise fall victim to attack mediated by the Fc receptors of these cells. The immediate onset of the effect when it works can buy time as other more long-term interventions are put into place. With older patients in particular, care to avoid fluid overload and pulmonary edema is vital. The volume of immunoglobulin used is great and the oncotic pressure of the mixture tends to pull water into the intravascular space.

Immunomodulator agents have been a mainstay in the treatment of AIHA for years, and corticosteroids are the bedrock of that approach. Intravenous infusion of high doses of steroids often dampens the hemolysis and stabilizes the hemoglobin in people who are critically ill. Many people who respond to steroids continue to require the medication, but at lower doses and in oral form. Occasionally, steroid-dependent patients can subsist on as little as 10 mg of prednisone per day.

More recently, other agents have entered the therapeutic armamentarium that act directly on the antibody producing immune cells. Promising reports exist for the use of the monoclonal antibody rituximab, which was initially introduced for treatment of B-cell lymphoid malignancies.[11–13] Presumably the agent controls or eliminates a clone of B cells that are responsible for the renegade antibody. The safety of this agent is not established for children. More nonspecific efforts to control the aberrant production of autoantibody involve the use of chemotherapy agents.

Splenectomy is more unpredictable and often less effective in the control of AIHA than is the case when the procedure is applied to patients with immune thrombocytopenic purpura (ITP). Splenectomy produces particularly disappointing results in patients who lack some degree of splenomegaly. The procedure has a relatively low operative risk, however, and is a common approach in people with refractory AIHA.

COLD AGGLUTININ DISEASE

Cold agglutinin disease is characterized by hemolytic anemia that usually includes obstruction of the microcirculation due to an antibody that promotes red cell agglutination. The agglutination phenomenon is most striking near 4°C, but occurs at higher temperatures in cases with clinical manifestations. In children, the process most commonly follows infections such as *Mycoplasma pneumoniae* or influenza. Cold agglutinin disease arises in adults most commonly as an idiopathic condition or as a sequela to an underlying lymphoproliferative process. The childhood process is self-limiting while that seen in adults is often chronic.

Older adults are the chief victims of cold agglutinin disease with an approximate mean age at onset of 60 years. Cyanosis and pain involving peripheral regions of the body, such as the fingers, ears, nose, and cheeks, are the problems that often bring people to medical attention. Winter exacerbates the difficulties to the point that some people are confined to their homes until spring. Prolonged exposure to cold occasionally produces severe acrocyanosis and even gangrene.

Cold agglutinin disease result from IgM antibodies that agglutinate red cells into clumps too large to pass through small-bore blood vessels. This occluded blood flow is the basis of the cyanosis and pain related to the disorder (Raynaud's phenomenon). The temperature dependence of the binding often is exquisitely specific. The IgM does not bind to blood flowing through the core of the body, which maintains a constant 37°C temperature. Therefore, occlusion of renal blood flow, for instance, does not occur with cold agglutinin disease. Blood flowing through the skin in the digits often falls to temperatures of 30°C or 32°C, which can be sufficiently low for the antibody to bind and produce erythrocyte clumps.

The IgM involved in cold agglutinin disease is directed against the I antigen of the red cell I-i duality. A low titer of cold-active anti-I IgM is common in adults, but the titers are low and the temperature dependence is such that little red cell binding or agglutination occurs normally. People with cold-agglutinin disease have both higher titers of antibody as well as antibodies whose temperature binding range (thermal amplitude) allows substantial red cell binding at temperatures found in the skin over the extremities.

The anemia produced by cold agglutinin disease usually is modest. Hemoglobin values can fall in the winter, however. At times the diagnosis becomes obvious by observing the clumping of blood drawn into a tube of anticoagulant as the temperature falls. Occasionally, the agglutination issue is profound to the point that making blood smears is difficult because the sample clumps when placed on the cool slide. Working with warmed equipment can be the only way around the problem. Polychromasia usually exists due to the elevation in reticulocyte count. Instances of erythrophagocytosis involving circulating monocytes/macrophages are visible occasionally, although a buffy coat preparation is best for this observation since it concentrates the white cells for easier viewing.

The hemoglobin value often hovers in the range of 10 or 11 g/dL in people with cold agglutinin disease. A mild elevation in unconjugated bilirubin produces mild jaundice. Mild or modest splenomegaly develops in some patients with cold agglutinin disease. The management of the condition first involves eliminating the possibility of an underlying lymphoproliferative process. Should the condition prove indeed to be idiopathic in nature, measures to protect the extremities against cold are the best and most efficient intervention. Occasional patients with the disorder have moved to warmer climates for relief. Splenectomy or immunosuppressive regimens generally provide little benefit.

PAROXYSMAL COLD HEMOGLOBINURIA

Paroxysmal cold hemoglobinuria is an extremely rare form of autoimmune hemolysis whose primary importance lies in its informative clinical and laboratory characteristics produced by an unusual antibody. The pathological agent in this condition, the Donath-Landsteiner antibody, is an IgG molecule with the peculiar propensity to bind red cell membrane antigens at low temperature, fix complement components, and then dissociate from the newly formed complex when the temperature rises. With the return to a temperature of 37°C, the attached complement completes the process of red cell lysis with no trace of the inciting antibody.

Acute attacks of paroxysmal cold hemoglobinuria have a characteristic and defining pattern. Exposure to chilling conditions often involves only one limb or part of the body, as might occur with a walk in cool shallow water. The attack commences abruptly with pain in the back and extremities, abdominal cramps, and temperatures that sometimes reach 40°C. With severe episodes, the hemoglobin level falls, the reticulocyte percentage rises, and free hemoglobin appears both in the plasma and urine. Although the attack is violent and abrupt in nature, the hemoglobin value fortunately falls only to levels that are modest at worst and usually not life-threatening.

Paroxysmal cold hemoglobinuria often follows infections. Early reports connected the disorder most commonly with syphilis, particularly the congenital variety. Today, paroxysmal cold hemoglobinuria occurs as a very rare sequela of common infections, such as infectious mononucleosis or parvovirus B19 infection.[14] The basis of these rare incidents is a mystery.[15] Protection from cold exposure during the active phase of the disease is the only effective intervention. Fortunately, the Donath-Landsteiner antibody fades over time along with its pathological features.

■ TRANSFUSION-RELATED HEMOLYSIS

Hemolysis following transfusion most commonly reflects the action of antibody (2) in Figure 19-1. Two natural sets of sentinel antibodies always exist and can produce hemolysis with a transfusion. The first group is the intrinsic strong antibodies directed against the ABO blood group. The second set of antibodies is aimed at the Rh blood groups. Matching for these antibodies is a mandatory part of the typing and screening for transfusion. Reactions involving these antibodies are rare and most often represent clerical or other errors during blood administration.

A violent and potentially deadly reaction occurs when a patient receives blood that contains an incompatible ABO blood group. Back pain, substernal discomfort, dyspnea, flushing, fever, nausea, vomiting, and shock can occur in fewer than 30 minutes following the start of transfusion. Lysed red cells bombard the circulation with stromal material that has particularly nocuous clinical effects. The material triggers DIC with all its attendant problems, including respiratory and renal failure. Renal tubular necrosis can supersede acute renal insufficiency, necessitating dialysis both in the short term and over the long term should the patient survive the episode. The abruptness of the event fortunately prompts the attendant staff to stop the transfusion before the entire quantity of blood is transferred. The morbidity is high nonetheless and the death rate is at least 10%.

The transfusion of Rh-incompatible blood is a serious problem, but not the unmitigated disaster of ABO incompatibility. Chills and fever commonly are the first toxsins indicating that the transfusion is going awry. Hemoglobinemia is common while hemoglobinuria is less frequent owing to the relatively small amount of hemoglobin released into the circulation. The bilirubin level rises over a period of 10–24 hours and patients often manifest some degree of jaundice or scleral icterus. The neutrophil count follows an interesting pattern of transient leukopenia followed by leukocytosis. Renal insufficiency is rare with Rh-incompatible transfusions. Antipyretics usually control the discomfort produced by fever and patients recover with few if any long-term deficits.

DELAYED HEMOLYTIC TRANSFUSION REACTIONS

Delayed hemolytic transfusion reactions occur in patients who receive chronic or intermittent transfusions that over time induce antibodies against one or more of the many score minor red cell antigens (alloimmunization). Repeated transfusions lead to the generation of low titer antibody against one or more of these minor antigens for which typing is not routinely performed since they rarely interfere with standard transfusions. Antibody levels fall and become undetectable between transfusions. However, the next exposure triggers a rapid rise in titers 4–7 days after transfusion.

The initial reactions are minor, with low-grade fever often as the most prominent symptom. When measured, either the rise in hemoglobin value is less than anticipated or the fall from the peak value is more marked than expected. Malaise, pallor, and jaundice afflict some patients in the course of a delayed transfusion reaction. Repeated exposure to the offending antigen can produce antibody titers sufficient to induce more severe responses, including fever, hemoglobinemia, and hemoglobinuria. Bilirubin levels rise while haptoglobin values fall dramatically. The LDH value typically is high, while hepatic enzyme values including the ALT, AST, and alkaline phosphatase are normal. Renal insufficiency fortunately is uncommon even with severe reactions. Ninety percent of sporadic cases of delayed hemolytic transfusion reactions derive from incompatibilities involving the Rh antigens, specifically the D (Rh_0) and CD (Rh_1) determinants.

Alloimmunization against minor red cell antigens is a major problem for patients whose disorders require frequent transfusion, such as people with thalassemia or sickle cell disease. Kell, E, and C are the most problematic minor antigens in these instances. The rate of alloimmunization approaches 40% in some reports. Occasionally, patients

TABLE 19-4 | **KEY DIAGNOSTIC POINTS OF IMMUNE HEMOLYTIC ANEMIAS**

Issue	*Manifestation*	*Approach*
Immune hemolysis with a negative DAT	Clinical and laboratory picture consistent with AIHA. Negative DAT	• ELISA-based test for red cell surface immunoglobulin or complement. • FACS analysis for red cell surface immunoglobulin or complement.
AIHA possibly secondary to immune-mediated disorder such as SLE	Often mild or no symptomatic manifestations of underlying disorders	• Screen for collagen vascular disease.
AIHA possibly secondary to CLL	Increased lymphocyte count on CBC, although the increment can be small	• Screen for circulating CLL cells.
Cold-induced red cell agglutination	Hemolysis, Raynaud's phenomenon	• DAT for C3 on red cell membrane.

develop such severe problems with alloantibodies that transfusion becomes nearly impossible.

Limited phenotype matching for these antigens markedly reduces the incidence of alloimmunization. The procedure involves screening for minor red cell antigens known to be problematic for chronically transfused patients. The problem of alloimmunization is a particular issue for people with sickle cell disease because the statistical distribution of minor red cell antigens differs between people of African and European ancestry. People with sickle cell disease are from the former group while in the United States blood donors are largely of European background.

Limited phenotype matching increases the cost of transfusion for patients with sickle cell disease. Avoidance of subsequent alloimmunization and the need for extensive screening entailed by this complication ultimately saves the transfusion service money both in manpower and materiel, however.[16] Most importantly, the approach abrogates possible danger to patients from transfusion time delays necessitated by extensive crossmatching for alloantibodies.

TRANSFUSION-INDUCED AUTOIMMUNE HEMOLYSIS

Transfusion-induced erythrocyte autoimmune responses are a poorly appreciated phenomenon in the medical community that occurs fairly commonly but fortunately produces significant problems only rarely. Although the mechanism of transfusion-induced autoimmunity is unclear, events that predispose to the problem are now better

TABLE 19-5	KEY MANAGEMENT POINTS OF IMMUNE HEMOLYTIC ANEMIA
Issue	*Comments*
Possible drug-induced AIHA	Some drugs such as ceftriaxone have a known association with AIHA. Most people are on medications lacking a known clear association. Empirically stop drugs or substitute with alternate medications where possible.
DIC versus AIHA	Mild DIC can present with few schistocytes and a relatively normal platelet count. At times, initial confusion with AIHA is possible. A low titer autoantibody with a weakly positive DAT can further confuse the picture. DIC screening helps to distinguish the two conditions.
Transfusion-induced autoantibodies	These commonly develop in patients who receive repeated transfusions. Alloantibodies develop prior to autoantibodies. Repeated challenges with red cells not matched for minor antigens can trigger severe autoimmune hemolysis.

recognized.[17,18] Alloimmunization against minor red cell antigens often precedes (or at least coexists with testing) the onset of an autoantibody. Autoantibodies develop in between 5% and 10% of who receive chronic transfusion. The first indication that autoantibodies have developed sometimes is difficulty in the crossmatching reaction. On rare occasion, the autoantibody is of a titer and activity that low-grade hemolysis is clear both from a clinical and laboratory standpoint.

Patients with alloantibodies in whom efforts at transfusion continue despite the barrier introduced by alloimmunization sometimes develop high titer and very active autoantibodies that can severely complicate a patient's clinical status. People with a chronic anemia, such as sickle cell disease, can suffer a fall in hemoglobin values to dangerously low levels. The interventions cited above for the treatment of autoimmune hemolysis sometimes are needed to stem the tide. These patients are refractory to virtually all blood transfusion products, creating a precarious clinical situation. Over time, the titer and activity of the autoantibody wane to the point that an acceptable steady state resumes. The risk of an anamnestic response to future transfusions is a specter that is difficult to shake. Meticulous records regarding the specificity of both the alloantibodies and autoantibodies must remain with the patient for life (Tables 19-4 and 19-5).

References

[1]   Diehl LF, Ketchum LH. 1998. Autoimmune disease and chronic lymphocytic leukemia: Autoimmune hemolytic anemia, pure red cell aplasia, and autoimmune thrombocytopenia. Semin Oncol 25:80–97.

[2]   Black AJ, Eisinger AJ, Loehry CA, Johnson GD. 1969. Ulcerative colitis with autoimmune haemolytic anaemia. Br Med J 2:31–32.

[3]   Shashaty GG, Rath CE, Britt EJ. 1977. Autoimmune hemolytic anemia associated with ulcerative colitis. Am J Hematol 3:199–208.

[4]   Ramakrishna R, Manoharan A. 1994. Auto-immune haemolytic anaemia in ulcerative colitis. Acta Haematol 91:99–102.

[5]   Elhajj II, Sharara AI, Taher AT. 2004. Chronic hepatitis C associated with Coombs-positive hemolytic anemia. Hematol J 5:364–366.

[6]   Ohsawa I, Uehara Y, Hashimoto S, Endo M, Fujita T, Ohi H. 2003. Autoimmune hemolytic anemia occurred prior to evident nephropathy in a patient with chronic hepatitis C virus infection: Case report. BMC Nephrol 4:7.

[7]   Ramos-Casals M, Garcia-Carrasco M, Lopez-Medrano F, et al. 2003. Severe autoimmune cytopenias in treatment-naive hepatitis C virus infection: Clinical description of 35 cases. Medicine (Baltimore) 82:87–96.

[8]   Seltsam A, Salama A. 2000. Ceftriaxone-induced immune haemolysis: Two case reports and a concise review of the literature. Intensive Care Med 26:1390–1394.

[9]   Ehmann WC. 1992. Cephalosporin-induced hemolysis: A case report and review of the literature. Am J Hematol 40:121–125.

[10] Murphy WG, Kelton JG. 1988. Methyldopa-induced autoantibodies against red blood cells. Blood Rev 2:36–42.

[11] Ramanathan S, Koutts J, Hertzberg MS. 2005. Two cases of refractory warm autoimmune hemolytic anemia treated with rituximab. Am J Hematol 78:123–126.

[12] Mantadakis E, Danilatou V, Stiakaki E, Kalmanti M. 2004. Rituximab for refractory Evans syndrome and other immune-mediated hematologic diseases. Am J Hematol 77:303–310.

[13] Robak T. 2004. Monoclonal antibodies in the treatment of autoimmune cytopenias. Eur J Haematol 72:79–88.

[14] Chambers LA, Rauck AM. 1996. Acute transient hemolytic anemia with a positive Donath-Landsteiner test following parvovirus B19 infection. J Pediatr Hematol Oncol 18:178–181.

[15] Wodzinski MA, Collin RC, Booker DJ, Stamps R, Bellamy JD, Sokol RJ. 1997. Delayed hemolytic transfusion reaction and paroxysmal cold hemoglobinuria: An unusual association. Immunohematol 13:54–57.

[16] Tahhan H, Holbrook C, Braddy L, Brewer L, Christie J. 1994. Antigen-matched donor blood in the transfusion management of patients with sickle cell disease. Transfusion 34:562–569.

[17] Aygun B, Padmanabhan S, Paley C, Chandrasekaran V. 2002. Clinical significance of RBC alloantibodies and autoantibodies in sickle cell patients who received transfusions. Transfusion 42:37–43.

[18] Young PP, Uzieblo A, Trulock E, Lublin DM, Goodnough LT. 2004. Autoantibody formation after alloimmunization: Are blood transfusions a risk factor for autoimmune hemolytic anemia? Transfusion 44:67–72.

INDEX